Assessm...
and Support in Clinical Practice

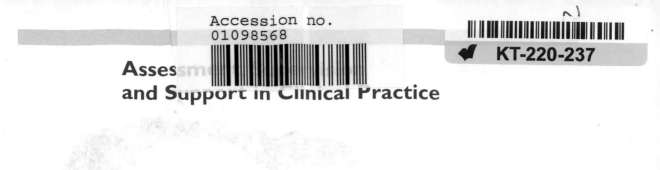

For Churchill Livingstone:

Senior Commissioning Editor: Sarena Wolfaard
Project Development Manager: Karen Gilmour
Project Manager: Gail Wright
Design Direction: Judith Wright
Illustrator and Cartoonist: John Marshall

Assessment, Supervision and Support in Clinical Practice

A Guide for Nurses, Midwives and other Health Professionals

Ci Ci Stuart BAppSci MEd RN RM MTD
City & Guilds Work Based Assessors' Awards D32 & D33

Lecturer in Nursing and Midwifery, School of Nursing and Midwifery, University of Sheffield, Sheffield, UK

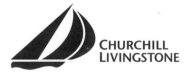

CHURCHILL
LIVINGSTONE

CHURCHILL LIVINGSTONE
An imprint of Elsevier Science Limited

First published 2003

ISBN 0 443 07065 2

British Library Cataloguing in Publication Data
A catalogue record for this book is available from the British Library

Library of Congress Cataloging in Publication Data
A catalog record for this book is available from the Library of Congress

Note
Medical knowledge is constantly changing. As new information becomes available, changes in treatment, procedures, equipment and the use of drugs become necessary. The author and the publishers have taken care to ensure that the information given in this text is accurate and up-to-date. However, readers are strongly advised to confirm that the information, especially with regard to drug usage, complies with the latest legislation and standards of practice.

The
publisher's
policy is to use
**paper manufactured
from sustainable forests**

Printed in China by RDC Group Limited

Contents

Preface

What helps students learn and develop into the professionals we desire them to be? Clinical settings provide unique learning experiences and opportunities for students – these need to be planned, structured, managed and coordinated (ENB and DoH 2001) so that students undergo professional socialization positively, and develop the competencies for professional practice that cannot readily be acquired elsewhere. The clinical experience for students should be much more than just learning what to do and how to do it: it should be about the education of students who will one day be our professional peers, colleagues and co-learners. This means that during clinical placements, learning needs to be actively facilitated and evaluated; it should not be left to chance.

Curriculum reforms in pre-registration nursing and midwifery education require both theory and practice to be subject to continuous assessment. While on clinical placements, students are supported, supervised and assessed by practitioners acting as mentors and assessors. The facilitation and assessment of learning in clinical settings are particularly challenging as these arenas are dynamic and teem with myriad non-stop activities. Both students and practitioners need to think on their feet during care delivery. While doing so, students are expected to learn and practitioners are expected to teach and assess.

The supervision and assessment of clinical practice are significant responsibilities and can be both challenging and time-consuming. Clinical practice is about engaging in human experiences: the human experiences of the individual health care practitioner arising predominantly from interactions with, and while caring for, patients and clients. Human experiences involve not only acting and thinking but also feeling, and it is only when all three are considered together that individuals can be empowered to enrich the meaning of their experiences. The world of the clinical setting provides the exclusive context in which learners can be empowered to learn not only the clinical skills vital for competent practice, but also the thinking and feeling behind the enaction of these clinical skills. These forms of learning can best take place if learners are carefully supervised, supported and assessed for such personal and professional development.

One of the key reasons for the existence of the educational system is to facilitate the development of students. Robertson et al (1997:174) point out that a 'major metamorphosis that must occur in the student clinician is the transformation from dependent, non-skilled, apprenticed technician into an independent, responsible, skilled, self-evaluating professional'. In participating in clinical education, the practitioner who is mentor and assessor to learners is challenged to empower the learner to reach those goals.

This book is written for all the mentors and assessors of clinical practice in the nursing, midwifery and other health care professions who have the onerous, and crucial, task of ensuring that the clinical practice of students attains the standard required for professional registration. This book is also for those clinical mentors and assessors who believe that the facilitation of the learning of students during their clinical practice, and the concomitant use of the process of the continuous assessment of practice, are worthwhile professional roles and responsibilities. Although this book is written primarily for all the mentors and assessors of clinical practice in the nursing and midwifery professions, it is seen that the principles of the facilitation of learning and assessment in the clinical setting are equally applicable to all mentors and assessors of other health care professions. Students of health care may also find some of the learning and assessment strategies useful for empowering their own learning.

Clinical practice and its assessment are challenging and rewarding professional activities. I hope you enjoy using this book and gain in your expertise as mentor or assessor to the very many students of health care who will pass your way. To the student readers, I hope you are empowered to manage your own learning and professional development.

Sheffield 2002   Ci Ci Stuart

REFERENCES

English National Board for Nursing, Midwifery and Health Visiting and Department of Health (2001) *Placements in Focus*. London: ENB and DoH.

Robertson S, Rosenthal J and Dawson V (1997) Using assessment to promote student learning. In: McAllister L, Lincoln M, McLeod S and Maloney D (eds) *Facilitating Learning in Clinical Settings*. Cheltenham: Stanley Thornes (Publishers), 154–184.

Nota bene

At the time of going to press, the newly formed Nursing and Midwifery Council (NMC), which took office on 1 April 2002, was in the process of taking over the functions of the UKCC and the four National Boards. During this transitional period, the majority of UKCC publications remained valid under the NMC (Registrars letter 9–2002, from UKCC to NMC, 18 March 2002, PH/JK). Those UKCC publications to be reprinted with the NMC's corporate identity, with the content remaining essentially unchanged, were then not available. References to UKCC publications throughout the book are made in the light of this information.

Acknowledgements

One never achieves solely by one's own efforts. There are many significant others, friends and colleagues who have made invaluable and invisible contributions to the development of this work. I would like to thank all the people, too numerous to name individually, who have helped in one way or another in bringing this book into existence. Prime thanks go to the many colleagues, clinical mentors, assessors and students who have contributed to my understanding and thoughts on the assessment, supervision and support of learners during clinical practice.

A particular thank you is extended to Professor Mavis Kirkham, Department of Midwifery and Children's Nursing, The University of Sheffield, for her constructive comments on the outline of the book. Thank you Mavis, for your implicit and explicit encouragement and support. Another particular thank you is extended to Emeritus Professor WA Hampton, of the then Division of Adult and Continuing Education, The University of Sheffield, for his constructive comments on the outline of the book and some invaluable 'home tips' on book writing. Thank you Bill, for always having the time, somehow!

I owe much to my 'faithful' partner who has spent many many lonely hours in solitude, waiting patiently for the fruition of this book, while I hammered away at the keyboard. Thank you, Frank, for having been behind me and believing that 'it' will happen.

The scope of the book

There are many books that deal in great depth with how the learning of theory should be assessed. There are also many books about facilitating student learning in academic settings. There are, however, few books that specifically address the uniqueness and complexity of learning in clinical settings, and how such learning can be facilitated and assessed. This is a 'how to do it' book with a solid theoretical base and considerable empirical research behind the clinical learning and assessment strategies. The purpose is to provide workable strategies to help busy practitioners supervise, support and assess learners with validity and reliability.

The book starts by exploring four broad categories of the purpose of assessment in nursing and midwifery education and the nature of assessment of clinical practice in the health care professions. The point is made that we need to review critically why we assess so that we may consider more carefully whether our assessment procedures are reasonable and just. Chapter 1 considers the conflicting values of these purposes, the impact on learners of our assessment procedures, and the complex nature of clinical practice and assessment.

In Chapter 2, the point is made that the very purposes of assessment we set out to achieve may not be fully realized if we do not pause to consider our professional responsibilities and accountability as mentors and assessors. This chapter explores the issues of responsibility and accountability surrounding assessment in nursing and midwifery education and professional practice. It includes an examination of the professional, statutory and institutional regulations governing the assessment of practice. Attempts are made to answer two key questions surrounding the assessment of clinical practice: What are mentors and assessors responsible and accountable for? Who are mentors and assessors responsible and accountable to? This latter question is considered in conjunction with the role, responsibilities and accountability of students for learning and assessment. The powerful influence of the mentor as a role model for learning, which raises accountability issues, is considered. Very frequently, a practitioner is mentor as well as assessor to the same student. This may cause dilemmas for such a practitioner when assessment decisions are made. Some of the dilemmas created by the mentor and assessor interface are explored.

In 1999 the UKCC recommended refocusing pre-registration education on 'outcomes-based competency principles' (UKCC 1999). In exploring what we assess, in Chapter 3, the case is made for the use of an integrated, competency-based approach for assessing nursing and midwifery practice. Arguments are put forward that a competency-based approach to education and training potentially provides a framework for bringing together professional policies for training and employment requirements, and that competencies provide consumers and professionals with some common understanding of standards expected of professionals. The nature of competencies, what it means to be clinically competent and the assessment of competencies in professional practice are explored. The competency-based model of assessment is critically evaluated as an assessment tool for assessing professional practice.

A range of forms of evidence (Bedford et al 1993) is required to enable assessors to make sound inferences that learners can perform competently in the variety of clinical situations in which they can find themselves. In Chapter 4, the uses and merits, and limitations, of a range of assessment methods that can be used in the competency-based approach for the assessment of clinical practice are explored and debated. The use of the strategy of triangulation to obtain the breadth and depth of assessment evidence to enhance the validity and reliability of assessment is discussed.

We rely on assessments to make some quite specific but also far-ranging judgements about our students' future behaviour as registered practitioners. A fundamental question we need to ask is this: Do our assessments enable us to make such judgements soundly? Deciding whether or not an assessment lives up to this task is not straightforward. In Chapter 5, there is an examination of those issues we need to consider in order to make sound judgements in assessments. Issues surrounding the questions of validity, reliability, feasibility and discriminating powers of assessment are explored. Those factors that can affect validity and reliability are considered, and measures to attain objective assessments and avoid subjective assessments are suggested so that we can begin to work towards assessments that are fairer to all students.

As discussed in Chapters 3 and 4, in a competency-based system, assessment has the key function of obtaining evidence of competence. Chapter 6 discusses the constructive focus of assessment where the aim is to help rather than sentence the individual (Gipps 1994). Learning is facilitated as part of the assessment process. In this chapter, the continuous assessment process is explored as the key assessment strategy to facilitate assessment as a learning process. It is suggested that integral to the continuous assessment of clinical practice is the strategy of using a learning contract with its concomitant assessment plan, formative assessment and summative assessment processes. These are examined with respect to the successful management of the continuous assessment of practice in order to realize the positive impact of assessment. Suggestions are made on how to manage constructive feedback.

Monitoring progress, managing feedback and making assessment decisions are interrelated activities that are integral to the continuous assessment of practice. These activities are central to, and essential in, helping students learn through their practice to develop clinical competence. If assessment is to be a learning process as discussed in Chapter 6, the student should be an equal partner in these activities: progress is monitored jointly through the formative assessment process set up, and the student participates actively during feedback and assessment decision-making sessions. In Chapter 7, a model comprising four assessment activities is suggested for monitoring the progress of learners. This is followed by a discussion of making formative and summative assessment decisions. Suggestions are made on how to manage some assessment problems such as students experiencing problems learning during clinical practice and the situation where a student has to be failed.

The clinical experience of students of health care is widely acknowledged as being one of the most important aspects of their educational preparation (ENB and DoH 2001). The clinical environment must therefore also be an environment where learning can take place, thus becoming an educational environment.

Marton et al (1984) make the important observation that learning is a function of the relationship between the learner and the environment and is never something determined by one of these elements alone. Learners do not respond merely to tasks assigned; rather, they adapt to, and work within, the environment taken as an interrelated whole. Chapter 8 examines those human and material factors contributing to a positive clinical learning environment. Strategies are suggested for creating this environment and for maintaining the quality and standards of clinical placements through educational audit. The centrality of the mentor in supporting learners and facilitating learning is emphasized.

The ideal clinical learning environment may not have any fruition if the complexities of learning through experience are not recognized and acknowledged. Learning from experience is not a simple rational process; not only do we need to know *what* and *how* to do, we also need to know *what* and *how* to think. Impacting on and influencing these psychomotor and cognitive processes are our feelings, values and beliefs. Chapter 9 proposes and explores the use of a *model for learning from experience* as the framework for considering experience-based learning, and how learners can be assisted to interact with the clinical environment in order to learn through practice and unearth meaning from experiences. This model, which is seen as a holistic model for the initial preparation and the continuing professional development of health care practitioners, has clinical experiences as one of its key focuses. It is also suggested that as professional knowledge and practices change constantly, the use of this holistic model will enable the practitioner to refine and update knowledge and practices so that professional expertise, and thus practice wisdom (Hull 1998), are continually developing.

Throughout the book, there are self-directed activities. These take the form of questions for you to answer or to discuss with colleagues. Do try to spend some time on them as they are intended to assist you consider more comprehensively the multifaceted roles of the practitioner who is also the clinical mentor, assessor and/or preceptor.

REFERENCES

Bedford H, Phillips T, Robinson J and Schostak J (1993) *Assessment of Competencies in Nursing and Midwifery Education and Training*. London: English National Board for Nursing, Midwifery and Health Visiting.

English National Board for Nursing, Midwifery and Health Visiting and Department of Health (2001) *Placements in Focus*. London: ENB and DoH.

Gipps CV (1994) *Beyond Testing: Towards a Theory of Educational Assessment*. London: The Falmer Press.

Hull C (1998) Open learning and professional development. In Quinn FM (ed) *Continuing Professional Development in Nursing*, pp 182–204. Cheltenham: Stanley Thornes (Publishers).

Marton F, Hounsell D and Entwistle N (1984) *The Experience of Learning*. Edinburgh: Scottish Academic Press.

United Kingdom Central Council for Nursing, Midwifery and Health Visiting (1999) *Fitness for Practice*. London: UKCC.

Abbreviations

CMB   Central Midwives Board

CPD   continuing professional development

DH   Department of Health

ENB   English National Board

GNC   General Nursing Council

HEI   higher education institution

NCVQ   National Council for Vocational Qualifications

NHS   National Health Service

NMC   Nursing and Midwifery Council

NVQ   national vocational qualification

PPC   Preliminary Proceedings Committee

PREP   Post-registration Education and Practice

RCN   Royal College of Nursing

UKCC   United Kingdom Central Council for Nursing, Midwifery and Health Visiting

1 The purposes and nature of assessment and clinical assessment

INTRODUCTION

In this chapter, I shall consider why we assess at all in the nursing and midwifery professions. As the purposes of assessment are explored, some of the common impact of our assessment procedures are examined. In considering the context of assessment in this book, this chapter will also take a look at the complexities of clinical assessment. The assumption made here is that, for many readers of this book, the nature of learning and being assessed in the clinical setting will be close to their hearts as a direct result of significant and meaningful personal experiences of having learnt and worked in that setting.

In this chapter, 'assessment' is used as a global term incorporating tests and examinations (whether oral or written), the judgement of clinical performance and any other method of measuring learning. Assessors may be anyone who assesses the student's work – clinical nurse or midwife or the lecturer from the higher education institution.

THE NATURE OF ASSESSMENT

We all are keenly aware of the importance of assessment and the influence it has on our lives. As Rowntree (1987:xii), perhaps in one of his lighter moments, points out:

> Assessment will remain with us from the cradle to beyond the grave. Scarcely have we taken our first breath before we have a label fastened to our wrists, giving weight at, and method of, birth, and, somewhere, our first file (medical) has already been opened. . . . And even in death we cannot escape the assessors – obituary-writers for the famous; just family, workmates and friends for the rest of us.

And don't Rowntree's sentiments strike a strong chord! Consciously or subconsciously, we are assessing most of the time, be it at work, at home or even when out walking in the countryside. 'Assessment is a central feature of social life' wrote Broadfoot (1996:3).

Passing judgement on people, on events, on ideas and on things and on values is part of the process of making sense of the world around us and where we stand in any given situation. Sometimes we judge to reassure ourselves – *I am glad I am not as selfish as she is* – (and we might be rather lacking in self-awareness)! We are all assessors; even very young children are capable of making assessments – ask a young child whether she or he likes her/his new school and, of course, the response will be either a 'yes' or a 'no'. The ability to respond implies that the child has activated the mental processes involving a mental review of perhaps the teachers, the other children, the events and the activities – that she or he likes or dislikes and has applied more or less conscious criteria to what would constitute, for instance, a like or dislike of the teacher. In social settings and during social interactions we may not be asked to justify our judgements and, indeed, may be most taken aback and even feel embarrassed if required to do so. However, in educational and professional settings, such justification is frequently required as the process of assessment is overt, formalized and controlled. The criteria we use are often subject to scrutiny and we are required to make our assessment decisions on the basis of available evidence.

Much has been written about educational assessment as it is a legitimate concern of practitioners, learners, teachers and those responsible for the development and accreditation of courses. Rightly or wrongly, assessment is assumed to be the nexus of learning. It might seem to be common sense, and indeed, is the 'custom and practice' today that students undertaking a course of training should be assessed. It is easy to polarize to the position of unquestioning acceptance of the necessity for assessment as we have all been subject to some form of educational assessment ourselves, such as sitting a timed, invigilated written examination or a multiple-choice paper, carrying out a practical procedure or enduring the agonies of an oral examination (you may argue that enduring the driving test is equally or more agonizing!). Assessment can reduce us to experience extremes of emotions.

During our training as nurse or midwife we have been observed, tested and questioned in the clinical setting: e.g. while giving patient/client care, performing procedures in conjunction with care delivery and carrying out tasks such as preparing a trolley or sterilizing a piece of equipment. A comprehensive list will be long. Many of us may also recall that, on our 'good' days, after completion of a span of duty we leave the clinical area feeling glad to have been on duty and to have had a positive and productive day. Our contributions to care and feedback from our mentor had helped our development as nurse or midwife. Patients had thanked us and conveyed to us how comfortable they had felt after our care. Conversely, on our 'bad' days, we may cry and threaten to hand our notice in!

An intramuscular injection technique that day had been given 'poorly' and the patient had complained severely; the ward was very busy and by the end of that shift, we were emotionally and physically drained. After that episode with the injection, we had concentrated and worked hard by ourselves so as not to make any more silly mistakes. The staff had been too busy to help us.

Those experiences we had on 'bad' days have not changed today. Mentors and assessors in Bedford et al's (1993) study reported experiencing role strain, and teaching and assessing students was an additional burden. Consequently, students' learning and assessing needs were marginalized and placed in opposition to client care needs, with students having to fend for themselves. This problem is not new. In 1989, Watts reported that, after an initial period of supervision, student nurses on a first clinical placement were left to practise independently. If they sought supervision and feedback, it was given. Students who were unaware of incorrect practice would continue to practice incorrectly without seeking help. The assumption made was that if no help was required, 'all was well'. Even assessment was carried out by inference – trained staff would assume safe and competent practice from students' expressions of confidence.

Learning and assessment in clinical practice seem to be rather 'hit and miss affairs'. Why then do we bother to assess students in clinical practice? during training in general? What are the purposes of assessment? It is perhaps appropriate to explore these at this point. The next section will explore the overall purposes of assessment in nursing and midwifery education. You may wish to try Activity 1.1 before you proceed.

THE PURPOSES OF ASSESSMENT

The nursing, midwifery and medical professions have required their 'trainees' to be examined since the 19th century. The medical profession was the first profession to institute qualifying examinations in 1815 in order to determine competence (Broadfoot 1979). In 1872, the London Obstetrical Society took the initiative to set up its own examination board to examine women between the ages of 21 to 30 who wanted to be certified as a 'skilled Midwife, competent to attend natural labours' (Donnison 1988:85). This examination comprised a written and oral examination (Sweet and Tiran 1997). In the case of nurses, the first examination was held with the establishment of a School of Nursing at the London Hospital in 1880 (Seymer 1949). Students had to sit an examination consisting of a paper, a viva voce and a practical test in the wards, at the end of their first and second years of training (Bendall and Raybould 1969). Certificates were awarded on successful completion of the 2-year course.

With the passing of The Midwives Act in 1902 and The Nurses Registration Act in 1919, it became a statutory requirement to be registered on the Midwives Roll and the Nurses Register in order to practise. Statutory registration was instituted to raise standards of care. In the early years of the Acts, one route to registration was to fulfil set conditions of practice and pass state examinations. Professionally then, we have been impressed with the necessity to be assessed and most of us have internalized this value.

To accept the necessity for assessment unthinkingly denies a complex debate concerning the purposes of assessments. It may also make us overlook the effects of the assessment on the learner as an individual, and its impact on the curriculum, teaching and learning. Critically reviewing 'why' we assess may make us consider more carefully whether our assessment procedures are reasonable and just. As professionals, we like to think that we know why we are doing what we are doing most, if not all, of the time. However, Foucault (1982:182) has this to say: 'People know what they do; they frequently know why they do what they do; but what they don't know is what what they do does'.

Klug (1975) acknowledged that one of the many difficulties of discussing the theme of assessment lies in the tangle of issues involved: even its explicit and acknowledged functions are multifarious and conflicting. In an earlier publication (Klug 1975 in Rowntree 1987), Klug gathered 32 reasons for formal assessment. Here, I shall concentrate on what I see are the four main reasons commonly advanced for assessment in nursing and midwifery education.

Assessment as a form of quality control

Students in training

The Nursing and Midwifery Council's (NMC) *Code of Professional Conduct* for nurses, midwives and health visitors (NMC 2002a) states that:

> As a registered nurse or midwife, you are personally accountable for your practice. In caring for patients and clients, you must: respect the patient or client as an individual; obtain consent before you give any treatment or care; protect confidential information; co-operate with others in the team; maintain your professional knowledge and competence; be trustworthy and act to identify and minimise risk to patients and clients.

The NMC is clearly concerned with maintaining a standard of practice such that high-quality care is provided to the recipients of health care at all times.

As discussed earlier, the issue of a 'licence' to practise by a professional statutory body offers some measure of public protection. The public have a fundamental right to expect competence from the qualified professional in health care, and protection against unsafe practice. The mechanism of statutory registration is designed to ensure that those legally entitled to call themselves 'midwife', 'nurse', 'physiotherapist', 'occupational therapist', 'doctor' and so on, possess the outcomes and competencies described in statute. For nurses and midwives, the kind and standard of pre-registration nursing and midwifery programmes leading to registration on the UKCC register are currently set out in Statutory Instrument 1989 No. 1456 (UKCC 1992).

More recently, the UKCC mandated that pre-registration nursing and midwifery programmes must be designed to prepare the student to provide the nursing and midwifery care that patients/clients require, safely and competently, and so assume the responsibilities and accountabilities necessary for public protection (UKCC 2000). Underpinning this mandate are four guiding principles:

1. *Preparation: fitness for practice* – The primacy of practice underpins the competencies and must be reflected in all programmes of preparation for entry to the register.

2. *Service: fitness for purpose* – Nursing and midwifery must relate to the changing needs of the health services and the communities which they serve, responding to current and future need.

3. *Recognition: fitness for award* – Education for practice must be established at the level and pace of learning commensurate with the demands of complex and professional practice. It must be designed to meet the needs of the health services and communities and be structured to meet the specific needs of the profession.

4. *Responsibility: fitness for professional standing* – The UKCC valued the rights implicit in the social contract between the profession and society to participate in the health care of individuals, families and communities. Such rights also carry obligations. These include not only the responsibility to provide competent, safe and effective care but also responsibility for the highest standards of professional conduct and ethical practice.

Professional nursing and midwifery education, then, is aimed at developing competent practitioners who are fit for practice. The educational and professional outcome is a nurse or midwife who is able to apply knowledge, understanding and skills to perform to the standards required in employment (UKCC 1998). The development of appropriate attitudes and values should be added to the above outcome. As practice takes place in the real world of health care delivery, fitness for practice is inextricably linked to other aspects of fitness: i.e. fitness for purpose, professional academic awards and professional standing. As professionals, we need to facilitate the achievement of these aims and to ascertain whether they have been achieved through our assessment of the student. Valid and reliable assessments will provide objective data upon which assessment decisions are made. We may need to remind ourselves that the UKCC is reliant on this assessment decision for conferring professional registration upon the nurse or midwife.

Take a few moments to consider Activity 1.2.

If we accept that one of the purposes of assessment is as a form of quality control of the standards and outcomes of nursing and midwifery education, the sobering answer to the question posed in Activity 1.2 is that this quality control

ACTIVITY 1.2

How well are we preparing nurses and midwives to be competent practitioners who are fit for practice as required by the UKCC? Be objective in your considerations.

is not fully realised (Bradshaw 2000, Glen and Clark 1999, UKCC 1999a, Runciman et al 1998). The following point was made by the UKCC Education Commission on nursing and midwifery education (UKCC 1999a):

> . . . there is concern that newly-qualified nurses, and to a certain extent midwives, do not possess the practice skills expected of them by employers, and public perceptions about levels of preparedness for practice are sometimes negative.

Reasons for this are wide ranging (Glen and Clark 1999). Amongst the most notable is the confusion in the terminology of 'competence' (Bradshaw 2000, Fraser et al 1997, Bedford et al 1993). With the publication of the report *Fitness for Practice* (UKCC 1999a:35), the UKCC defined 'competence' for the first time. The Council used the term 'competence' to describe the skills and ability to practise safely and effectively without the need for direct supervision.

To achieve the above purpose of assessment, we need to examine more carefully how we can better manage nursing and midwifery education, including the assessment of clinical practice, so that when students qualify they can meet service needs and requirements. Within this framework more concerted efforts are required to make valid assessments of students' clinical practice. Amongst the radical agenda set by the UKCC to refocus nursing and midwifery education is the use of an outcomes and competencies framework in developing nursing and midwifery curricula. An outcomes-based competency approach to the management of clinical assessment is explored in Chapter 3.

Qualified nurses and midwives

The NMC maintains a register of practitioners who have met the standards for entry to the professions. This is central to the Council's role in protecting the

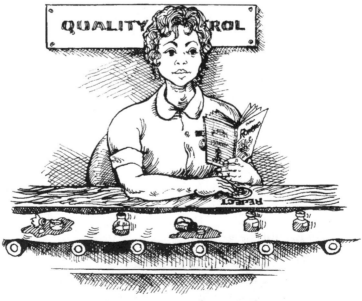

Assessment as quality control?

public. Being on the NMC register demonstrates to the public that we have accepted the responsibilities which go along with registration, and that we will abide by the professional standards set by the NMC. This is done through professional self-regulation. Professional self-regulation means that in exercising our professional accountability, we use our professional knowledge, judgement and skill to interpret and apply professional standards in practice. Although the NMC – as the current regulatory body for nursing, midwifery and health visiting – administers the system of professional self-regulation, it is through us, as individual accountable practitioners, that professional standards are maintained in the workplace.

The NMC's *Code of Professional Conduct* is the basis of the regulatory framework. We are required not only to monitor and maintain our own professional standards but that of our colleagues. Clause 6.4 of the Code requires us to assist professional colleagues to develop their professional competence in order to contribute safely to care. When we assist colleagues thus, we will directly or indirectly be supervising and assessing care given. In exercising our individual professional responsibility and accountability, the Code requires us to report to an appropriate person or authority, circumstances which may put patients and clients at risk. The NMC's position on this is explicit:

> You must act quickly to protect patients and clients from risk if you have good reason to believe that you or a colleague, from your own or another profession, may not be fit to practise for reasons of conduct, health or competence. . . . Where you cannot remedy circumstances in the environment of care that could jeopardise standards of practice, you must report them to a senior person with sufficient authority to manage them and also, in the case of midwifery, to the supervisor of midwives (NMC 2002a: Clauses 8.2; 8.3).

The UKCC's 1990 *Post-Registration Education and Practice* (PREP), endorsed by the NMC (NMC 2002b), is a set of UKCC standards which practitioners must meet to demonstrate that their professional knowledge and competence have been developed and maintained. Practitioners must undertake and record their continuing professional development (CPD) over the 3 years prior to renewal of their registration in a personal professional profile. The NMC will audit compliance with the PREP (CPD) standard (NMC 2002b). The NMC will be assessing directly that practitioners have maintained this standard by monitoring a sample of registrants who will be asked to provide the NMC with evidence of their learning activity and the relevance of this learning to their work.

In its paper titled *A First Class Service* (Department of Health 1998), the government stated that clinical governance will provide a framework through which National Health Service (NHS) organizations will be accountable for continuously improving the quality of their services and safeguarding high standards of care by creating an environment in which excellence in clinical care will flourish. For the first time, NHS organizations and individuals will have a statutory duty to achieve quality improvement. NHS organizations are required to develop processes for monitoring and improving clinical quality.

Like professional self-regulation, clinical governance is all about promoting high standards of care in order to protect the public. The government sees clinical governance as the main vehicle for continuously improving the quality of patient care and developing the capacity of the NHS to maintain high standards, including dealing with poor professional performance. The established professional self-regulation of nursing, midwifery and health visiting can thus make a major contribution to clinical governance.

For qualified practitioners, the quality control purpose of assessment starts at the point of entry into the profession and terminates on exiting the profession. Assessment is a means of answering the demands of public accountability. Assessment takes the forms of self-assessment through professional self-regulation and clinical governance as systems of monitoring clinical quality are developed through its framework.

Assessment for entry into the profession

Closely related to the quality control purpose is this second purpose. The quality control purpose acts as the 'entry gate' into, and staying in, the profession. However, assessment for entry into the profession starts at the point of application for training. Candidates are screened for the required 'academic' qualifications, their ability to complete the course and the potential qualities of a nurse or midwife. In the United Kingdom, typical academic qualifications required for entry to pre-registration nursing and midwifery programmes include five GCSE/GCE 'O' levels, grade C or above; the General National Vocational Qualification Advanced level or an Access course for Higher Education (NMAS 2000). Candidates have to prove that their ability to contribute to the profession is greater than that of others. One of the assumptions implicit in this selection procedure is that only those who are deemed capable of successfully completing the training are funded for the training. Disappointingly, the correlation between fulfilment of selection criteria and successful completion of training is low. Levels of discontinuation from pre-registration nursing and midwifery courses are a source of concern. Detailed statistics published by the English National Board (ENB) for Nursing, Midwifery and Health Visiting are used here as a case study. Figures 1.1–1.4 (ENB 2002) show the statistics for the period 1996–2001 of all pre-registration student nurses who commenced and completed or discontinued the Branch part of the programme in England. Figure 1.5 shows the statistics for the period 1996–2001 of all pre-registration

FIGURE 1.1   *General/adult 1996/97–2000/01 (reproduced with permission from ENB 2002).*

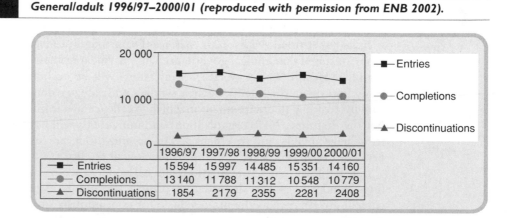

	1996/97	1997/98	1998/99	1999/00	2000/01
Entries	15594	15997	14485	15351	14160
Completions	13140	11788	11312	10548	10779
Discontinuations	1854	2179	2355	2281	2408

FIGURE 1.2   *Mental health 1996/97–2000/01 (reproduced with permission from ENB 2002).*

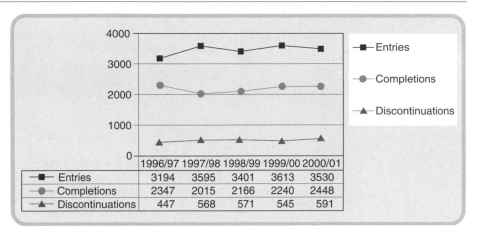

	1996/97	1997/98	1998/99	1999/00	2000/01
Entries	3194	3595	3401	3613	3530
Completions	2347	2015	2166	2240	2448
Discontinuations	447	568	571	545	591

FIGURE 1.3   *Children's 1996/97–2000/01 (reproduced with permission from ENB 2002).*

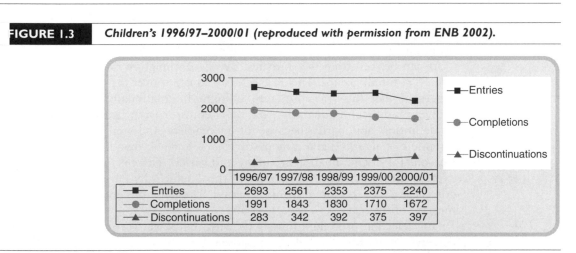

	1996/97	1997/98	1998/99	1999/00	2000/01
Entries	2693	2561	2353	2375	2240
Completions	1991	1843	1830	1710	1672
Discontinuations	283	342	392	375	397

FIGURE 1.4   *Learning disability 1996/97–2000/01 (reproduced with permission from ENB 2002).*

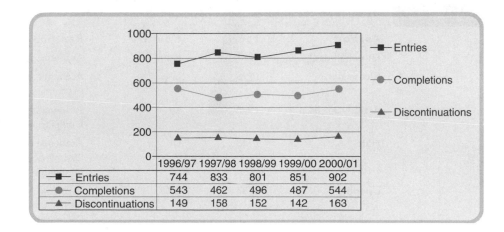

	1996/97	1997/98	1998/99	1999/00	2000/01
Entries	744	833	801	851	902
Completions	543	462	496	487	544
Discontinuations	149	158	152	142	163

FIGURE 1.5	*Midwifery 1996/97–2000/01 (reproduced with permission from ENB 1999, 2002).*

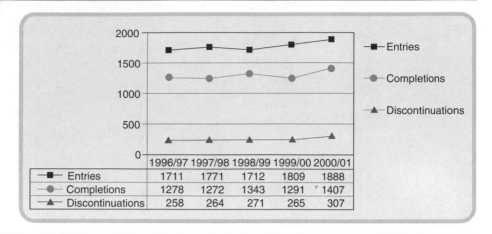

	1996/97	1997/98	1998/99	1999/00	2000/01
■ Entries	1711	1771	1712	1809	1888
● Completions	1278	1272	1343	1291	1407
▲ Discontinuations	258	264	271	265	307

student midwives who commenced and completed or discontinued the total programme.

As can be seen from the statistics, the discontinuation rate is between 15% and 18% for all groups. This rate is fairly constant over the 5-year period. It is suggested that this 'casualty' rate is high. Internationally, the scale of the problem is difficult to quantify from the literature, partly because of differences in definition and partly because of incomplete and non-comparable data. Ehrenfeld et al (1997) give a figure of 23.5% for their own institution in Israel. Reasons for discontinuation are many and varied. There is no intention here to explore these fully but to refer only to those which, by our stringent selection criteria, we seek to prevent from occurring. These reasons are listed in Table 1.1 for ease of reference.

Our selection procedure invests us with the power to reject those who we perceive do not fulfil our selection criteria. Prior academic achievement may be seen as an objective measure for assessment for entry to nursing and midwifery education, and ultimately the profession. As can be seen in Table 1.1, academic

TABLE 1.1	*Reasons for the discontinuation of nurse training*			
	Author	*Year*	*Country*	*Reasons*
	Ehrenfeld et al	1997	Israel	Academic failure – 50%
	Richardson	1996	UK	Academic failure – 20% Misconduct
	Braithwaite et al	1994	UK	Academic failure Disciplinary proceedings
	Hutt	1988	UK	Academic failure Disciplinary proceedings Unsuitable for the training
	Lindop	1987	UK	Unsatisfactory performance Not suited to nursing Personality disorders

failure is cited as a key reason for discontinuation of training in all the studies. This certainly casts great doubt over the assumption that those who perform best in current examinations are those who would become most capable as a result of our educational investment. Perhaps such factors as maturity, personality and motivation have more or less influence on success in nursing and midwifery education. As discussed, even the relevance and usefulness of this perceived 'objective measure' has serious shortcomings. Thomas Love Peacock (1860 in MacLeod 1982:7) railed against the preponderance of examinations which would 'infallibly have excluded Marlborough from the Army and Nelson from the Navy'! The other selection criteria are predominantly subjective and therefore open to the personal biases of the selectors. Of the candidates we reject, we will never know how many would have become the sensitive and caring nurse or midwife – their potential may never be realized. The academic high-flyer may not be the better nurse or midwife if she/he does not possess qualities such as compassion and empathy.

Assessment for the motivation of students

Assessments serve as a powerful motivating force for students – were it not for the carrot of success or stick of failure created by summative assessments, many students, it is claimed, would lack any real incentive to work. With motivation, we are talking of using assessment in order to encourage the student to learn. From this standpoint, assessments are seen as a form of positive help to students. Rowntree (1987:23), however, reminds us in no uncertain terms that 'assessment can be used as an instrument of coercion, as a means of getting students to do something they might not otherwise be inclined to do – especially if unfavourable

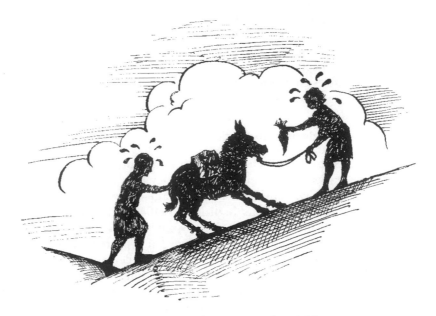

Assessments – the carrot or the stick?

assessments can have unpleasant consequences'. He goes on to say that the line between coercion and encouragement is hard to draw. Let us take the case of nursing and midwifery education – one key aim of these programmes of education must be to prepare practitioners who are safe and competent. Of necessity then, students are assessed for their achievement of statutory competencies. How else can we measure such learning? Failure to pass these competencies results in being discontinued from the course. The reader may wish to decide whether assessments in this instance are used to coerce or encourage the student!

It is important not to take too simplistic a view of motivation and assessment, as motivation is a complex concept. A high level of motivation is not a sufficient condition, but is a necessary one for learning (Gipps 1994). The importance of motivational factors influencing learning was succinctly stated by Howe (1987:142):

> I have a strong feeling that motivational factors are crucial whenever a person achieves anything of significance as a result of learning and thought, and I cannot think of exceptions to this statement. That is not to claim that a high level of motivation can ever be a sufficient condition for human achievements, but is undoubtedly a necessary one. And, conversely, negative motivational influences, such as fear of failure, feelings of helplessness, lack of confidence, and having the experience that one's fate is largely controlled by external factors rather than by oneself, almost certainly have effects that restrict a person's learned achievements.

In an extensive review of the impact of classroom evaluation on students, Crooks (1988) found that research repeatedly demonstrated that the responses of individual students to educational experiences and tasks are complex functions of their abilities and personalities, their past educational experiences, their current attitudes, self-perception and motivational states, together with the nature of the current experiences and tasks. Crooks' review also revealed just how important assessment is in defining the attitude students take towards their work, their sense of ownership and control of their own learning, the strategies they employ in learning and their confidence and self-esteem, all of which impact profoundly on the quality of learning achieved. The significant effects of assessment on motivation for learning (Crooks 1988) and their implications for assessment in nursing and midwifery education are discussed here.

Student self-efficacy

Self-efficacy refers to students' perceptions of their capability to perform certain tasks. Perceptions of self-efficacy have a strong influence on effort and persistence with difficult tasks, or after experiences of failure: under such circumstances, students high in self-efficacy usually redouble their efforts, whereas students low in self-efficacy tend to make minimal efforts or avoid such tasks. Self-efficacy can be developed if repeated success is experienced. Success at tasks perceived to be difficult or challenging is more influential than success on easier tasks: conversely, repeated failures lead to lowered self-efficacy.

Self-efficacy is best enhanced if longer-term goals are supported by a carefully sequenced series of sub-goals with clear criteria that students find attainable. In addition, standards must be clearly specified. The setting of clear and attainable goals has significant implications for strategies used by clinical assessors in relation to the level and type of work which is aimed at individual students. These important points are discussed further in Chapters 6 and 7.

Intrinsic motivation and continuing motivation

Intrinsic motivation to learn (defined as a self-sustaining desire to learn) and continuing motivation (defined as a tendency to return to and continue working on tasks away from the instructional context in which they were initially confronted) are highly related concepts. Both, in turn, are closely related to interest in the material that is being studied. Where students initially lack intrinsic motivation in a particular subject area, a carefully planned programme of positive educational experiences accompanied by extrinsic motivation can lead to the development of interest in the area, and thus to intrinsic motivation. On the other hand, where students are initially intrinsically motivated, attempting to stimulate learning through extrinsic motivation usually leads to decreased intrinsic motivation, especially on challenging tasks.

These findings have obvious implications for teachers and assessors of nursing and midwifery students when learning experiences are designed for the students. Crooks' description of what effective education should be (Crooks 1988:460) may help us focus more carefully on how, through our educational endeavours, which include assessment strategies we use, we can help our students develop and/or maintain intrinsic and continuing motivation:

> Effective education requires the fusing of 'skill and will', and intrinsic interest and continuing motivation to learn are educational outcomes that should be regarded as at least as important as cognitive outcomes.

This aspect of learning and assessment is explored in Chapter 6.

Assessment anxiety

The fact that clinical experience is stressful for many students is well documented (see, for example, Phillips et al 2000, Williams 1993, Kleehammer et al 1990, Parkes 1985). These authors also report that anxiety can contribute to decreased learning. To be subject to assessment in the face of this negative emotion can only compound the situation. Crooks (1988) found that the debilitating effects for high-anxiety students are greater when the student perceives good performance to be particularly important, when the test is expected to be difficult and when the testing conditions are particularly intrusive, e.g. rigid timing. Although extrapolations must be made with extreme caution, it seems possible to draw parallels between these findings and the circumstances faced by nursing and midwifery students during clinical practice. The performance of students in the clinical setting must meet the required standards within the time frame of the clinical placement. The achievement of some aspects of care can be difficult, such as being able to perform cardiopulmonary resuscitation, communicating with the very ill/dying client/patient and managing the care of a group of clients/patients. For some students, experiences of assessment may then be rather dispiriting and demotivating.

As can be seen from this presentation of the possible impact of assessment on motivation, there are many factors to be considered if we wish to realize this purpose of assessment. A comprehensive review of the motivational aspects relating to assessment can be found in Crooks (1988).

Assessment to support teaching and learning

Knowledge of performance in an assessment exercise, such as during clinical practice or a written assignment, will help the student benefit educationally from the assessor's response to the work that has been done. The importance of this type of feedback is probably captured by Rowntree (1987:24) when he stated that 'feedback, or "knowledge of results", is the life-blood of learning'. Student nurses and student midwives work at getting helpful feedback (O'Neill and McCall 1996, Spouse 1996, Bedford et al 1993). In O'Neill and McCall's study, student nurses found face-to-face feedback a very positive aspect of their learning, helping them to identify strengths and weaknesses so that they improved where they were weak and built upon what they did best.

For this form of feedback to be effective, assessment needs to be used as a 'diagnostic aid' to learning throughout the course so that it becomes an integral part of the educational process, continually providing both 'feedback' and 'feed-forward' (Torrance 1993:334) for both the student and the assessor. This formative element of the assessment process will then have a positive impact on learning, particularly if it focuses on helping the student to achieve short-term goals and specific feedback on progress is provided. A detailed discussion of unhelpful forms of feedback such as the award of marks, grades, a pass or fail can be found in Rowntree (1987). In summary, being awarded just a mark or a pass or a fail does not indicate to the student how well or badly he may have performed in aspects of the assessment exercise. Such grades are meted by the teacher at the end of a term or a course. Students may therefore not know how to improve future performance. Rowntree (1987) believes that such feedback can only begin to be useful when it includes verbal comments.

Insofar as the assessment evidence reveals strengths and weaknesses in the student's learning, the assessor may be able to identify what has been taught well, what has not been so well explained and therefore may have confused the issue for the student, what further experiences are required, and so on. In the clinical setting, such information will further enable the assessor to plan the clinical experiences and teaching sessions the student will require to achieve learning outcomes and competencies. The use of the formative assessment process is explored in Chapter 6, where the process of the continuous assessment of clinical practice is discussed.

Torrance and Pryor (1998:10) contend that 'all assessment practices have an impact on [student] learning'. As revealed by Crooks' review of 1988, our teaching arrangements, notably the assessment approaches used, is particularly potent in influencing how students go about studying and learning. Marton and Säljö (1984) reported that students' approaches to learning tasks could be categorized into two broad categories that they labelled as *deep* or *surface* approaches. Deep approaches involve an active search for meaning in order to understand material for oneself. The content is interacted with vigorously and critically. Organizing principles are used to integrate ideas. Surface approaches, in contrast, rely primarily on attempts to memorize course material, treating the material as if different facts and topics were unrelated.

Our assessment strategies should encourage deep learning, higher-order thinking and self-monitoring, alongside the acquisition of knowledge, from the earliest stages of professional education to develop the practitioner who is 'fit for practice' (UKCC 1999a). Higher-order learning is retained longer and encourages the development of intrinsic motivation and positive attitudes to continued learning (Gipps 1994). The nursing and midwifery professions can only stand to benefit given the professions' aim to develop and foster the attitude of lifelong learning in its practitioners (UKCC 1999a; ENB 1995) in order to strive constantly to improve standards and quality of client/patient care (Department of Health 1999).

ASSESSMENT IN CLINICAL PRACTICE

The nature of clinical assessment

You may be able to recall your experiences of being assessed when you were a student nurse or student midwife. Some of these memories may no doubt be rather vivid! Not only were you required to sit written tests and be subjected to oral and practical examinations but also you were assessed while you were 'working'. In the classroom, your teacher gave you feedback on your test papers and assignments. In the clinical area, your mentor gave you feedback, thus implying that some form of assessment of your practice had taken place. You were either pleased or dissatisfied with your performance – you had therefore assessed yourself. Patients gave you feedback on the care you had given – you were subject to yet further assessment!

All in all, you may have frequently felt quite overwhelmed as you knew that what you said or did or the way you behaved or even the way you dressed was under scrutiny. If we reflect on our experiences of being assessed as nurse or midwife, some of us may even begin to say that we experienced assessment as though we had experienced a 'phenomenon'. What is the nature of this *phenomenon*? Pause for a moment to consider the questions posed in Activity 1.3.

In most of the instances in the sketch, feedback you received about your performance and abilities or otherwise was based on another person's inferences and estimations of your actions and behaviours. In other words, you had been judged by someone else. Rowntree (1987:4) says that when we assess, we enter into human encounters whereby we make attempts to know that person. He explains further:

> . . . assessment in education can be thought of as occurring whenever one
> person, in some kind of interaction, direct or indirect, with another, is

ACTIVITY 1.3

From the above sketch of assessment, what inferences can be drawn about the nature of assessment in general? about assessment in the clinical setting? How were you affected by the many occasions when you were assessed?

conscious of obtaining and interpreting information about the knowledge and understanding, or abilities and attitudes of that other person.

In our position as assessors of students in the clinical setting, we make judgements about how students are integrating into the ward team, how they are developing as nurses or midwives, what they are learning and what they have accomplished. We hope that the assessments may reveal to us the changes in the student's knowledge and understanding, abilities and attitudes as a result of our supervision and guidance, the practical experiences, influences and effects of the clinical milieu on the student. The nature of clinical practice, and the clinical milieu itself, places multiple demands on the skills of the mentor as practitioner, teacher and assessor. The dynamic clinical setting is ever-changing and unstructured. It provides a range of clients whose conditions are varied and changeable. Learning experiences for students are therefore not consistent. Each of these situations has to be dealt with in different ways. Real people in the real world of practice do not see things in a uniform way. Bedford et al (1993) make the point that assessors are individuals who are not automatons, but people who interpret and make sense of what they encounter in terms of their own experience. Our own values will also influence the interpretations we make of situations. The subjectiveness of the clinical world will inevitably mean that assessments we make are likely to be influenced by our own personal and professional experiences and perceptions of the situation.

The diversity of context and the differing demands of each context also mean that we can only assess the student's knowledge, understanding, abilities and attitudes within those contexts that the student has encountered. In Rowntree's terms then, assessments of our students during clinical practice are truly *only attempts* to know our students. We may have worked with the student for the maximum number of shifts possible within the student's allocation but will only have been able to form such opinions of the student's learning on the basis of what we observed of the student's performance. While we are observing, we cannot be sure that we have picked up every aspect of performance – there may have been some aspect of care or nuances that we have missed or we may interpret ability to perform or otherwise based on our personal biases for, or against, the student. During clinical placements then, finding out about a student's abilities to perform is done mainly through informal processes and as opportunities arise. As our assessments are likely to be based on these 'snapshots' of practice (Bradshaw 1989), we need to question how well we truly know our student. Knowledge of our student's achievements is of course important when we make assessment decisions, whether they are formative or summative.

As the student works alongside us, we hope that they are learning through observation of our practices. Throughout the student's placement, we are also facilitating their learning through instruction, guidance and supervision as they participate in care delivery. While they are adjusting to clients, staff and other personnel and also learning to perform care, we are assessing and giving them feedback on their performance. This means that while the student is learning she is being assessed. Wood (1982) says that this situation is less than ideal and it would be better to separate learning and assessment. Working in the demanding clinical setting may prevent us from carrying out our roles of mentor and assessor as effectively as we would wish to. From their study, one conclusion that Bedford et al (1993) drew was that at the grass roots, the first responsibility of nurses and midwives is to care for clients. As discussed earlier, even the extremely important activity of teaching and assessing students comes second to this. Fretwell's study in 1980 showed that student nurses were taught and supervised for 11.6–36.9% of the time. In a lengthy and detailed study of all aspects of student nurses' clinical experience, Jacka and Lewin (1987) reported that learners spent more than 50% of their time, with some spending more than 75% of their time, working alone. The results of these studies indicate that teaching and assessing activities are left to chance. If this is the case, how then can we be sure that our students are learning what they should in order to achieve professional competence? Strategies to facilitate more effective learning and assessment are made in Chapters 7 and 9.

The complexities of clinical assessment

From the above discussion, it is clear that the nature of clinical assessment is complex. There is much in the nursing literature which says that assessment of students in clinical practice is a continuing problem (While 1991, Wood 1972, 1982, Woolley 1977), and one which 'will not go away' (Chambers 1998:201). The basic issues complicating clinical assessments discussed by Wood in 1982 are as real today. Try Activity 1.4.

From your experience both as a student and a mentor, the problems you most commonly identified are likely to be similar and could also be shared by your colleagues. Problems you experienced might be as follows:

- Clinical assessment is based predominantly on direct observation of practice. Human observation inevitably possesses inherent biases and subjectivity and is therefore a subjective process. Interpretations of standards of performance are therefore inconsistent and unreliable.

- Over the course of the training programme, the student has to adapt to new and differing clinical areas on a regular basis, with some clinical placements lasting only 4 weeks. During each placement, the student has to adjust and adapt to a multitude of personalities. The student has to interact with other students, the nurses and midwives, the doctors and other health professionals such as the physiotherapist and dietician who are also attending the client/patient. The student also has to adjust to, and learn to care for, a range of clients/patients with their differing illnesses and needs, possibly attempting to apply what has been learnt in the classroom to the real-life situation of the clinical world. As already mentioned earlier, the student is assessed while she is adapting, coping and trying to learn and achieve the competencies of being a nurse or a midwife. It is therefore important to remember that students are

ACTIVITY 1.4

Think of the clinical experiences in the different placements you experienced, either as a student or a mentor. From these experiences, identity the problems which arose as you attempted to learn to care for clients/patients or when teaching students.

assessed in their capacity as students at the pre-specified level. This point is discussed in more detail in Chapter 7.

- The attainment of behavioural skills forms one essential element of learning in the clinical environment (Department of Health 1999, While 1991). The unpredictability of the clinical learning environment means that there can be little educational control over the clinical learning experiences for students. Patient turnover and patient dependency changes mitigate against consistency of experience. Jacka and Lewin (1987) noted the variation in the quality and quantity of practical experience on apparently similar wards. The diverse experiences mean that the demonstration of behavioural skills may vary from occasion to occasion (Boreham 1978). Boreham cited the example of explaining a procedure to an articulate English-speaking patient as compared to achieving the same level of understanding in an anxious non-English-speaking patient. The second student was assessed on her ability to communicate with an anxious non-English-speaking patient. Should this student be judged to be more skilful than the first student? Given the multicultural society of Great Britain, should all students be expected to be able to communicate likewise? And can clinical experiences be provided to enable the development of these skills? If the second student is unable to achieve the same level of understanding in her patient, should she be given a fail grade?

  The Department of Health (1999) requires nurses and midwives to be trained to 'broadly the same standards and have the same skills' – wherever they are trained. Is this an 'order' that is achievable? The reality of being able to achieve this requirement is perhaps summed up in the following statement by Young (1994:47):

  > Even for students following the same course, the variations in clinical experience ensure that no two people's trainings, and therefore learning outcomes, are ever identical. For example, a student may not be involved in cardiac resuscitation at all during a three-year training, while a colleague on the same course may have assisted with resuscitation on a number of occasions. This means that even with detailed training criteria, it is impossible to specify precisely in what skills a registered nurse will be competent.

  The issues of uniformity, consistency and fairness of clinical assessment have remained contentious over the years (Chambers 1998, Girot 1993, While 1991, Wood 1982). These issues are addressed in more detail in Chapters 4 and 5, where strategies to try to achieve fairness of assessment are discussed.

- Clinical areas are under pressure for increasing periods of the year. Large student intakes and staff shortages mean that even the most committed of nurses and midwives, and these are the majority, are hard pressed to support and supervise students adequately (UKCC 1999a). Bedford et al (1993) reported that total assessment demands within many placement areas had increased. Many nursing staff were involved in assessing other health care personnel such as health care assistants and paramedics. This may result in a mentor supervising several students simultaneously. The assessment of an individual student's performance is likely to be based on a sample of the student's total experience, as it would be impossible to achieve a constant 1:1 supervision and observation of the student. In White et al's (1994:103) study, students cited examples where assessments of their practice were made in the absence of any witness of it! One student blatantly said that it was virtually impossible to fail the practical part of the course and there would always be ways of getting round a weak area of practice. Herein lies a grave concern – if we accept that one of the purposes of assessment is to ensure that the student has achieved professional competencies prior to professional registration, the above way of making assessment decisions clearly indicates that this purpose is not fulfilled.

■ The advent of Project 2000 (UKCC 1986) courses emphasizes the supernumerary status of students. Clinical placements are also shorter in many instances. Opportunities to develop substantive relationships between trained nurses/midwives and students are not as prevalent. Mentors are therefore unable to provide an adequate level of support and supervision of students (Earnshaw 1995, Girot 1993). This further contributes to assessments being made on the basis of 'snapshots' of practice, with the potential of making inaccurate assessment decisions.

■ There is much rhetoric on the theory–practice gap in nursing. Few people would doubt its existence, and supporting evidence is available from many studies and official reports (see, for example, McCaugherty 1991 for a review). Patients and clients are individuals with individual needs. Thus, nursing and midwifery practice cannot be exact sciences: there needs to be more than one way of meeting patient and client needs. In attempts to describe nursing and midwifery care, the unique psychological and social dimension of each patient and client cannot be captured. Theory gleaned can only paint incomplete and generalized pictures of the realities of practice. However good classroom and textbook theory may be, clinical practice may not always correlate, making it difficult for the student to apply theory to practice. From the student's viewpoint, clinical practice can appear quite different from theory learnt during lectures and from books (McCaugherty 1991).

The student has to learn to integrate knowledge learnt in a context away from the world of practice with the real world of clinical practice. Many students may find this very difficult, as cognitive processes indicate that there is an intimate connection between the acquisition of knowledge and the context in which it is used (Gipps 1994). Educationally, this suggests that we cannot teach theory in one setting and expect it to be applied automatically in another. Studies in educational research confirm that facts cannot be learnt in isolation and then used in any context, as skills and knowledge are now understood to be dependent on the context in which they are learnt (Gipps 1994).

Clinical assessors are frequently not party to theoretical instruction in the classroom. White et al (1994) found that practitioners were not well-informed about the Project 2000 course, which militated against assisting students in successfully integrating theory to practice. If students encounter such difficulties in relating theory to practice, they will not be as likely to develop the clinical competencies required of them. In these circumstances, we need to question the validity of our assessment processes.

In the face of the complexities of learning and assessment in the clinical setting, it would appear that it is difficult to realize fully the purposes of assessment of clinical practice in the nursing and midwifery professions. Perhaps this is not surprising. Our students have been set the onerous task of becoming 'fit for practice' in what I would suggest is a short period of 3 years – short, because the nature of nursing and midwifery education and practice today is making increased demands on students. Students now also have to achieve the academic demands of study at an institution of higher education. Other factors, to name but a few, such as the dynamic health care setting with its changing patient/client needs, the reduced number of clinical areas to attain clinical experiences, the constantly changing and increased demands made on the nurse and the midwife, an increasing number of specialities, technological innovations and an ever-increasing knowledge base stretch students' resources much more today. And if the support that many students require is not readily available, many may fall by the wayside. Without an adequate level of support and supervision of the students during clinical practice, the very purposes of assessment we set out to achieve will not be fully realized.

CONCLUSION

Four broad categories of purpose in nursing and midwifery education have been outlined. These are not entirely without overlap and conflict. In our role as assessors of learners in the nursing and midwifery professions, we need to consider carefully the learning that must be achieved and balance this against the needs of the learner as an individual, which may conflict on occasions. Our personal philosophy of what teaching and learning in clinical practice is about is powerful in determining our attitudes to the assessment of clinical practice, which in turn influences our use of any assessment system, tools and procedures. As we examine the nature of clinical assessment, we might begin to analyse the reasons underpinning our attitudes towards learning and assessment in clinical practice.

Reilly (1980:2–3) poses the following questions of us as accountable self-regulating professionals:

> Do our educational offerings stand the test of accountability? Can we demonstrate that the nurses [and midwives] sent into the health care system have made a difference for the better in the quality of health care provided in proportion to the scope of their educational preparation?

Who is responsible and accountable? After you have examined the issues of responsibility and accountability surrounding assessment in nursing and midwifery education and professional practice in the next chapter, you may be in a better position to contribute to the wider debate surrounding the achievement of the purposes of assessment in the health care professions.

REFERENCES

Bedford H, Phillips T, Robinson J and Schostak J (1993) *Assessment of Competencies in Nursing and Midwifery Education and Training*. London: The English National Board for Nursing, Midwifery and Health Visiting.

Bendall ERD and Raybould E (1969) *A History of the General Nursing Council for England and Wales: 1919–1969*. London: H.K. Lewis and Co.

Boreham NC (1978) Test-skill interaction errors in the assessment of nurses' clincal proficiency. *Journal of Occupational Psychology*, **51**, 249–258.

Bradshaw A (2000) Editorial. *Journal of Clinical Nursing*, **9**, 319–320.

Bradshaw PL (ed) (1989) *Teaching and Assessing in Clinical Nursing*. Hemel Hempstead: Prentice Hall.

Braithwaite DN, Elzubeir M and Stark S (1994) Project 2000 student wastage: a case study. *Nurse Education Today*, **14**, 15–21.

Broadfoot P (1979) *Assessment, Schools and Society*. London: Methuen.

Broadfoot PM (1996) *Education, Assessment and Society*. Buckingham: Open University Press.

Chambers MA (1998) Some issues in the assessment of clinical practice: a review of the literature. *Journal of Clinical Nursing*, **7**(3), 201–208.

Crooks TJ (1988) The impact of classroom evaluation practices on students. *Review of Educational Research*, **58**(4), 438–481.

Department of Health (1999) *Making a Difference*. London: Department of Health.

Department of Health (1998) *A First Class Service, Quality in the New NHS*. London: Department of Health.

Donnison J (1988) *Midwives and Medical Men*, 2nd edn. London: Historical Publications Ltd.

Earnshaw GJ (1995) Mentorship: the students' views. *Nurse Education Today*, **15**, 274–279.

Ehrenfeld M, Rotenberg A, Sharon R and Bergman R (1997) Reasons for attrition on nursing courses: a study. *Nursing Standard*, **36**(8), 393–396.

ENB (2002) *Student Statistics Report: 1996/97–2000/2001*, 3rd edn. London: English National Board for Nursing, Midwifery and Health Visiting.

ENB (1995) *Creating Lifelong Learners: Partnerships for Care*. London: English National Board for Nursing, Midwifery and Health Visiting.

Foucault M (1982) Letter quoted in Dreyfus HL and Rainbow P (eds) *Michael Foucault: Beyond Structuralism and Hermeneutics*. Brighton: Harvester.

Fraser D, Murphy R and Worth-Butler M (1997) *An Outcome Evaluation of the Effectiveness of Pre-registration Midwifery Programmes of Education*. London: English National Board for Nursing, Midwifery and Health Visiting.

Fretwell JE (1980) An inquiry into the ward learning environment. *Nursing Times*, **76**(16), 69–75.

Gipps CV (1994) *Beyond Testing: Towards a Theory of Educational Assessment*. London: The Falmer Press.

Girot E (1993) Assessment of competence in clinical practice: a review of the literature. *Nurse Education Today*, **13**, 83–90.

Glen S and Clark A (1999) Nurse education: a skill mix for the future. *Nurse Education Today*, **19**, 12–19.

Howe MJA (1987) Using cognitive psychology to help students learn how to learn. In Richardson TE, Eysenck MW and Piper DW (eds) *Student Learning: Research in Education and Cognitive Psychology*. Milton Keynes: Open University Press and Society for Research into Higher Education.

Hutt R (1988) Lasting the course, Part IV: findings and conclusions. *Senior Nurse*, **10**(3), 4–8.

Jacka K and Lewin D (1987) *The Clinical Learning of Student Nurses*. NERU Report No. 6, Dept of Nursing Studies. London: King's College.

Kleehammer K, Hart AL and Keck JF (1990) Nursing students' perceptions of anxiety producing situations in the clinical setting. *Journal of Nursing Education*, **29**(40), 183–187.

Klug B (ed) (1975) *A Question of Degree: Assorted Papers On Assessment*. A report by the group for research and innovation in higher education. London: The Nuffield Foundation.

Lindop E (1987) Factors associated with student and pupil nurse wastage. *Journal of Advanced Nursing*, **12**, 751–756.

McCaugherty D (1991) The theory–practice gap in nurse education: its causes and possible solutions. Findings from an action research study. *Journal of Advanced Nursing*, **16**, 1055–1061.

MacLeod R (1982) Science and examination in Victorian England. In MacLeod R (ed) *Days of Judgement*, pp 2–24. Driffield, N. Humberside: Nafferton Books.

Marton F and Säljö R (1984) Approaches to learning. In Marton F, Hounsell D and

Entwistle N (eds) *The Experience of Learning*, pp 36–55. Edinburgh: Scottish Academic Press.

Nursing and Midwifery Admissions Service (NMAS) (2000) *Applicant Handbook 2000*. Cheltenham: NMAS.

Nursing and Midwifery Council (2002a) *Code of Professional Conduct*. London: Nursing and Midwifery Council.

Nursing and Midwifery Council (2002b) *The PREP Handbook*. London: Nursing and Midwifery Council.

O'Neill A and McCall J (1996) Objectively assessing nursing practitioners: a curricular development. *Nurse Education Today*, **16**, 121–126.

Parkes R (1985) Stressful episodes reported by first year student nurses: a descriptive account. *Social Science and Medicine*, **20**(9), 945–953.

Phillips T, Schostak J and Tyler J (2000) *Practice and Assessment in Nursing and Midwifery: Doing it for Real*. London: The English National Board for Nursing, Midwifery and Health Visiting.

Reilly DE (1980) *Behavioural Objectives – Evaluation in Nursing*, 2nd edn. Norwalk: Appleton-Century-Crofts.

Richardson J (1996) Why won't you stay? *Nursing Times*, **92**(32), 28–30.

Rowntree D (1987) *Assessing Students: How Shall We Know Them?* 2nd edn. London: Kogan Page.

Runciman P, Dewar B and Goulbourne A (1998) *Employers' Needs and The Skills of Newly Qualified Project 2000 Students*. Edinburgh: National Board for Nursing, Midwifery and Health Visiting for Scotland.

Seymer LR (1949) *A General History of Nursing*, 2nd edn. London: Faber and Faber.

Spouse J (1996) The effective mentor: a model for student-centred learning in clinical practice. *Nursing Times Research*, **1**(2), 120–133.

Sweet BR and Tiran D (1997) History and development of the midwifery profession. In Sweet BR and Tiran D (eds) *Mayes' Midwifery: A Textbook for Midwives*, 12th edn, pp 1005–1010. London: Baillière Tindall.

Torrance H (1993) Formative assessment: some theoretical problems and empirical questions. *Cambridge Journal of Education*, **23**(3), 333–343.

Torrance H and Pryor J (1998) *Investigating Formative Assessment*. Buckingham: Open University Press.

UKCC (2000) *Requirements for pre-registration nursing programmes*. London: United Kingdom Central Council for Nursing, Midwifery and Health Visiting.

UKCC (1999a) *Fitness for Practice*. London: United Kingdom Central Council for Nursing, Midwifery and Health Visiting.

UKCC (1999b) *Register*, Spring 1999, No. 27. London: United Kingdom Central Council for Nursing, Midwifery and Health Visiting.

UKCC (1998) *Guidelines for Higher Education Institutions on Registration for Newly-Qualified Nurses and Midwives*. London: United Kingdom Central Council for Nursing, Midwifery and Health Visiting.

UKCC (1992) *Statutory Instrument 1989 No. 1456. The Nurses, Midwives and Health Visitors (Registered Fever Nurse Amendment Rules and Training Amendment Rules) Approval Order 1989*. London: United Kingdom Central Council for Nursing, Midwifery and Health Visiting.

UKCC (1990) *The Report of the Post-registration Education and Practice Project*. London: United Kingdom Central Council for Nursing, Midwifery and Health Visiting.

UKCC (1986) *Project 2000, UKCC: A New Preparation for Practice*. London: United Kingdom Central Council for Nursing, Midwifery and Health Visiting.

Watts G (1989) Students' feedback from practical learning. *Nursing Times*, **85**(18), 63.

While AE (1991) The problem of clinical evaluation – a review. *Nurse Education Today*, **11**, 448–453.

White E, Riley E, Davies S and Twinn S (1994) *A Detailed Study of the Relationship between Teaching, Support, Supervision and Role Modelling in Clinical Areas within the Context of the Project 2000 Courses*. London: The English National Board for Nursing, Midwifery and Health Visiting.

Williams RP (1993) The concerns of beginning nursing students. *Nursing and Health Care*, **14**(4), 178–184.

Wood V (1982) Evaluation of student nurse clinical performance – a continuing problem. *International Nursing Review*, **29**(1), 11–18.

Wood V (1972) Evaluation of student nurse clinical performance: a problem that won't go away. *International Nursing Review*, **19**(4), 336–343.

Woolley AS (1977) The long and tortured history of clinical evaluation. *Nursing Outlook*, **25**(5), 308–315.

Young AP (1994) *Law and Professional Conduct in Nursing*, 2nd edn. London: Scutari Press.

2

The legal and ethical issues of assessment

INTRODUCTION

For the many busy nursing and midwifery practitioners, having the additional role of mentor and/or assessor to students adds to the role strain (Phillips et al 1993, 2000). Teaching and assessing are add-on activities and the adjuncts that are attended to when time permits. Practitioners who are in this unenviable position frequently feel unhappy that the supervision and support of students cannot be made more of a priority. What students learn may be left to chance. Positive assessment decisions about performance may have been made without the concrete evidence of having observed the student in action (White et al 1994). Practitioners may, or may not, be aware of the many legal and ethical ramifications of making assessment decisions in this manner, and providing an insufficient level of supervision and support for learners.

This chapter explores the issues of responsibility and accountability surrounding assessment in nursing and midwifery education and professional practice. There is a discussion of the meanings and implications of the concepts of responsibility and accountability in professional practice. This is followed by an exploration of two key questions surrounding the assessment of clinical practice:

- *What* are mentors and assessors responsible and accountable *for*?
- *Who* are mentors and assessors responsible and accountable *to*?

This latter question is considered in conjunction with the role, responsibilities and accountability of students for learning and assessment. Very frequently, a practitioner is mentor as well as assessor to the same student. Some of the dilemmas of this dual role are also explored.

ACCOUNTABILITY AND PROFESSIONALISM

As nursing and midwifery strive for professional status, the term 'account-ability' has assumed increasing importance in the last two decades (Ormerod 1993, Emerton 1992, Bergman 1981). In 1981, Bergman said that nursing worldwide was concerned with accountability. Accountability was chosen as the watchword for the International Congress of Nurses for the 1977–81 quadrennium. Bergman believed that one of the main reasons for that choice was to make accountability an integral part of nursing practice and not mere lip service, making the point that:

> Nurses must move beyond 'talking about' accountability, and more into building specific measures, tools, periods and systems of reporting and implementing accountability.

Accountability as an integral part of nursing and midwifery practice has been high on the agenda of the United Kingdom Central Council for Nursing, Midwifery and Health Visiting (UKCC). The position taken by the UKCC will be discussed later. The Royal College of Nursing (RCN) of the United Kingdom (1990) pointed out that a wide range of skills are required in the complex and varied settings in which nurses work. Nurses are required to consider and observe – often simultaneously – ethical, psychological, ethnic and human rights aspects in the discharge of their duties. Society places a high value on the nursing and midwifery professions. The confidence and trust in which nurses and midwives are held are measures of the special relationship between them and the vulnerable patients and clients in their care.

In the United Kingdom (UK), until April 2002, the responsibility for the regulation of nursing, midwifery and health visiting was vested with the UKCC under the Nurses, Midwives and Health Visitors Act of 1979. This Act set out the constitution, establishment and functions of the UKCC. These were adopted by the amended Act of 1992. The Act of 1992 stated that:

> The principal function of the Central Council shall be to establish and improve standards of training and professional conduct for nurses, midwives and health visitors.

All nurses, midwives and health visitors had to register with the UKCC in order to practise in the UK. This professional register maintained by the UKCC was the principal agency for the regulation of nurses, midwives and health visitors.

From April 2002, under the Nurses and Midwives Order 2001, SI 2002 No 253, the Nursing and Midwifery Council (NMC) replaces the UKCC and the four National Boards for Nursing, Midwifery and Health Visiting in each of the countries of the UK. The NMC inherits from the UKCC and the National Boards the standards already set and will apply them until such time as it determines new standards. In all its work, the NMC will have a statutory duty to safeguard the welfare of patients and to act in collaboration with others, including statutory and professional bodies, education providers, employers and education commissioners.

In 1992, the UKCC published the third edition of the *Code of Professional Conduct* for nurses, midwives and health visitors. This has been replaced by the first edition published by the NMC in 2002 (NMC 2002a). The Code is intended to assist individual practitioners, in addition to safeguarding standards and principles for patients and clients, by an expression of the components of acceptable professional practice and related ethical considerations. The NMC's *Code of Professional Conduct* sets out the responsibilities and accountability of the registered practitioner and is the basis of the regulatory framework. It stresses the personal accountability of each practitioner for her/his own practice, and that accountability may not be delegated or transferred to another person.

The Code expressly requires that the interests of patients and clients should take precedence over all other considerations. Accountability becomes strikingly real when set in the context of clinical situations where professional knowledge and competence are exercised when caring for the diverse range of patients and clients. It is evident that professional accountability in the nursing and midwifery professions is a complex matter. It includes 'ethical, societal and public duty and protective elements for patients and clients' (RCN 1990:4).

ACCOUNTABILITY AND RESPONSIBILITY

There are many questions that we can ask ourselves about accountability in general. You may wish to carry out Activity 2.1 before progressing with an exploration of the concept of accountability.

It is not possible to enter into an extensive philosophical discussion of the concepts of accountability and responsibility. The discussion is therefore limited to aspects of what I see is relevant to our educational role as mentors and assessors. Responsibility is linked inextricably with accountability. We talk of a 'responsible person' as one who accepts and executes an undertaking so long as it is within her/his capabilities (Champion 1991). To be responsible implies being answerable to either another or oneself for some act – it implies a moral accountability for one's actions as one is capable of rational conduct and fulfilling obligations for vested trust (Brykczynska 1995). Brykczynska goes on to point out that a responsible person is reliable and can justify a trust. Bergman (1981) believes that responsibility is the key component of accountability. However, it is only a part of accountability, as accountability is more inclusive than responsibility. Before one can be accountable, several preconditions have to be present. These preconditions (Figure 2.1) are shown in the model used by Bergman (1981:55).

The basic precondition is to have the ability (knowledge, skills, values) to decide and act on a specific issue. Next, one must be given, or take, the responsibility to carry out that action. One also needs the autonomy to carry the responsibility. Champion (1991) describes two forms of autonomy: personal and structural autonomy. Personal autonomy refers to the expertise, the knowledge and skills related to the defined area of work, the understanding of

ACTIVITY 2.1

What is meant by accountability? What is the relationship between responsibility and accountability?

FIGURE 2.1	*Model of the preconditions leading to accountability (reproduced with permission from Bergman 1981).*

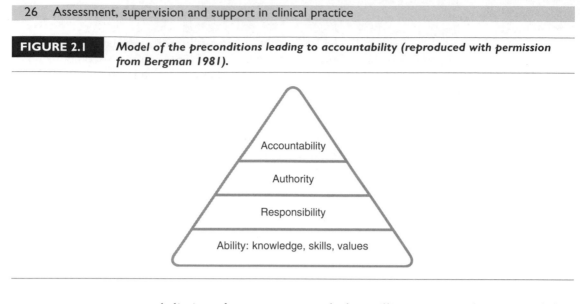

personal limits of competence and the willingness to take responsibility. Structural autonomy is the 'authority to act' given by the organization. When these preconditions are present, one can then be held accountable for the actions one takes.

Professional accountability involves accepting responsibility for professional decisions. Stated more simply, practitioners are 'entrusted with, answerable for, take the credit and blame for and can be judged within legal and moral boundaries' (Castledine 1991). The RCN (1990:4) suggests this working definition of professional accountability for nurses and midwives:

> It is that obligation on the practitioner that binds her [sic] to a code of conduct, based on the expectations of society that she will use her discretion and skill to safeguard her patients and act in every way to uphold professional standards. This obligation, and the values of the profession [contained in the Code], provide a framework for professional and ethical behaviour within which nurses [and midwives] must personally and professionally conduct themselves and within which the primacy and vulnerability of those served is observed and protected.

In view of the substantial clinical role of practitioners, the *Code of Professional Conduct* (NMC 2002a) appropriately focuses on professional accountability to patients and clients. Generally, nurses and midwives are in little doubt about their professional accountability towards their patients and clients. What may not be so clear is accountability for student learning and assessment of clinical practice. Although accountability in the nursing and midwifery professions has been examined extensively, its implications for nursing and midwifery education has not received the same attention and interest (Marks-Maran 1995, Harding and Greig 1994). Of all the clauses in the Code which provide the guiding principles for professional conduct, only one clause, to be explored later, makes a direct reference to the support and supervision of learners. Any other aspects of accountability to the learner are inferred from the general references to the accountability of the practitioner to the patient/client.

There can be few nurses and midwives who are not in some way involved in the training and supervision of others. Increasingly, these roles are part of the contract of employment. In England, the mentoring and assessing roles of nurses and midwives were formalized by the English National Board (ENB) in 1997 and 1988 and the ENB and the Department of Health in 2001 (ENB and Department of Health 2001, ENB 1997, 1988). In 1997 and 1988, the Board defined the *mentor* as an appropriately qualified and experienced first-level nurse who, by example and facilitation, guides, assists and supports the student in learning new skills, adopting new behaviours and acquiring new attitudes. The *assessor* is an appropriately qualified and experienced first-level nurse who has undertaken a course to develop skills in assessing or judging the students' level of attainment relating to the stated learning outcomes. The role of the assessor is a formal one. Each student is required to have a named assessor. The ENB and Department of Health (2001:9) made it clear that mentors are 'responsible for the formative and summative assessment of student learning in practice'. They acknowledged that the practitioner who is the assessor performed roles of the mentor, saying that:

> The term '*mentor*' is used to denote the role of the nurse, midwife or health visitor who facilitates learning and supervises and assesses students. The term 'assessor' is often used to denote a role similar to that of the mentor . . .

The UKCC accepted the post-registration education and practice (PREP) proposals in 1994. One major requirement of PREP is that a period of support should be provided for newly registered practitioners under the guidance of a preceptor (UKCC 1995). Within the PREP guidelines a *preceptor* is a first-level nurse or midwife who is a 'role model and support' for the newly registered practitioner for about the first 4 months of practice.

The above requirements for training, supervision and support, and the concomitant assessment of learning, mean that more and more nurses and midwives must take on these roles. Dimond (1994:272) says that 'for the most part this is unlikely to give rise to many legal issues'. However, an awareness of the potential dangers and problems associated with these roles may prevent grief from arising. The rest of the chapter therefore examines accountability issues surrounding the assessment of clinical practice and shows that assessors have moral and legal obligations to fulfil and learners have rights and legal means of redress.

ACCOUNTABILITY FOR THE ASSESSMENT OF CLINICAL PRACTICE

Before going on to explore this section, consider the questions given in Activity 2.2

ACTIVITY 2.2

What are mentors and assessors responsible and accountable **for**?
Who are mentors and assessors responsible and accountable **to**?

Many of the problems associated with current pre-registration programmes relate quite specifically to the issue of competence to practise at the point of registration (Gilmore 1999). Newly qualified nurses, and to a lesser extent new midwives, have a need for a high level of support and may lack practical skills literacy. In its document *Making a Difference* (Department of Health 1999:24), the government makes it clear that it wants practitioners who are fit for purpose, with excellent skills and the knowledge and ability to provide the best care possible in a modern National Health Service (NHS). One priority set in this document is to 'increase the level of practical skills within the training programme'. It goes on to say that 'every practitioner shares responsibility to support and teach the next generation of nurses and midwives'. The government's vision will stand a better chance of being fulfilled when mentors and assessors are fully cognizant of their responsibility and accountability for the supervision and assessment of clinical practice. The following section examines WHAT the mentor/assessor is responsible and accountable for when supervising and assessing learners.

Responsibility and accountability FOR WHAT?

Direct reference is made to professional accountability for the support and supervision of learners, and by inference, the assessment of standards of practice, in the *Code of Professional Conduct* (NMC 2002a). Clause 6.4 of the Code states:

> You have a duty to facilitate students of nursing and midwifery and others to develop their competence.

In Clause 1.3 of the *Code of Professional Conduct*, the NMC makes it clear that no one else can answer for you and it will be no defence to say that you were acting on someone else's orders, thus:

> You are personally accountable for your practice. This means that you are answerable for your actions and omissions, regardless of advice or directions from another professional.

The Code also makes it clear that if you delegate work to someone who is not registered with the NMC, your accountability is to make sure that the person who does the work is able to do so and that appropriate levels of supervision and support are provided. When these NMC requirements for professional practice are applied to assessment, it can be seen that the practitioner has professional responsibility and accountability to fulfil in her/his role as a mentor/assessor. It is suggested here that the mentor/assessor can be answerable for the following aspect of personal professional practice with its inevitable impact on learning, and the following aspects of supervision and assessment:

- personal standards of practice
- standards of care delivery by learners
- what is taught, learnt and assessed
- standards of teaching and assessing
- professional judgements about student performance.

Personal standards of practice

It is discussed in Chapter 1 that one purpose of assessment in nursing and midwifery education is as a form of quality control of the outcome of the educational process. The educational and professional outcome is a nurse or midwife who is able to apply knowledge, understanding and skills to perform to the standards required in employment (UKCC 1998a). The full realization of this outcome is dependent on the successful achievement of both theoretical and clinical learning measured by assessment. Assessment is an integral part of professional health care training. The processes of clinical teaching, learning and assessment are complex. The committed input of clinical mentors and assessors is required to plan and implement these processes if learning outcomes are to be achieved successfully. I would suggest that this commitment starts with the individual practitioner's competence and standard of practice as a nurse or a midwife. Eraut et al (1995) strongly state that if aspects of clinicians' practice are ill-defined, lack quality or make insufficient use of scientific knowledge, the next generation of practitioners will suffer.

Much of the learning which takes place in professional education does so in the practice setting (Baskett and Marsick 1992, Schon 1983). Role modelling is an important (Spouse 1998, Wood 1987), and an almost inevitable learning strategy in this environment. Within social learning theory, Bandura (1977) suggests that, in role modelling, one person sets a pattern of behaviour which is then copied by another. Learning takes place constantly from observing role models deliver care – these practices are subsequently emulated (Charters 2000). Davies' (1993) study of role modelling showed that major aspects of nursing were learnt by students when they observed role models providing direct patient care. Students who worked alongside knowledgeable and respected practitioners developed an enthusiasm and commitment to their professional development that was unparalleled by any other learning experience (Spouse 1998). It is therefore important for the mentor/assessor to adhere to high standards of professional practice so that students learn this high standard of care and are assessed against these professional practices. We cannot expect a high standard from students if this is not role modelled. We will not be fulfilling one aspect of professional and moral accountability without modelling high standards of practice.

Nicklin and Kenworthy (1995:72) say that 'assessment inevitably takes place in a role-relationship'. The usual relationship that exists between a student and a mentor/assessor is hierarchical in nature. Neary (2000) pointed out that many mentors or assessors take for granted their position of power in the assessment relationship. Her study in 1996 (in Neary 2000) showed the extent to which this 'taken-for-granted' power relationship became explicit at early stages of the relationship when assessors quickly confirmed their expertise and established the subordination of their students. The authority of the mentor/assessor over the student is exercised, frequently without question, as happens when summative assessment decisions are made and when feedback is given of practice without soliciting the opinion of the student. Within this hierarchical situation, one assumption made of the practitioner as a mentor/assessor is that she/he possesses the requisite professional qualities and can recognize these in the learner (Harding and Greig 1994). This assumption is of course open to debate. Hepworth (1991:46) expressed her disagreement when she said that:

the assessor of a student's clinical nursing skills can only assess the student in the light of her own perceptions of the nursing situation, and her own nursing expertise.

Our assessments, then, are likely to be based on our own standards of practice and perceptions of the situation. Therefore, as practitioners who are also assessors, we have the responsibility for maintaining competent practice so that our measurements are made against these standards. Furthermore, in exercising professional accountability, the NMC (2002a) requires its practitioners on the professional register to maintain and improve professional knowledge and competence. One point arising from debates on competence is the requirement for the practitioner to keep up-to-date to claim that practice is competent (Hager and Gonczi 1996, McGaghie 1991). The ENB (1995) states that assessors 'must be able to demonstrate a sound knowledge of, and skills in, contemporary nursing practice'. Notwithstanding professional requirements, the bottom line in the argument for keeping up-to-date must be the legal requirement that professional health care practitioners can exercise contemporary professional practices as the law expects current practice to be the accepted practice (Young 1994). The practitioner thus has the legal duty to update knowledge and practice.

Young (1994) states that the legal implication of the instructor omitting certain information, or of giving wrong information, is potential negligence. This potential exists whenever a failure in instruction jeopardizes the safety of the nurse being instructed, or of the patient in her care. I would also suggest that unless a mentor/assessor is also a competent practitioner, training requirements may not be fulfilled due to the inability to teach what is competent practice. The mentor/assessor thus has a legal duty, as well as moral and professional accountability to fulfil, in terms of keeping up-to-date and maintaining competent practice.

Standards of care delivery by learners

The mentor/assessor has a dual responsibility: to the patient/client and to the student. Mentors and assessors must meet a standard of care with respect to the patient/client and a standard of conduct with respect to the student. Assessors must ensure that students have the necessary clinical experiences to develop professional competencies in such a way so that the patient/client is not harmed in any way while the student is giving the care. The NMC (2002a) states that patient safety must always take precedence above all else. The *Code of Professional Conduct* (NMC 2002a) makes sure that practitioners put the interests of patients, clients and the public before their own interests and those of professional colleagues: i.e. accountability to the patient is always more important than to the student.

In the eyes of the law, the student's performance must be equal to that of a registered practitioner (Young 1994). The law is quite clear that a lack of experience or knowledge is never an excuse for incompetent care. Student nurses and student midwives are thus required to provide care equivalent to that of the registered nurse or midwife. One judge (in Young 1994:56) adopted the following view:

The law requires the trainee or learner to be judged by the same standard as his more experienced colleagues. If it did not, inexperience would frequently be urged as a defence to an action for professional negligence.

Another judge linked the expected standard of care to that of the post rather than to the status of the person performing the care, saying:

> To my mind the notion of a duty tailored to the actor, rather than to the act which he elects to perform, has no place in the law of tort.

Therefore, in a highly specialized clinical setting, the standard must be 'not just that of the averagely competent and well-informed [nurse] but of such a person who fills a post in a unit offering a highly specialized service' (Wilsher v Essex AHA 1988, in Young 1994).

For the student to deliver care to a standard equivalent to that of a registered nurse or midwife, that care to be given to the patient/client must be within the student's capabilities. As far as the NMC (UKCC 1998c) is concerned, it is the registered practitioner working with the student who is professionally responsible for the consequences of the actions and omissions of that student. A pre-registration student, or any other unqualified staff, who is not on the professional register cannot be called to account for her/his actions or omissions by the NMC. This is made explicit in the following clause in the Code:

> You may be expected to delegate care delivery to others who are not registered nurses or midwives. . . . You remain accountable for the appropriateness of the delegation, for ensuring that the person who does the work is able to do it and that adequate supervision or support is provided.

Delegation of responsibility to unqualified staff generated a lot of debate at the UKCC (UKCC 1996b). There have been a number of cases where qualified staff have been reported to the UKCC for inappropriate delegation of responsibilities. One case, which was closed by the Preliminary Proceedings Committee (PPC) of the UKCC, concerned the delegation by a nurse to a care assistant of the task of administering an insulin injection. The case was reported on the basis that such administration by a care assistant was prima facie wrong. The issue considered by the PPC was not whether the care assistant could not give the injection but whether the person to whom the responsibility was being delegated was competent to carry out the task. The UKCC concluded that the issue was about supervision, the appropriateness of the delegation and the instruction of unqualified staff, not about the rigid demarcation of work into tasks to be done by one group or another.

It is therefore important to know *when* and to *whom* it is safe to delegate. In order to delegate safely and to avoid negligent delegation, the practitioner must be satisfied that the person performing the delegated task is competent to carry it out (Young 1994). Making the following two checks may help you to decide when it is safe to delegate. Assess:

■ The extent of the person's knowledge and understanding of the task. This requires skilful questioning of the person. This point is developed in Chapter 4.
■ How skilful the person is in the task delegated. This may require observation and close supervision of the person initially. It is important to provide ongoing supervision. The amount and extent of the supervision will vary from person to person. However, Wood (1987) holds that students must be under strict supervision at all times. This point on supervision of students will be developed in Chapter 6 when management of the continuous assessment process is discussed.

The learning and assessment programme for the student must therefore be planned so that the patient/client is protected from harm while enabling the student to develop and achieve the professional competencies required by the NMC.

Clause 4.1 of the Code requires the practitioner to recognize and respect the involvement of patients/clients and their families and informal carers in the planning and delivery of care. The practitioner has to be concerned about standards when care is undertaken by relatives. The legal position, once again, involves the possible negligence of delegating care inappropriately to a relative or an informal carer (Young 1994). If the relative takes on this care voluntarily and the care is that normally undertaken by the relative at home, then legal outcomes should be unlikely. Nevertheless, where the care given requires nursing skill that has to be learnt, training and supervision must be provided. In addition, senior management should be consulted as to the appropriateness of the delegation, as the employing authority has to carry vicarious liability for the practitioner's actions (Young 1992).

What is taught, learnt and assessed

The mentor/assessor has the responsibility for ensuring that the learning environment is conducive to learning. A wide range of high-quality learning opportunities should be arranged and provided to enable the student to achieve learning outcomes and competencies. The Nurses, Midwives and Health Visitors Act 1997 Section 2(3) requires the NMC, by means of rules, to determine the standard, kind and content of training to be undertaken with a view to registration. The kind and standard of pre-registration nursing programmes leading to registration on Parts 12, 13, 14 or 15 of the NMC's register are currently set out in Statutory Instrument 1989 No. 1456, The Nurses, Midwives and Health Visitors (Registered Fever Nurse Amendment Rules and Training Amendment Rules) Approval Order 1989. Rule 33 of the Midwives Rules (UKCC 1998b) sets out the outcomes of programmes leading to entry to Part 10 of the NMC's register. Following the publication of the report of the UKCC's Education Commission, *Fitness for Practice* (UKCC 1999b), the UKCC adopted the competency-based approach to pre-registration nursing and midwifery education. Pre-registration nursing and midwifery programmes now require students to achieve national competencies (UKCC 2000a, 2000b – Appendices 1 and 2). It is a requirement that pre-registration programmes shall be designed to enable students to apply knowledge, understanding and skills when performing to the standards required in employment and to provide the care that patients/clients require, safely and competently, in order to assume, on registration, the responsibilities and accountability necessary for public protection. The UKCC made it clear that these competencies are achieved under the direction of the mentor/assessor. In accepting the roles of mentor/assessor as defined by the ENB and the Department of Health (see earlier discussion), the practitioner is responsible for ensuring that teaching and learning activities, including clinical experiences, assist the student in achieving these competencies. This requires practitioners to have a sound knowledge of the learning needs of the students they are mentoring and assessing. The ENB (1995) stated that assessors 'must be able to demonstrate a full understanding of the appropriate aspects of the curriculum'. This will enable the mentor/assessor identify and plan appropriate teaching and learning activities and clinical experiences. As in any practice discipline, it is not enough just to have a 'knowledge of' – one needs to know what to do with that knowledge. This leads us into the next 'what for' aspect of accountability of the mentor/assessor: namely that of facilitating and measuring that learning.

Standards of teaching and assessing

The student is entitled to the best instruction available (Young 1994, Wood 1987). Failure to instruct properly could be construed as a negligent act (Goclowski 1985). The standard of teaching and learning that an academic institution is expected to provide for its students is generally stated in the institution's 'student charter'. For example, the *Student's Charter* of the University of Sheffield states that the 'University will provide in all its Faculties a high standard of teaching, guidance, supervision and academic facilities' (University of Sheffield 2001a). Service providers for patient/client care enter into contracts with higher education institutions to provide clinical experience for students. Within such contracts is an agreement to provide a standard of teaching and learning in the clinical setting commensurate with that set by the educational institution. To achieve the required standards of the teaching and assessment of clinical practice, mentors and assessors need to attain and maintain competent practice in these roles. It is recognized that clinical staff exercise a major influence on the quality of pre-registration programmes (Eraut et al 1995). They do much of the teaching, supervision and assessment of students, and as it is likely that this will continue, it is imperative that they are capable of fulfilling these roles (Clifford 1995, White et al 1994). Activities that mentors/assessors are expected to provide will include planning learning opportunities for and with students to enable them to achieve their individual learning needs; facilitating and supporting the learning process; assessing learning; and providing feedback to students on their performance (Neary 2000, Eraut et al 1995). To support these educational processes in the clinical setting, higher education institutions generally include a policy for the management of the assessment of clinical practice in its curriculum document. For example, at the University of Sheffield (2000), the assessor is required to carry out an initial interview with the student to negotiate and formulate a learning contract in order that the learning outcomes may be achieved. Subsequently, an intermediate interview must take place half way through the placement to review the student's progress and achievement, and formal feedback is given and documented. A final interview allows the assessor to make a summative assessment of whether the student has achieved the learning outcomes of the placement.

Assessors must be aware of, and be careful that, any policy regulating the assessment of practice is followed, as any deviation from such regulations could give rise to students appealing against any unfavourable assessment decision on the grounds of not having received the supervision, guidance and support to which they are entitled. Cases of students suing nursing institutions in the courts using the above grounds as educational malpractice are well documented in the North American literature (see for example Halstead 1998a, Graveley and Stanley 1993, Goclowski 1985, Spink 1983). Courts have recognized that by virtue of their training, assessors are uniquely qualified to observe and judge all aspects of their students' performance. Court decision ruling in favour of the student has been on the basis of assessors not following established guidelines for the supervision of the student.

Mentors and assessors require adequate preparation to enable them to manage the educational activities to support learning and assessment. Subsequently, regular updates are important to inform mentors and assessors of developments in the curriculum and the assessment process. These sessions can be used as opportunities to discuss assessment problems which can contribute to the enhancement of the mentoring/assessing roles. Unfortunately, there is current unease about the expertise of mentors and assessors. Research shows that the initial preparation and continuing development of mentors and assessors are inadequate, particularly with respect to knowledge of programmes and assessment of practice (Gerrish et al 1997). In order to address and overcome these urgent problems, the Department of Health (1999) and the UKCC (1999b) strongly recommend that there should be joint responsibilities between service providers and higher education institutions for the preparation, support and updating of mentors and assessors. Whereas mentors and assessors are personally accountable for their practice of the supervision and assessment of students (NMC 2002a), service providers and higher education institutions are responsible for ensuring that training, support and updating opportunities are provided for practitioners to develop their mentoring and assessing roles.

Professional judgements about student performance

By virtue of their role, assessors have the right, and are indeed vested with the onerous responsibility of making professional judgements about the performance of students (ENB and Department of Health 2001; ENB 1997, 1988). These professional judgements require the assessor to make and report on two important professional decisions: first, they are reporting on the degree to which a student has met the programme learning outcomes and standard; secondly, they are reporting on the ability of the student to provide professionally competent and safe care to the public. It is important for the assessor to remember that professional judgements not only assess the student's current competence but also provide a prediction of the student's potential ability to practise as a professional nurse or midwife. Therefore, the conclusion about a student's performance should attempt to elicit predictive validity and reliability. These important criteria of sound assessments are developed in Chapter 5.

Literature on the assessment of clinical practice abounds with discussions about the subjective nature of this process. Ashworth and Morrison (1991:260) stated that:

> . . . assessing involves the perception of evidence about performance by
> an assessor, and the arrival at a decision concerning the level of
> performance of the person being assessed. Here there is enormous,
> unavoidable scope for subjectivity especially when the competencies being
> assessed are relatively intangible ones.

Assessments about a student's performance frequently reflect the assessor's personal perception of what performance constitutes professional nursing or midwifery practice. Such an assessment is based on both objective and subjective criteria. There is, therefore, a danger that some decisions about student performance may be biased and unfair. Assessors should be aware that many factors, some of which they are unaware of, can interfere with fair and equitable professional judgements, resulting in the student being treated unfairly.

As noted earlier, students have the right to expect that they will be notified of any deficiencies in their performance. The mentor/assessor is behaving unfairly and unethically if the student is not informed about unsatisfactory performance (Orchard 1994). Furthermore, mentors and assessors who fail to evaluate a student's unsatisfactory performance accurately, either through reluctance to expose the student to the experience of failure or through a fear of potential redress by the student, are guilty of misleading the student, potentially jeopardizing patient/client care and placing the higher education institution in a difficult situation. It is much fairer to students to inform them of unsatisfactory performance as soon as such performance is identified. Informing students of deficiencies in a caring and constructive way allows students the opportunity to improve their performance; not to inform them denies them this opportunity and right (Halstead 1998a).

I have put forward what I see are the main aspects that mentors and assessors are responsible and accountable for when they supervise and assess learners. The next section examines the 'TO WHOM?' aspects.

Responsibility and accountability TO WHOM?

As discussed earlier, one position that the RCN takes in relationship to professional accountability is that it comprises ethical, societal and public duty and protective elements for patients and clients. These elements of professional accountability may also be applied to the supervision and assessment of learners. With professional registration, each practitioner is vested with personal autonomy. A contract of employment gives the structural autonomy for the authority to act in the best interests of patients and clients. This contract frequently also requires the nurse or midwife to take on the role of mentor and/or preceptor – this gives the mentor/preceptor the authority to act in the best interests of the learner.

Based on the above context of accountability, and extrapolating from the work of mainstream education, mentors and preceptors responsible for the supervision and assessment of clinical practice can be seen to assume the three aspects of educational accountability described by Becher et al (1981):

- professional accountability: responsibility to self, colleagues and the profession
- contractual accountability: accountability to the employer or someone in authority
- moral accountability: answerability to students and their parents.

Teachers are accountable for their professional conduct, such as the selection and implementation of appropriate forms of practice. Contractually, they are under an obligation to report to, and be partly directed by a specific person or group of persons. A teacher in mainstream education is contractually accountable to the head teacher. Moral accountability is of special importance in education as it pervades the teacher–pupil relationship. These aspects of

ACTIVITY 2.3

Make a list of the individuals and bodies that you consider you are responsible and accountable to when you supervise and assess students. Why do you think you are responsible and accountable to them?

accountability will now be used to examine the *to whom* aspects of responsibility and accountability when supervising and assessing the clinical practice of students. Before you proceed, you may wish to try Activity 2.3.

After the fairly extensive discussion of professional responsibility and accountability required of the practitioner by the NMC, the most obvious individual to be named would be the patient/client. Other 'stakeholders' are:

■ the student
■ yourself as the professional
■ your professional colleagues
■ your profession and the NMC
■ your trust or employing authority
■ the higher education institution.

Each of the above individuals and bodies will now be considered in an examination of why you might be responsible and accountable to them. This will be developed in four sections, namely that of responsibility and accountability to:

■ the patient/client
■ the student
■ the trust/employing authority and the higher education institution
■ yourself, colleagues and your profession.

The patient/client

The practitioner on the NMC professional register has both a legal and a professional duty of care for patients and clients. In law, the courts could find a registered practitioner negligent if a person suffers harm because the practitioner has failed to care for the patient/client properly. Professionally, the NMC's Professional Conduct Committee could find a registered practitioner guilty of misconduct and remove the practitioner from the register if he or she failed to care properly for a patient/client, even though the patient/client suffered no harm (NMC 2002a, 2002b). The practitioner's accountability and duty of care to the patient/client when supervising students has been discussed at some length in the previous section (see responsibility and accountability for standards of care delivery by learners). It will be reiterated here that the pre-registration student cannot be called to account by the NMC for any actions and omissions. It is the registered practitioner with whom the student is working who is professionally responsible and accountable for the consequences of the student's actions and omissions.

When making arrangements for the student to care for patients and clients, the wishes of the patients and clients should be respected at all times. Under the *Patient's Charter*, patients/clients have the right to choose whether or not to take part in medical research or student training (Department of Health 1995).

This right should be made clear to them when they are first given information about care they will receive from the student. Their rights as patients or clients supersede at all times the student's rights to knowledge and experience (UKCC 1998c).

The student

Students have rights: these need to be respected, while at the same time professional standards and expectations of their performance are maintained. Students also have obligations and responsibilities to fulfil. It is important for the mentor/assessor to recognize what these rights, obligations and responsibilities are so that the student may be assisted in the most appropriate ways to succeed during clinical practice. The mentor/assessor also needs to recognize that there are legal, professional and moral obligations towards students under supervision.

Student rights, obligations and responsibilities.   Higher education institutions have the right to set academic standards for students. They have the responsibility to communicate those standards to students. Institutions usually have written policies that govern student progression, grading and discipline. These policies are typically made available to students through the student handbook, which serves as a contract between the student and the institution (Halstead 1998a). The policies that individual schools of nursing and midwifery or courses have regarding progression, grading and dismissal of students must be in agreement with the institution's policies. Any student who has enrolled in a course has agreed to abide by the policies of the course and those of the higher education institution. Within assessment regulations (Halstead 1998a) students have the following rights:

- to know the behaviours and competencies that are expected of them to pass the clinical placement successfully
- to receive timely feedback about their performance and the opportunity and support to correct behaviour that is considered unsatisfactory
- to be made aware that their performance is not meeting the criteria that have been set for satisfactory performance before being failed
- to work under the supervision of a qualified practitioner who has been appropriately trained to be a mentor/assessor.

Within any scheme of the continuous assessment of practice, there must be formalized meetings between the student and the mentor/assessor to guide student learning, which will also enable these rights to be met. Assessment regulations relating to the continuous assessment of practice at the University of Sheffield (2000, 2001b) require clinical mentors/assessors to conduct a minimum of three documented formal interviews with student nurses and student midwives. Failure to do so could give rise to grounds for student appeal against an unfavourable assessment decision.

All higher education institutions have established policies for hearing student grievances and appeals. These policies exist to protect the student's rights and to provide student recourse to appeal assessment decisions previously made (Halstead 1998a). The grievance and student appeal process provides the opportunity for the original assessment decision to be reassessed. An example of the appeals process of one higher education institution can be found in Appendix 3.

As stated above, any student who has enrolled in a course has agreed to abide by the policies of the course and those of the higher education institution. Additionally, nursing and midwifery students need to abide by the standards set out in the UKCC document *A UKCC Guide for Students of Nursing and Midwifery* (UKCC 1998c). Several responsibilities are thus conferred on the student. Higher education institutions can expect students:

■ to fulfil regulations governing the progress of students
■ not to behave in ways which can be alleged as misconduct.

Appendices 4 and 5 contain one higher education institution's regulations governing the progress and discipline of students. These regulations serve to safeguard standards of training and conduct. Failure to fulfil and/or comply with these regulations could result in the student being dismissed from the course. Students are thus directly accountable to their higher education institution. In my professional experience, I have known students to be disciplined by the higher education institution for falsifying their assessors' signatures in the assessment of practice records. This misconduct has resulted in those students being dismissed from their course. Mentors and assessors have the responsibility of assisting higher education institutions to uphold these regulations.

The UKCC (1998c) and higher education institutions make it clear to students that they must always work under the direct supervision of a registered nurse, midwife or health visitor. Furthermore, students should not participate in any procedure for which they have not been fully prepared or in which they are not adequately supervised (UKCC 1998c). The University of Sheffield (2000, 2001b) allows its students to practise only to the level of competence consistent with course requirement. Within this regulation, when it is unclear whether engagement in an aspect of care delivery could be beyond the student's usual scope of practice, it becomes incumbent upon the student, and her mentor/assessor, to seek guidance from the School of Nursing and Midwifery.

The student can also be called to account by the law for the consequences of her actions or omissions as a pre-registration student (UKCC 1998c). The student must behave in a reasonable way (Castledine 2000). What is reasonable? The case of Bolam v Friern Hospital Management Committee produced the 'Bolam Test' of what is reasonable (UKCC 1996a). The test derives from a case heard in 1957 where a psychiatric patient was given electroconvulsive therapy without any relaxant drugs or restraint. He suffered several fractures and claimed compensation. The judge, in deciding how to determine the standard which should have been followed, said:

> When you get a situation which involved the use of some special skill or competence, then the test as to whether there has been negligence or not is the standard of the ordinary skilled man exercising and professing to have that special skill. A man need not possess the highest expert skill; it is well established that it is sufficient if he exercises the ordinary skill of an ordinary competent man exercising that particular art.

> He is not guilty of negligence if he has acted in accordance with a practice accepted as proper by a responsible body of medical men skilled in that particular art.

> (in Dimond 1994:115).

Although the case concerned a doctor, the Bolam Test can be used to examine the actions of any professional person. The case of Wilsher v Essex AHA (1988 in Young 1994) sets the standard of reasonable care to be expected of students and junior staff. The standard is that of a reasonably competent practitioner and not that of a student or junior.

A student must be of 'good character' before being admitted to the UKCC professional register. The *Declaration of Good Character* form (see Appendix 6), issued by the UKCC, has to be signed by the course director of the higher education institution prior to registration (UKCC 1998c). Generally, within assessment structures and processes, mentors and assessors contribute evidence to enable the higher education institution to judge whether the student is suitable for professional practice. There are occasions where directors do not support the declaration because of gross misconduct or criminal convictions during the training (Castledine 2000).

Professional and legal responsibility and accountability to the student.
Professional accountability to the student requires the practitioner to respect and uphold student rights and the higher education institution's regulations as discussed above. It also requires the practitioner to be aware of those aspects of accountability when supervising and assessing students. These have been discussed in the section Responsibility and accountability FOR WHAT?

The practitioner has a legal duty to care not only for patients/clients but also for others under her/his care, such as students (UKCC 1996a, NMC 2002a). In law, the courts could find a registered practitioner negligent if a person suffers harm because she or he failed to care for them properly. Lord Atkin (House of Lords 1932 in UKCC 1996a:10) defined the duty of care when he gave judgement in the case of Donoghue v Stephenson:

> You must take reasonable care to avoid acts or omissions which you can reasonably foresee would be likely to injure your neighbour. Who, then, in the law is my neighbour? The answer seems to be persons who are so closely and directly affected by my act that I ought to have them in contemplations as being so affected when I am directing my mind to the acts or omissions which are called in question.

This means that a practitioner has a duty in relation to colleagues to ensure that they are reasonably safe from her/his actions (Dimond 1994). This important duty to safeguard the health and safety of other persons who may be affected by the practitioner's acts or omissions also comes under Health and Safety at Work regulations (Young 1994). For example, if work is delegated, a failure to supervise can lead to the practitioner who delegates being sued for negligence by the less experienced person if she/he (rather than the patient) suffers harm (Young 1994:58). In addition, under the Health and Safety at Work Act 1974, a practitioner could be prosecuted for any such acts or omissions.

Under health and safety at work regulations the employer has a statutory duty to keep employees informed, as well as provide training, on topics that are likely to affect health and safety (Young 1994). Examples of training are the provision of information on particular diseases that have health implications to the practitioner, such as HIV infection and AIDS, and treatments that carry risks to those administering them, such as the toxic effects of certain drugs.

Practitioners working in some areas will often face particular risks. For example, the community nurse will need specialist training to enable her to move and handle clients safely in their homes and the nurse in the psychiatric or learning disability areas may need a greater input on preventing and dealing with aggression and violence. Careful record-keeping of any training is important under the Health and Safety at Work Act for the protection of both the employer and employee.

Training needs to be given to both qualified and unqualified personnel. This means that students must also receive such training. The higher education institution must ensure that a student receives sufficient training on health and safety prior to the start of clinical practice. This is to protect the student as well as patients and others. Areas of particular concern are moving and handling, the handling of aggression and violence, firefighting regulations and safety and the control of infection. Subsequently, when the student starts the clinical placement, it is the joint responsibility of the mentor/assessor and the student to ensure that the following training takes place on the student's first working day:

- the student understands her/his responsibilities in the event of a fire, cardiac arrest and any other emergency
- the student has been shown the layout of the clinical area, including fire exits and fire and resuscitation equipment
- the student knows her/his responsibilities with regard to health and safety at work
- the student has been instructed in moving and handling patients/clients in the clinical area.

The training should be documented in the student's records. This is to protect the student, the service provider and the higher education institution in case of any later legal action for negligence.

Students with special needs. Rowntree (1987:60) says that to 'treat people equally is not necessarily to treat them fairly. Indeed, people being so different, equal treatment probably means injustice for most'. This is more so for students with special needs than for the majority who are sufficiently fortunate to be classed as 'normal'. Students with particular health problems, e.g. diabetes, should be allocated the appropriate meal breaks to assist in maintaining the desired control over the diabetic condition. Students who have dyslexia should be accorded the due regard for their condition and be provided with any extra support and time they may require in order to learn (Wright 2000). The reader is directed to the work of Halstead (1998b) for a further discussion of teaching students with special needs.

Moral responsibility and accountability to the student. Moral responsibility and accountability are of special importance as they pervade the mentor/assessor–student relationship. Several of the ENB standards (ENB 1997) for the approval of higher education institutions and programmes call for clear lines of support to be developed to enable students to achieve the learning outcomes of the educational programmes. Cox (1982) makes the point that unless students are adequately supervised and supported on the wards, they are getting short-changed in educational terms. What actions can mentors/assessors take so that they do not fall short of fulfilling moral responsibilities and accountability owed to the student?

During the early days of working in a clinical area, the student is a 'guest' in that area. Special efforts should be made to make students feel welcomed initially and to help them settle into the area as quickly as possible. A common anxiety of students starting new placements is to feel unwelcomed and unwanted (Phillips et al 2000). If students feels safe and that they belong, they will begin to relax and be in a better position to start learning (Maslow 1954). In the hierarchy of human needs, Maslow (1954) postulates that the basic needs must be met first in order for the higher needs to be achieved. Many students lack confidence in their ability to learn and need to be empowered to believe in their ability to succeed (Halstead 1998a).

The clinical area is anxiety-provoking for students (Halstead 1998a, Parkes 1985). The mentor/assessor can help reduce levels of anxiety and stress for the student by being aware of situations which may be stressful to students. Action can then be taken to assist the student to cope with these stressors. The quality of student–mentor/assessor interactions has the potential to have either positive or negative effects on the outcomes of the educational process by affecting student performance in the clinical setting (see, for example, Spouse 1996, Earnshaw 1995, Darling 1984). The mentor/assessor has the responsibility to befriend the student so that a positive relationship can start to be fostered. Other qualities of the mentor/assessor that a student seeks, and which directly affect learning and performance and hence the outcomes of assessment, are discussed by Neary (2000). The mentor/assessor owes it to the student to know what these are so that the student may be assisted in the most effective ways of achieving learning outcomes.

As we have seen in Chapter 1, the power for making assessment decisions is firmly in the hands of the assessor. The law also emphasizes the authority of the roles of the teacher and assessor (Young 1992). A student has the right to appeal only against the conduct of the assessment but not the verdict. Within this assessment practice, several assumptions are made about the assessor (Harding and Greig 1994):

- The assessor is aware of personal limitations and can always be objective in assessment. The discussion in Chapter 5 will show that our assessments can be greatly influenced by personal biases and prejudices. This makes many assessment decisions far from the objectivity we like to espouse.

- There is a universally agreed standard of practice by which to judge a student's practice. However, standards of clinical practice vary amongst practitioners. Some students therefore, may be subject to assessments which have been made based on standards of practice falling at either end of the continuum of high to low standards. In either case, the student is treated unfairly.

- Assessors possess the necessary knowledge, skills and attitudes for the supervision and assessment of learners who may be undertaking a course of training different from their own. However, many research studies have found that assessors frequently do not understand the learning needs of students they are assessing (Fraser et al 1997, May et al 1997, Eraut et al 1995, White et al 1994, Bedford et al 1993).

- Students receive sufficient quality teaching and supervision from their mentors and assessors to enable them to achieve learning outcomes so that they pass their assessments. Again, findings from the above studies indicate that

ACTIVITY 2.4

If a student fails a placement, has the placement and by inference the mentor/assessor, failed in their duties towards the student, or has the student failed the placement?

this is not the case. The student is generally in competition against the patient/client for the practitioner's time and the student loses out. The *Code of Professional Conduct* (NMC 2002a) makes it clear that the duty of care to the patient/client must always take precedence over all else.

By virtue of the authority and assumptions vested in assessors, students are owed a high level of moral responsibility and accountability. Lello (1979:6) makes the point that 'if people are working closely together they have a continuing and permanent answerability to each other'. Who, then, is on trial, asks Rowntree (1987:9). The mentor/assessor or the student? Ponder this question posed by Rowntree in Activity 2.4.

Even if a student has been openly disinterested and has made no effort to learn, Rowntree cautions against laying the entire responsibility for the failure upon the student. There may be no straightforward answers to the question. It is up to the mentor/assessor to confront the answers after considering the moral responsibilities and accountability owed to the student. Issues surrounding the legal and professional responsibility and accountability of assessment are less tangible and it is perhaps easier for the student to obtain redress if she or he is unfairly treated. Moral responsibility and accountability, however, rest very much with the individual's moral code. It may not be possible for the student to obtain any form of redress if unfairness is the result of failure to exercise a level of moral responsibility and accountability towards the student.

The trust/employing authority and the higher education institution

Higher education institutions enter into contracts with their students to provide such educational experiences as are required to fulfil the aims of the programme. In the case of nursing and midwifery students where clinical experience is a requisite component of pre-registration programmes, higher education institutions in the United Kingdom require to enter into contracts with service providers such as National Health Service Trusts and private organizations such as nursing homes to provide the clinical experiences. Such contracts are typically written and specify the management of the educational process for the student during clinical practice. The specifications of the service agreement between the University of Sheffield and a National Health Service Trust (University of Sheffield 2001c) is provided in detail here as an example. The agreement specifies that the Trust will provide the following:

- A high standard of teaching, learning and assessment.
- A designated supervisor who is responsible for supervising, teaching and assessing student performance.
- The supervisor is also responsible for assigning the relevant duties to the student, so that the student is given opportunities to work with a range of patients/clients.

- A liaison officer for the placement area who will liaise directly with the designated clinical link lecturer.
- Advising students of all local internal protocols, policies and reporting procedures relevant to the area of work.
- Ensuring that the University is notified of any accident or illness sustained by a student on placement within a timescale appropriate to the seriousness of the situation.
- Advising or instructing students to leave clinical areas, if in the Trust's view, the student is at risk or the student's health status is putting colleagues or patients at risk.
- Informing students of the specific approaches and practices for moving and handling people.
- Liability for students during the period of their placement, extending to matters of employers/occupiers liability and public liability and in respect of acts or omissions of its own employees.
- When undertaking specific procedures, the student will be provided with all protective clothing or equipment necessary for the maintenance of health and safety.
- In the event where there are reasonable grounds to suspect that a student may have committed a criminal offence or an act of serious misconduct, the Trust may immediately suspend, without prejudice, the attachment of the student and remove the student from the work area. Any such suspension must be reported to the University within 24 working hours.
- Where a student is involved in any Trust disciplinary proceedings, the University will be informed.
- There is no discrimination against any student on grounds of race, creed, gender, sexual orientation or disability and the Trust will apply its equal opportunity policy to students as it does its own employees.
- Should service developments and changes impact on the placement educational environment in respect of both quality and capacity, the Trust will inform the University in advance of any service changes.
- The Trust will allow access to placement areas for University staff for the purposes of educational audit.

The specifications of these agreements have been provided here in detail to inform mentors and assessors of their direct lines of responsibility and accountability to the Trust, and indirectly to the higher education institution, when supervising and assessing students. The list of specifications may appear onerous. However, if the mentor/assessor exercises the requisite duty of care owed to students as discussed above, and follows assessment regulations laid down by the higher education institution, there will then be no necessity for concern.

Yourself, colleagues and your profession

The NMC's responsibilities are set out in the Nurses, Midwives and Health Visitors Acts of 1979 and 1992. The Council's main responsibility is to protect the interests of the public. To do this, standards for education, training and professional conduct are set for its practitioners. The NMC (2002a) and the law make it clear that standards of clinical practice must be upheld at all times. As an assessor then, failure to uphold standards of clinical practice may compromise not only yourself professionally and legally but also your colleagues and the profession, as your personal standard of practice is frequently reflected in your assessment decisions. Stated simplistically, a lower standard of clinical practice may result in the assessor expecting a lower, maybe even unsafe, standard of performance of their student. You would not have fulfilled moral and professional responsibilities and accountability towards your colleagues and the profession if these compromised standards are not recognized, resulting in a failure to correct such deficits or to remove the student from training. Such unsafe students are likely to become registered practitioners on the NMC's professional register. As practitioners and assessors, we need to uphold the role of the NMC in protecting the public by maintaining a register of people who are recommended to be suitable practitioners and who have demonstrated knowledge and skill through a qualification registered with the NMC. Fowler and Heater (1983:404) stated very strongly that assessors are:

> . . . bound by a moral responsibility to the profession of nursing to give passing grades to only those students who have demonstrated clinical competence.

In accepting the role of clinical assessor, the practitioner implicitly accepts the responsibility and accountability for maintaining standards of supervision and assessment in order that the standards of professional colleagues and the profession are protected.

ISSUES AND DILEMMA OF THE MENTOR–ASSESSOR INTERFACE

Holloway (1985) found that moral accountability to students (see discussion above) emphasizes the importance of a 'special relationship' between teacher and student. This 'special relationship' is permeated by empathy, trust and affinity, which in turn facilitate the learning process. Good mentoring practices (discussed in Chapters 8 and 9) on the part of the practitioner require the development of this 'special relationship'. At the same time, the practitioner has professional accountabilities to fulfil. Professional accountability stresses the importance of maintaining standards of professional practice to safeguard patient/client care. The practitioner working with a student is thus required to be an assessor – to judge the student's clinical competence. Can both moral accountability to students and professional accountability be fulfilled without causing anguish to both parties? In developing a 'special relationship' the practitioner as mentor is a 'friend' to the student (Neary 1997, Darling 1984). Enacting the role of assessor requires the practitioner to be a 'judge' (Neary 1997). Is a friend capable of being an objective judge? Students in Neary's (1997) study saw the assessor as not forming any 'special relationship' with them but as having the formal tasks of assessing skills and progress, completing assessment booklets and keeping records. They thought that mentors took responsibility for students and provided guidance, gave support, assisted the student in setting learning outcomes and subsequently acted as facilitator for learning and created learning opportunities.

Whereas it is already accepted in many practice settings that mentors do act as assessors and vice versa (Andrews 1999, Neary 1997), should a mentor and an assessor be the same person? The student nurses interviewed in Neary's study had opinions which ranged from being happy with the same practitioner as both mentor and assessor to the other extreme of preferring the mentor and assessor to be two different people. Many did not wished to be assessed summatively by their mentor, especially if the relationship was not a comfortable or relaxed one. Many students referred to the necessity of a good relationship for the assessment to be fair. When the relationship developed into friendship, some students felt that the mentor could not remain unbiased. Students in White et al's (1994) study also thought that the nature of the relationship between mentor and student affected the assessment process – positively in the event of a good relationship or negatively in the event of a poor relationship. However, there were students in Neary's study who expected all practitioners to remain 'professional' and to be able to assess against agreed criteria without bias or prejudice. Such is the idealistic world! The practitioners in Neary's study were more definite in their view about being both mentor and assessor – many found it difficult to 'wear two hats' and experienced role conflict. They obviously preferred not to be in this position.

Recent guidelines from the ENB and the Department of Health (2001) state clearly that the mentor has the responsibility to supervise, support and guide students in practice as well as implement approved assessment procedures and assess competencies to demonstrate the extent to which learning outcomes have been met. The mentor is now expected to be the assessor as well. Prior to these guidelines, mentors were not required to assess – rather, their roles and responsibilities related directly to guiding, assisting and supporting student learning (ENB 1988, 1997). Neary (1997:37) made this succinct point:

> . . . [rather] than to continue the debate on what is a 'mentor' and what is an 'assessor', it is perhaps more important for nurses to work together at local level and reach a common understanding of what is expected of the qualified staff in practice placement . . .

Furthermore, it is my contention that if assessment processes are to assist learning (see Chapter 6) the practitioner who is both mentor and assessor is best placed to fulfil this function of assessment. Assessment of clinical practice is a complex activity and has always been fraught with difficulties – is it ever possible to remain 'professional' and to be able to assess against agreed criteria without bias or prejudice? What is important is that assessment processes assist learning while retaining a focus on procedures (Torrance and Pryor 1998). If learning is facilitated through our assessment processes, the products of assessment are more likely to be positive.

CONCLUSION

Inherent in professional practice are professional responsibilities and accountability. The nursing and midwifery professions, along with other professional groups serving our society, are increasingly held accountable for the quality of service they provide. Is society receiving the care it needs, or is it receiving the care we think it needs or deserves (Reilly 1980)? This requires an assessment of our goals, our actions, resources and outcomes of care in light of society's needs. As mentors and assessors in whatever setting we practise, we too will be held more and more accountable for our actions. We must answer to the student, to society, to our profession, to our colleagues, to our employer, to the higher education institution offering the programme, and to ourselves.

The student is the direct consumer and beneficiary of our educational programmes. Is the student getting the kind of learning that is needed or is the student getting short-changed in educational terms? Before we claim that the student is indeed the beneficiary, we should try to answer the following question posed by Reilly (1980:3): 'How well do we meet our contract with the learner?'

Assessment of clinical practice is a significant responsibility and can be both challenging and time consuming. It also carries professional, contractual and moral accountability. Lello (1979) acknowledges the burden of being answerable and responsible. The strain results from the amount of responsibility shouldered rather than from the amount of work done. To achieve the purposes of clinical assessment, we need to recognize and accept the responsibilities and accountability of an assessor. Reilly (1980:3) challenges us most succinctly by posing the following questions:

> We are the gatekeepers of our profession, with the power to determine who enters the profession and to define the nature of nursing [and midwifery] practice. How well are we using the power bestowed upon us?

> How well do we meet the test of accountability to ourselves? Are we authentic individuals? Have we formalised for ourselves values and beliefs that guide our actions? Are we true to those values, and are we real and genuine human beings?

Reilly raised these questions to remind nursing educators and clinical assessors involved with the evaluation of nursing and midwifery programmes that to achieve quality in any plan for accountability, they must incorporate the concept of responsibility. We have the ultimate responsibility – that of ensuring that only nurses and midwives who are competent are allowed to register with the NMC so that the public is safeguarded against unsafe and incompetent practice.

REFERENCES

Andrews M (1999) Mentorship in nursing: a review of the literature. *Journal of Advanced Nursing*, **29**(1), 201–207.

Ashworth P and Morrison P (1991) Problems of competence-based nurse education. *Nurse Education Today*, **11**, 256–260.

Bandura A (1977) *Social Learning Theory*. Englewood Cliffs, NJ: Prentice Hall.

Baskett M and Marsick V (1992) *Professional Ways of Knowing*. San Francisco: Jossey-Bass.

Becher T, Eraut M and Knight J (1981) *Policies for Educational Accountability*. London: Heinemann Educational Books.

Bedford H, Phillips T, Robinson J and Schostak J (1993) *Assessment of Competencies in Nursing and Midwifery Education and Training*. London: The English National Board for Nursing, Midwifery and Health Visiting.

Bergman R (1981) Accountability – definition and dimensions. *International Nursing Review*, **28**(2), 53–59.

Brykczynska G (1995) Working with children: accountability and paediatric nursing. In Watson R (ed) *Accountability in Nursing Practice*, pp 147–160. London: Chapman and Hall.

Castledine G (2000) Professional misconduct case studies: nursing students' accountability. *British Journal of Nursing*, 9(15), 965.

Castledine G (1991) Accountability in delivering care. *Nursing Standard*, 5(25), 28–31.

Champion R (1991) Educational accountability – what ho the 1990s! *Nurse Education Today*, 11, 407–414.

Charters A (2000) Encouraging student centred learning in a clinical environment. *Emergency Nurse*, 7(10), 25–29.

Clifford C (1995) The role of the nurse teachers: concerns, conflicts and challenges. *Nurse Education Today*, 15, 11–16.

Cox C (1982) The seeds of time. *Nurse Education Today*, 2(6) 4–10.

Darling LAW (1984) What do nurses want in a mentor? *The Journal of Nursing Administration*, **October**, 42–44.

Davies E (1993) Clinical role modeling: uncovering hidden knowledge. *Journal of Advanced Nursing*, 18(4), 627–636.

Department of Health (1999) *Making a Difference*. London: Department of Health.

Department of Health (1995) *The Patient's Charter*. London: Department of Health.

Dimond B (1994) *The Legal Aspects of Midwifery*. Cheshire: Books for Midwives Press.

Earnshaw GJ (1995) Mentorship: the students' views. *Nurse Education Today*, 15, 274–279.

Emerton A (1992) Professionalism and the UKCC. *British Journal of Nursing*, 1(1), 25–29.

ENB and Department of Health (2001) *Preparation of Mentors and Teachers*. London: The English National Board for Nursing, Midwifery and Health Visiting and the Department of Health.

ENB (1997) *Standards for Approval of Higher Education Institutions and Programmes*. London: The English National Board for Nursing, Midwifery and Health Visiting.

ENB (1995) *Creating Lifelong Learners: Partnerships for Care*. London: English National Board for Nursing, Midwifery and Health Visiting.

ENB (1988) *Institutional and Course Approval/Reapproval Process: Information Required, Criteria and Guidelines*. Circular 1988/39/APS. London: English National Board for Nursing, Midwifery and Health Visiting.

Eraut M, Alderton J, Boylan A and Wraight A (1995) *An Evaluation of the Contribution of the Biological and Social Sciences to Pre-registration Nursing and Midwifery Programmes*. London: The English National Board for Nursing, Midwifery and Health Visiting.

Fowler GA and Heater B (1983) Guidelines for clinical evaluation. *Journal of Nursing Education*, 22(9), 402–404.

Fraser D, Murphy R and Worth-Butler M (1997) *An Outcome Evaluation of the Effectiveness of Pre-registration Midwifery Programmes of Education*. London: The English National Board for Nursing, Midwifery and Health Visiting.

Gerrish K, McManus M and Ashworth P (1997) *Levels of Achievement: A Review of the Assessment of Practice*. London: English National Board for Nursing, Midwifery and Health Visiting.

Gilmore A (1999) *Report of the Analysis of the Literature Evaluating Pre-registration Nursing and Midwifery Education in the United Kingdom*. London: United Kingdom Central Council for Nursing, Midwifery and Health Visiting.

Goclowski J (1985) Legal implications of academic dismissal and educational malpractice for nursing faculty. *Journal of Nursing Education*, 24(3), 104–108.

Graveley EA and Stanley M (1993) A clinical failure: what the courts tell us. *Journal of Nursing Education*, 32(3), 135–137.

Hager P and Gonczi A (1996) Professions and competencies. In Edwards R et al (eds) *Boundaries of Adult Learning*, pp 246–260. London: Routledge.

Halstead JA (1998a) The academic performance of students. In Billings DM and Halstead JA (eds) *Teaching in Nursing: A Guide for Faculty*, pp 35–57. Philadelphia: WB Saunders.

Halstead JA (1998b) Teaching students with special needs. In Billings DM and Halstead JA (eds) *Teaching in Nursing: A Guide for Faculty*, pp 57–66. Philadelphia: WB Saunders.

Harding C and Greig M (1994) Issues of accountability in the assessment of practice. *Nurse Education Today*, 14, 118–123.

Hepworth S (1991) The assessment of student nurses. *Nurse Education Today*, 11, 46–52.

Holloway D (1985) Accountability in further education: teachers' perceptions. *Journal of Further and Higher Education*, 9(2), 31–45.

Lello J (ed) (1979) *Accountability in Education*. London: Ward Lock Educational.

McGaghie WC (1991) Professional competence evaluation. *Educational Researcher*, **20**, 3–9.

Marks-Maran D (1995) Accountability in nursing education. In Watson R (ed) *Accountability in Nursing Practice*, pp 232–240. London: Chapman and Hall.

Maslow A (1954) *Motivation and Personality*. New York: Harper and Row.

May N, Veitch L, McIntosh J and Alexander M (1997) *Evaluation of Nurse and Midwife Education in Scotland: 1992 Programmes*. Edinburgh: The National Board for Nursing, Midwifery and Health Visiting for Scotland.

Neary M (2000) *Teaching, Assessing and Evaluation for Clinical Competence*. Cheltenham: Stanley Thornes (Publishers).

Neary M (1997) Defining the role of assessors, mentors and supervisors: part II. *Nursing Standard*, 11(43), 34–38.

Nicklin PJ and Kenworthy N (1995) *Teaching and Assessing in Clinical Practice*, 2nd edn. London: Baillière Tindall.

Nursing and Midwifery Council (2002a) *Code of Professionaal Conduct*. London: Nursing and Midwifery Council.

Nursing and Midwifery Council (2002b) *Complaints about Professional Conduct*. London: Nursing and Midwifery Council.

Orchard C (1994) The nurse educator and the nursing student: a review of the issue of clinical evaluation procedures. *Journal of Nursing Education*, 33(6), 245–251.

Ormerod JA (1993) Accountability in nurse education. *British Journal of Nursing*, 2(14), 730–733.

Parkes R (1985) Stressful episodes reported by first-year student nurses: a descriptive account. *Social Science and Medicine*, 20(9), 945–953.

Phillips T, Schostak J and Tyler J (2000) *Practice and Assessment in Nursing and Midwifery: Doing it for Real*. London: The English National Board for Nursing, Midwifery and Health Visiting.

Phillips T, Bedford H, Robinson J and Schostak J (1993) *Assessment of Competencies in Nursing and Midwifery Education and Training*. London: The English National Board for Nursing, Midwifery and Health Visiting.

RCN (1990) *Accountability in Nursing – a Discussion Document*. Royal College of Nursing of the United Kingdom. Harrow: Scutari Press.

Reilly DE (1980) *Behavioral Objectives: Evaluation in Nursing*. Norwalk: Appleton-Century-Crofts.

Rowntree D (1987) *Assessing Students: How Shall We Know Them?* 2nd edn. London: Kogan Page.

Schon D (1983) *The Reflective Practitioner*. New York: Basic Books.

Spink LM (1983) Due process in academic dismissal. *Journal of Nursing Education*, 22(7), 305–306.

Spouse J (1998) Learning through legitimate peripheral participation. *Nurse Education Today*, 18(5), 345–351.

Spouse J (1996) The effective mentor: a model for student-centred learning in clinical practice. *Nursing Times Research*, 1(2), 120–132.

Torrance H and Pryor J (1998) *Investigating Formative Assessment*. Buckingham: Open University Press.

UKCC (2000a) *Requirements for Pre-registration Midwifery Programmes/ Registrar's Letter 25/2000*. London: United Kingdom Central Council for Nursing, Midwifery and Health Visiting.

UKCC (2000b) *Requirements for Pre-registration Nursing Programmes/ Registrar's Letter 17/2000*. London: United Kingdom Central Council for Nursing, Midwifery and Health Visiting.

UKCC (1999a) *Register*, Spring 1999, No. 27. London: United Kingdom Central Council for Nursing, Midwifery and Health Visiting.

UKCC (1999b) *Fitness for Practice*. London: United Kingdom Central Council for Nursing, Midwifery and Health Visiting.

UKCC (1998a) *Guidelines for Higher Education Institutions on Registration for Newly-Qualified Nurses and Midwives*. London: United Kingdom Central Council for Nursing, Midwifery and Health Visiting.

UKCC (1998b) *Midwives Rules and Code of Practice*. London: United Kingdom Central Council for Nursing, Midwifery and Health Visiting.

UKCC (1998c) *A UKCC Guide for Students of Nursing and Midwifery*. London: United Kingdom Central Council for Nursing, Midwifery and Health Visiting.

UKCC (1996a) *Guidelines for Professional Practice*. London: United Kingdom Central Council for Nursing, Midwifery and Health Visiting.

UKCC (1996b) *Issues Arising from Professional Conduct Complaints*. London: United Kingdom Central Council for Nursing, Midwifery and Health Visiting.

UKCC (1995) *Registrar's Letter 3/1995. The Councils's Position Concerning a Period of Support and Preceptorship*. London: United Kingdom Central Council for Nursing, Midwifery and Health Visiting.

UKCC (1992) *Code of Professional Conduct*, 3rd edn. London: United Kingdom Central

Council for Nursing, Midwifery and Health Visiting.

University of Sheffield (2001a) *Student Handbook*. The University of Sheffield.

University of Sheffield (2001b) *Pre-registration Advanced Diploma in Midwifery Studies*. The University of Sheffield.

University of Sheffield (2001c) *Service Agreement for the Provision of Clinical Placement Services and Facilities*. The University of Sheffield.

University of Sheffield (2000) *Pre-registration Advanced Diploma in Nursing Studies*. The University of Sheffield.

White E, Riley E, Davies S and Twinn S (1994) *A Detailed Study of the Relationship between Teaching, Support, Supervision and Role Modelling in Clinical Areas within the Context of P2000 Courses*. London: The English National Board for Nursing, Midwifery and Health Visiting.

Wood V (1987) The nursing instructor and the teaching climate. *Nurse Education Today*, 7, 228–234.

Wright D (2000) Educational support for nursing and midwifery students with dyslexia. *Nursing Standard*, 14(41), 35–41.

Young AP (1994) *Law and Professional Conduct in Nursing*, 2nd edn. London: Scutari Press.

Young AP (1992) *Case Studies in Law and Nursing*. London: Chapman and Hall.

3 | What do we assess?

INTRODUCTION

There has been much accusation over the years that nursing and midwifery education do not produce competent nurses and midwives (Bradshaw 2000a, Castledine 2000). The recent UKCC Education Commission report (UKCC 1999) highlighted this concern when it reviewed pre-registration nursing and midwifery programmes. The nursing and midwifery professions have a responsibility to, and are accountable to, the public they serve to train nurses and midwives who are clinically competent. Fraser et al (1997:51) put it very simply:

> The public needs to be assured that those about to become midwife [and nurse] practitioners have developed the right blend of knowledge, skills and attitudes to become competent.

It is essential that student nurses and student midwives achieve the competencies that will satisfy the UKCC's training requirements (UKCC 2000a, 2000b – Appendices 1 and 2). We need to measure and assess competencies so that the practitioner who qualifies is clinically competent. The issue of being clinically competent is not just restricted to newly qualified practitioners. The UKCC

(1996a) reported that a significant number of cases referred for misconduct are for allegations which relate to the actual competence of the practitioner and not to professional misconduct. Registered practitioners are also accountable for maintaining and improving their professional knowledge and competence (NMC 2002a). It is therefore important to consider carefully what competencies are and what it means to be clinically competent.

In this chapter, the use of competency statements and a competency-based model of assessment are suggested as means to be clear about what we want to assess (Hager and Gonczi 1996). The key features of the national vocational qualification (NVQ) system are described to illustrate how a tight structure and format for assessment can be constraining but has the potential advantages of validity and reliability of assessment. The nature of competencies, what it means to be clinically competent and their assessment in professional practice are explored. The competency-based model of assessment is critically evaluated as an assessment tool for assessing professional practice.

PRE-REGISTRATION TRAINING REQUIREMENTS

The background

The fact that nursing and midwifery are professions protected by Acts of Parliament is the result of the intense political activity of militant women in the late 19th and early 20th centuries to obtain registration status for nurses and midwives (Baly 1995, Donnison 1988). Midwifery attained legal recognition as a profession with the passing of the first Midwives' Act in 1902 which made provision for the setting up of the Central Midwives Board (CMB) to regulate the training and registration of midwives. Likewise, nursing gained this recognition in 1919 when the Nurses' Registration Act was passed and a General Nursing Council (GNC) for England and Wales was established. Mrs Bedford Fenwick (1919 in Davis 1991:iv), editor of the *British Journal of Nursing* of 5th July 1919, described the achievement of nursing registration as:

> . . . placing in the forefront registration of nurses, for the standardisation and improvement of nursing education, for the protection of the sick, and for the improvement of economic status of trained nurses.

It is interesting to note that Florence Nightingale firmly opposed registration, writing that 'seeking a nurse from a Register is very much like seeking a wife from a Register, as is done in some countries' (in Abel-Smith 1960:65). Her principal concerns were that registration would involve the introduction of examinations for nurses and that the professional competence of a nurse could not be judged in this way. All an examination could test was knowledge, and a nurse could acquire all the knowledge she needed in 6 months (Abel-Smith 1960).

Fortunately, Florence Nightingale's fears were unfounded as training for nursing and midwifery competence from the early days until the mid-1980s relied on standardized, explicit, defined syllabi listing theoretical subjects, as well as specified practical skills (Bradshaw 2000b, Kent 2000). The GNC and the CMB prescribed the methods for training and examination of that training, and specified precisely the competencies – the knowledge, practical skills and attitudes – required to be achieved. The nurse's or midwife's competence and fitness to practice was tested by ward observation and practical and written examinations. A list of the detailed practical instruction and experience required within the GNC syllabus in 1970 can be found in Appendix 7. Appendix 8 gives the CMB syllabus of training for England and Wales.

Although student nurses and student midwives learnt through an apprenticeship model on the wards, they were also taught and assessed by experienced ward sisters. Nursing and midwifery training were not seen merely as the mechanistic passing of examinations but were designed to ensure individual achievement and competence. Ward reports and records of practical experience were tools by which the student was known individually to ward sisters, and also to matrons. Personal interviews with ward sisters and matrons meant that the work, skills, knowledge and attitudes of students were closely monitored. Historically, nursing competence was related to the nature of the nurse's role as a practical bedside nurse, generally in hospital. This system of competence presumed a clearly defined purpose: the bedside nurse whose primary function was to care for the sick person (Bradshaw 2000b). Midwives had to be competent to assume autonomous practice for the care of the majority of women experiencing a normal pregnancy, labour and puerperium (Kent 2000). For more detailed accounts tracing the development of midwifery and nursing education with the passing of the Midwives' Act of 1902 and the Nurses' Registration Act of 1919, readers are recommended to read the works of Kent (2000) and Bradshaw (2000b), respectively. Kent provides an account covering the period 1902 until recent times, whereas Bradshaw's account covers the period 1919 to 1977.

Until April 2002, nursing, midwifery and health visiting were regulated by the United Kingdom Central Council for Nursing, Midwifery and Health Visiting (UKCC). This body was established under the 1979 Nurses, Midwives and Health Visitors Act that sought to bring control of the professions in all parts of the United Kingdom under one body. Its aim was to 'make new provision with respect to the education, training and regulation and discipline of nurses, midwives and health visitors and the maintenance of a single professional register' (Department of Health and Social Security 1979). Four national boards, one for each country of the UK, were established and the GNC and the CMB were dissolved.

Both the nursing and midwifery professions underwent a profound ideological shift concerning the preparation and qualification of nurses and midwives (Kent 2000, Bradshaw 1997). The UKCC introduced statutory pre-registration nursing 'competencies' in the training rule of 1983 (UKCC 1983). For the first time, nursing students had to achieve competencies during training (see Appendix 9). In that same Rule of 1983, midwifery students had to meet the requirements of the Midwives Directive and the theoretical, clinical and practical instruction in each of the subjects included in Schedule I. The training rules of both the nurses and midwives were reviewed in 1989 and 1990, respectively, resulting in the introduction of statutory learning 'outcomes' (UKCC 1989, 1990a) for pre-registration nursing and midwifery programmes. The 1983 Rule required nursing students to acquire nine broad 'competencies' and programmes 'shall provide opportunities to enable the student to accept responsibility for her personal professional development'.

The 1989 and 1990 rules require pre-registration programmes to prepare students to assume the responsibility and accountability that registration confers. These training rules also stipulated that students 'shall have supernumerary status'.

Nursing students have to achieve 13 broad outcomes (see Appendix 10) and midwifery students have to achieve the requirements of the Midwives Directive and 11 broad outcomes (see Appendix 11). Consequently, the curriculum content of courses is broad and nonspecific (Bradshaw 1997), involving the acquisition of outcomes such as appreciating the influence of social, political and cultural factors in relation to health care; understanding the ethical issues relating to health care and professional practice and the responsibilities that these may impose; and so on. The practical procedures and clinical skills which the GNC specified are excluded.

The UKCC's training rules for nurses (UKCC 1983, 1989) and the training rules for midwives (UKCC 1990a) were totally different in concept to the training rules framed by the GNC and the CMB. Within the training rules of the GNC and the CMB, the syllabi of pre-registration programmes were prescribed by these bodies and rigid details stipulating how theory was to be assessed and the amount and type of clinical experience were provided. As discussed above, from 1983 onwards the UKCC defined pre-registration preparation in general terms and individual nursing and midwifery institutions are free in their interpretation of these general guidelines provided by the rules. Responsibility for examination and assessment were devolved to educational institutions and no longer the responsibility of a central body. Continuous assessment of theory and practice was recommended. The UKCC, however, did not define competency or specify how the 'competencies' and outcomes were to be measured within this process to produce the new kind of nurse or midwife who is a 'knowledgeable doer'. Under the umbrella of *Project 2000: A New Preparation for Practice* (UKCC 1986), this 'knowledgeable doer' will be confident and politically, socially and economically aware. This practitioner will be equipped with the skills to be flexible and adaptable to manage the unpredictability of care within constantly changing professional and health care contexts. These are the skills most frequently associated with higher education. Colleges of nursing and midwifery were required to form collaborative links with higher education institutions (HEIs) in order to develop and validate Project 2000 courses to diploma level as a minimum standard. This has resulted in pre-registration courses giving an academic award as well as professional registration on the UKCC register.

The UKCC Commission for Education

One of the statutory responsibilities of the UKCC was to set standards for pre-registration education. The last revision of the standards for pre-registration nursing education was made in 1986 in Project 2000 (UKCC 1986). Since the implementation of Project 2000, there have been major changes in health care and public expectations of health and higher education. The UKCC considered the effectiveness of pre-registration education and made the decision that it should provide an authoritative stance on pre-registration education urgently. In 1998, the Council established a Commission for Education whose remit was to:

Prepare a way forward for pre-registration nursing and midwifery education that enables fitness for practice on health care need . . .

Current pre-registration training requirements

It is acknowledged that many current pre-registration programmes are still based on the standards set in 1986. This section discusses the UKCC's requirements for pre-registration nursing and midwifery programmes based on the recommendations made in *Fitness for Practice* (UKCC 1999). Following a period of intensive investigation, the UKCC Commission for Education (UKCC 1999) found overall that although the nursing and midwifery professions had achieved much over the previous 10 years, shortcomings exist in the current preparation for registration. There was concern that 'newly-qualified nurses, and to a lesser extent midwives, do not possess the practice skills expected of them by employers, and public expectations about levels of preparedness for practice are sometimes negative' (UKCC 1999:4). They went on to say that the 'knowledgeable doer' is right for the professions now and will continue to be so in the future. Future trends indicate that the needs of the health services will place greater demands upon nurses and midwives for technical competence and scientific rationality, coupled with the expectation that holistic care will continue to be provided (UKCC 1999). The Commission recommended refocusing pre-registration education on 'outcomes-based competency principles to ensure that students develop not only higher order intellectual skills and abilities but also the practice knowledge and skills essential to the art and science of nursing and midwifery' (UKCC 1999:4). As Bradshaw (2000a:320) points out most succinctly:

> The 'knowledgeable doer' needs to know what he or she is supposed to be 'doing'.

The process of conjoint validation between nursing/midwifery professional bodies and HEIs frequently brings competing sets of demands in relation to course assessment strategies (Bedford et al 1993). Professional bodies are concerned that assessment strategies are sensitive to the demands of professional practice. On the other hand, HEIs' concerns focus on academic credibility and the extent to which assessment strategies are sensitive to intellectual competence. In *Fitness for Practice*, the UKCC (1999) set out a radical agenda in order to refocus nursing and midwifery education to meet the needs of the rapidly changing health service by ensuring that nurses and midwives are fit for practice. By refocusing pre-registration education on outcomes-based competency principles, the UKCC believed that the needs of the three key stakeholders of pre-registration education – namely the UKCC, the prospective employers and the HEIs – were more likely to be met. These needs underpinned the UKCC's requirements for pre-registration programmes (UKCC 2000a, 2000b). The needs of each of the stakeholders are set out below:

Fitness for practice. The UKCC, endorsed by the NMC, is primarily concerned about fitness for practice – can the student register as a practitioner?

Fitness for purpose. Prospective employers are primarily concerned about fitness for purpose – is the newly qualified nurse or midwife able to function competently in clinical practice?

Fitness for award. Higher education institutions are primarily concerned about fitness for award: Has the student attained the appropriate level, breadth and depth of learning to be awarded a diploma or degree?

Gilbert Jessup, who is viewed as the most prominent English advocate of competency-based testing, argued that 'the measure of success for any education and training system should be what people learn from it, and how effectively. Just common sense you might think . . .' (Jessup 1991:3). The use of an outcomes-based competency approach allows the different stakeholders to agree a set of competencies and outcomes for pre-registration programmes to cover the knowledge, understanding, skills, abilities and values expected of newly qualified practitioners (UKCC 1999). Using these competencies and outcomes (see Appendices 1 and 2), the UKCC required pre-registration nursing and midwifery programmes to be designed to prepare the student to be a practitioner who can apply knowledge, understanding and skills to perform to the standards required in employment, and to provide care safely and competently, thereby assuming the responsibilities and accountability necessary for public protection (UKCC 2000a, 2000b). Jessup's measure of success may thus be fulfilled!

The Council used the term competence to describe the 'skills and ability to practise safely and effectively without the need for direct supervision' (UKCC 1999:35). It went on to say that this concept of competence is fundamental to the autonomy and accountability of the individual practitioner and, therefore, to the *Code of Professional Conduct* (UKCC 1992), *Guidelines for Professional Practice* (UKCC 1996b) and the *Midwives Rules and Code of Practice* (UKCC 1998). These references to the professional codes of practice means that the UKCC expected practitioners on the professional register to maintain and develop competence in the rapidly changing world of health care. In *Fitness for Practice*, the UKCC pointed out that fitness for purpose is not fixed: it depends on the commitment of practitioners to constant professional updating. In an earlier publication (UKCC 1990b:10), the UKCC stated that 'competence can only be maintained by continuing education and professional development'. This now brings us to a discussion of the Council's requirements for practice following registration.

UKCC REQUIREMENTS AND STANDARDS FOR PRACTICE FOLLOWING REGISTRATION

The UKCC recognized that continuing professional development is necessary to enable practitioners to maintain and develop their professional knowledge and competence. The main focus of the UKCC's standards for education and practice following registration (post-registration education and practice – PREP – UKCC 1994) is on this maintenance and improvement of knowledge and competence. In the *Report of the Post-Registration Education and Practice Project* (UKCC 1990b), the Council emphasized strongly that 'competence can only be maintained by continuing education and professional development'. These requirements are endorsed by the NMC (2002b). In the *Code of Professional Conduct* (NMC 2002a), the Council makes it clear that each registered practitioner is responsible and personally accountable for his or her own professional development, stating that:

As a registered nurse or midwife, you must maintain your professional knowledge and competence:

6.1 You must keep your knowledge and skills up-to-date throughout your working life.

6.2 To practise competently, you must possess the knowledge, skills and abilities required for lawful, safe and effective practice without direct supervision. You must acknowledge limits of your professional competence and only undertake practice and accept responsibilities for those activities in which you are competent.

6.3 If an aspect of practice is beyond your level of competence or outside your area of registration, you must obtain help and supervision . . .

Practitioners are thus ultimately responsible for determining their own individual competence. Bradshaw (1998:107–108) points out that the practitioner has 'no sure way of knowing whether she [sic] is in fact competent', going on to state that 'it must be known what makes the basic level of nursing [and midwifery] competency'. Jessup (1991) suggests that professional training frequently fails to make explicit statements as to what professionals should know, understand and be able to do. Practitioners need to know, with confidence, the 'right blend of knowledge, skills and attitudes to become competent' (Fraser et al 1997:51) and the standard of competency at which they are safe. This knowledge will enable mentors/assessors to conduct assessments and make assessment decisions with the assurance that students who qualify are fit for both practice and purpose – in other words, they have achieved the *competence*, as defined by the NMC. Two major concepts now require exploring: the nature of competence and the outcomes-based competency approach.

THE NATURE OF COMPETENCE

I start this discussion by posing the question: *What does it mean to be professionally competent?* The NMC (2002a) stipulates that competence is the individual practitioner's responsibility. On completion of a nursing updating course in order to return to practise after a career break, Bradshaw (2000a:319) came to this conclusion:

. . . I had no objective measures or standards by which to judge what I knew, what I *should* know, and most importantly, what I *did not* know . . . [it] left me unsure about my competence in the practicalities of caring for patients . . . gradually I realized that I had no idea whether I was competent in the new techniques and technology which I was expected to use [original emphases]

What, indeed, does it take to be a professionally competent nurse or midwife? You may wish to discuss with your colleagues the questions in Activity 3.1.

You may have discovered that the concept of professional competence resists straightforward answers or categorization. Debates I held with groups of nurses and midwives about the meaning of professional competence gave me much

ACTIVITY 3.1

What does professional competence mean and entail?
What does it mean to be professionally competent?
What does it take to be a professionally competent nurse or midwife?

room for thought. The main aspects elicited are shown in Figure 3.1. These aspects point to the multifaceted and complex nature of competence, and what it means to be a professionally competent nurse or midwife. Nursing and midwifery research by Bedford et al (1993) and Fraser et al (1997) concluded that there is no commonly-shared definition of a competent nurse or a competent midwife. Bedford et al (1993:40) think that there are:

> many different aspects of this wide-ranging and complex concept . . . there is more to competence than simply what can be easily observed and measured.

Wolf (1995), who is viewed as one expert in the field of competency-based assessment, wrote that 'competence' and 'competencies' are vexed terms – acres of print continue to be expended over their definitions. Rather than take the reader on a tedious trawl of these definitions, I have selected those which I see are pertinent to our discussion of competence in the nursing and midwifery professions.

Jessup (1991:26) defines both occupational and job competence. Note that his concept of occupational competence is broader:

> A person who is described as competent in an occupation or profession is considered to have a repertoire of skills, knowledge and understanding which he or she can apply in a range of contexts and organisations. To say that a person is competent in a 'job', on the other hand, may mean that their competence is limited to a particular role in a particular company.

Jessup's definition of competence is stated simply as 'the ability to perform to recognised standards' (1991:40). He goes on to say that 'these standards are those used to maintain or improve "quality" in the relevant occupation or profession'. Here, Jessup reiterates the expectation of the Manpower Services Commission

FIGURE 3.1   *The main aspects of professional competence.*

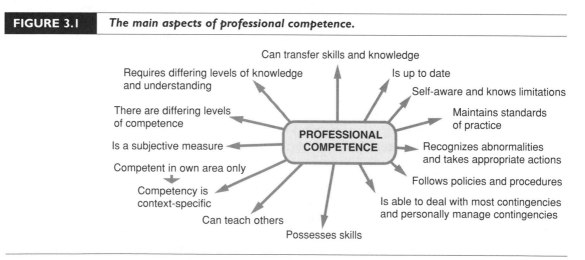

(1985 in Wolf 1995:31) of someone who is competent – 'by competent we mean performing at the standards expected of an employee doing the same job'.

The definition of competence that underpins the thinking of those professions in Australia that have established competency standards is as follows (Gonczi et al 1993:5):

A competent professional has the attributes necessary for job performance to the appropriate standards

The above definition of competence possesses three key components:

- attributes
- performance
- standards.

Attributes

Professionals are competent as a result of possession of a set of relevant attributes such as knowledge, understanding, skills, personal traits, attitudes and values. These attributes which jointly underlie and determine competence are referred to as *competencies*. A *competency* is therefore a combination of attributes underlying some aspect of successful professional performance.

Performance

In competency-based assessments, competence is focused on *performance* of a role or sets of tasks (Gonczi et al 1993). Performance is directly observable, whereas competence is not: rather, it is inferred from performance, which is why competency is defined as a combination of attributes that underlie successful performance. There are numerous professional roles, such as nurses, midwives, doctors, pharmacists, teachers and so on. Roles consist of a multitude of tasks which can be further divided into sub-tasks. The approach taken by the national vocational qualification (NVQ) movement in the UK focuses on the performance of discrete tasks and sub-tasks – each NVQ covers a particular area of work at a specific level of achievement (Wolf 1995). The professions in Australia have taken what Gonczi et al (1993) describe as the 'integrated approach' – analysis into tasks ceases at the level of relatively complex and demanding professional activities. Competency standards consider the complex combinations of attributes which are required for effective professional activities.

Gonczi et al (1993) stress that both the attributes of the practitioners and their performance of key professional tasks are essential to their definition of competence – this means that attributes of individuals do not in themselves constitute competence. Nor is competence the mere performance of a series of tasks. Rather, the notion of competence integrates attributes with performance.

Standards

The judgement of the performance of a role and its associated tasks is either competent or incompetent – competence therefore requires that the performance is judged against pre-specified 'standards'. Standards specify the skills, knowledge and understanding which underpin performance in the workplace' (Wolf 1995). The 'standards' embody and define competence in the relevant occupational context. A 'competency standard' consists of a unit of competence (representing a wide work function) which is subdivided into smaller elements of competence (tasks within the wider function) with their associated performance criteria (the standards by which the competence in the task will be judged) (Hager and Gonczi 1996). This is the framework in both England and Australia. This framework is illustrated in Figure 3.2.

An example of a unit of competency and its associated elements of competency is shown Box 3.1.

THE OUTCOMES-BASED COMPETENCY APPROACH TO PROFESSIONAL EDUCATION AND ASSESSMENT

An outline of the background of competency-based assessment

Modern competency-based assessment (in association with competency-based education) first became important in the early 1970s in the context of American teacher education and certification (Wolf 1995). In response to mounting public attacks on the quality of teacher education, the federal government became involved in education reform – competency-based teacher education was seen as a major panacea for the improvement of American education. In the late 1980s in Australia, there was considerable pressure from the national government on industry and the professions to adopt a competency-based approach to education, staff development and performance appraisal (Sutton and Arbon 1994). Consequently, most of the professions have developed competency-based standards (statements) and competency-based assessment strategies (Hager and Gonczi 1996). In the UK in the 1980s, following a Scottish lead, the government launched a huge programme of 'standards development' – this produced 'standards of competence' in around 200 occupational sectors, each with its associated NVQ award or in Scotland, the Scottish vocational qualification (SVQ). Although NVQs are accredited by a national body, the National Council for Vocational Qualifications (NCVQ), the actual processes of supervision and assessment are carried out by 'awarding bodies' such as the City and Guilds of London Institute. The reader is directed to the work of Wolf (1995), who gives a critique of competency-based assessment and the NVQ system.

FIGURE 3.2   *A competency standard.*

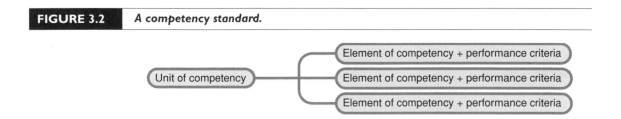

Competency-based assessment is a form of assessment that emphasizes the outcomes of achievement. These outcomes are specified to the point where they are clear and 'transparent', so that assessors, assessees and 'third parties' can all make reasonably objective judgements with respect to their achievement or non-achievement. Certification is made on the basis of demonstrated achievement of these outcomes (Wolf 1995).

Using competency-based assessment in nursing and midwifery education

Can a case be made for using the competency-based approach in the nursing and midwifery professions? Twenty years ago, Patricia Benner (1982:303) had this to say about using this approach in nursing education:

> The quest for competency statements and competency-based exams in nursing has led to what seems to be a premature faith in the current state of the art and capability of competency-based performance examinations in nursing. Carried along by a technological, measurement-oriented age, we have been convinced that many of our problems in nursing education and practice will be solved when we have mastered the current measurement technology available – when we can simply and unequivocally describe the competencies involved in the practice of nursing and measure them. Some of us have gone so far as to say that any area of practice that cannot be so defined, described, and measured does not legitimately belong in the arena of professional practice.

> Unfortunately, this faith in the feasibility of competency examinations does not come to grips with the difficulties and issues inherent in the methodology.

One recommendation made in the reports *Making a Difference* (Department of Health 1999) and *Fitness for Practice* (UKCC 1999) is to refocus pre-registration nursing and midwifery education on an outcomes-based competency approach. Are both the UKCC and the Department of Health justified in making this recommendation? What are the implications of using competency-based assessment of clinical practice? An examination of two particular ways of using competency-based assessment may provide some answers: these are the NVQ system in the UK and the 'integrated' approach used by the professions in Australia.

Competency-based assessment for NVQs

The NVQ framework represents a very particular application of competency-based assessment (Wolf 1995). This section will provide an outline of the basic structure of NVQs and discuss the principles underlying competency-based assessment for NVQs. The process of assessment within the competency-based framework is discussed in Chapter 6. Inferences will then be drawn about the appropriateness of the NVQ system for the assessment of professional practice, such as in the nursing and midwifery professions.

An NVQ comprises several units and their associated elements to be achieved at one of the five pre-specified levels (NCVQ 1991). A unit consists of a group of 'elements of competence' and their associated performance criteria. Each unit reflects a discrete activity or sub-area of competence – each is worthy of separate accreditation, much like an academic module in fact (NCVQ 1991). An element of competence is a description of something which a person who works in a given occupational area should be able to do: it encompasses some action, behaviour or outcome. Competency-based assessment for NVQs is made concrete through highly specified performance criteria. The element of competence is assessed and validated against these performance criteria. Box 3.1 provides

---

BOX 3.1

Sample unit with its elements and one element of competence with its associated performance criteria. Extract from NVQs in Care Level 2 – Unit U1 and Element U1.a (City and Guilds 1992)

Unit title: Contribute to the maintenance and management of domestic and personal resources

Elements of Competence:
U1.a: Maintain a supply of personal clothes and linen
U1.b: Clean individual rooms and surfaces
U1.c: Contribute to the maintenance of furnishings and fittings
U1.d: Prepare food and drink for clients

Element U1.a:
Maintain a supply of personal clothes and linen

Performance criteria:

■ Prior to any laundering or cleansing taking place, agreement is obtained from those concerned

■ The tasks which the client wishes to be undertaken are established with her/him

■ Soiled clothing and linen are collected as soon as possible in the appropriate containers

■ Any prescribed procedures for handling fouled or infected items are followed, consistent with maintaining the dignity and rights of the individuals concerned

■ Where the clothes and linen belong to an individual client, maintenance activities are carried out consistent with the client's preferences

■ Worn or damaged articles are repaired or discarded consistent with the client's choice and the agency's policies

■ Equipment is in safe working order and used consistent with manufacturer's instructions

■ Equipment is returned to storage after use and the work area is left clean and tidy

■ Any faults are clearly, accurately and promptly recorded and/or reported in the required format

■ Where the client, the worker or others have adverse reactions to cleaning materials, the appropriate action is taken without delay

an example of a unit, its associated elements and one element of competence with its performance criteria.

Assessment requires that the individual demonstrates successfully that he or she has met every one of the performance criteria, as these are the statements by which an assessor judges whether the evidence provided by the individual is sufficient to demonstrate competent performance (Wolf 1995). The NCVQ (1991) approach requires assessment to be centred on whether performance meets the pre-specified standards. Performance is judged to be either competent or not yet competent only – the individual has either consistently demonstrated workplace performance which meets the specified 'standards' or has not yet been able to do so. Grading is rejected – the individual either has or has not reached the required level of the NVQ.

Each element of competence and its associated performance criteria have an associated 'range'. The ranges officially 'elaborate the statement of competence by making explicit the contexts to which the element [of competence] and performance criteria apply. Also they put limits on the specification to ensure a consistent interpretation' (NCVQ 1991:14). Contextualizing the performance criteria identifies the different contexts in which the individual is expected to achieve competent performance. This means that competence must also be assessed 'across the range' and performance evidence is 'normally required for every performance criteria [sic] across as much of the range as possible' (City and Guilds 1992). Box 3.2 specifies the range statements for element U1.a detailed in Box 3.1.

In its early years, NVQs were criticized for producing people who might be able to demonstrate performance but would have no understanding of what they were doing (Norris 1991). To fend off mounting attacks on NVQs as undemanding, and to ensure that individuals have an understanding of what they are doing (Wolf 1995), NCVQ added a separate 'knowledge/understanding' list to every element of competence. City and Guilds (1992) requires its candidates to demonstrate that they understand all the items listed under knowledge evidence

| **BOX 3.2** | *Range statements for Element U1.a: Maintain a supply of personal clothes and linen. Extract from NVQs in Care Level 2 – Unit U1 and Element U1.a (City and Guilds 1992)* |

Range

Personal clothing and linen:
1. personal apparel (clothes, shoes and accessories)
2. domestic linen (such as sheets, towels, tea towels)

Maintenance of personal clothing and linen:
1. washing (hand and machine)
2. dry cleaning
3. cleaning and mending of shoes and leather goods
4. mending (such as sewing on a button)
5. ironing

Maintenance materials:
1. cleansing (e.g. washing powders and stain removers)
2. restorative (e.g. shoe polish)

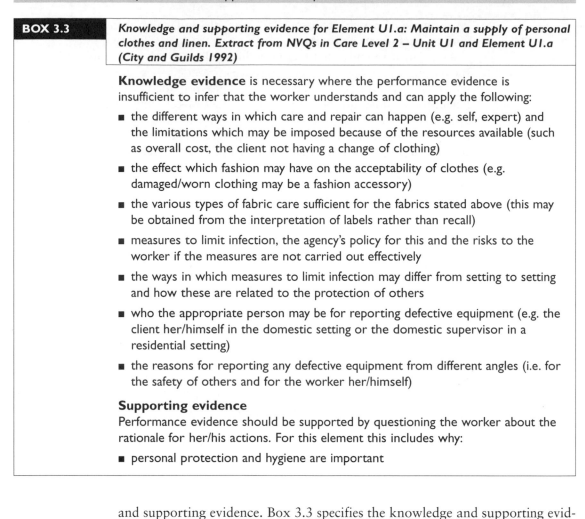

BOX 3.3 *Knowledge and supporting evidence for Element U1.a: Maintain a supply of personal clothes and linen. Extract from NVQs in Care Level 2 – Unit U1 and Element U1.a (City and Guilds 1992)*

Knowledge evidence is necessary where the performance evidence is insufficient to infer that the worker understands and can apply the following:

■ the different ways in which care and repair can happen (e.g. self, expert) and the limitations which may be imposed because of the resources available (such as overall cost, the client not having a change of clothing)

■ the effect which fashion may have on the acceptability of clothes (e.g. damaged/worn clothing may be a fashion accessory)

■ the various types of fabric care sufficient for the fabrics stated above (this may be obtained from the interpretation of labels rather than recall)

■ measures to limit infection, the agency's policy for this and the risks to the worker if the measures are not carried out effectively

■ the ways in which measures to limit infection may differ from setting to setting and how these are related to the protection of others

■ who the appropriate person may be for reporting defective equipment (e.g. the client her/himself in the domestic setting or the domestic supervisor in a residential setting)

■ the reasons for reporting any defective equipment from different angles (i.e. for the safety of others and for the worker her/himself)

Supporting evidence
Performance evidence should be supported by questioning the worker about the rationale for her/his actions. For this element this includes why:

■ personal protection and hygiene are important

and supporting evidence. Box 3.3 specifies the knowledge and supporting evidence for element U1.a.

NVQs are offered at five levels to cover progression from routine and predictable work activities to the complex and unpredictable (NCVQ 1991). The summary of each level is as follows:

■ Level 1: competence in a range of work activities which are primarily routine, or provide a broad foundation, primarily as a basis for progression.
■ Level 2: competence in a broader and more demanding range of work activities, involving greater individual responsibility and autonomy than at Level 1.
■ Level 3: competence in a broad range of varied activities performed in a wide variety of contexts, most of which are complex and non-routine. There is considerable responsibility and autonomy, and control or guidance of others is often required.
■ Level 4: competence in a broad range of complex technical or professional work activities performed in a wide variety of contexts and with a substantial degree of personal responsibility and autonomy. Responsibility for the work of others and the allocation of resources is often present.
■ Level 5: competence which involves the application of a significant range of fundamental principles and complex techniques across a wide and often

unpredictable variety of contexts. Very substantial personal autonomy and often significant responsibility for the work of others and for the allocation of substantial resources feature strongly, as do personal accountabilities for analysis and diagnosis, design, planning, execution and evaluation.

It can be seen that the NVQ system applies competency-based assessment in a very tightly defined format. It embraces the performance philosophy of competency-based systems to the very core (Wolf 1995). Thus, its notion of competence is 'the ability to perform the activities within an occupation' (Wolf 1995:31). While competency-based systems vary in their interpretation of what outcomes may be (see for example Gonczi et al 1993), the learning outcomes in NVQs relate directly to performance – what counts as an outcome is thus very highly constrained. An element of competence must encompass some action, behaviour or outcome which is contextually related to that occupational sector through its range statement. The elements of competence referred to in Unit U1 above are legitimate as being outcome-based because they involve an *active verb* and an *object* and relate directly to performance. Each element of competence is specified in such a way that there can be no doubt about what constitutes satisfactory performance. For example, competence in Element U1.a requires the person to be able to 'maintain a supply of personal clothes and linen'.

Arguments for and against the NVQ system for assessing professional practice

As stated earlier, the NVQ framework represents a very particular application of competency-based assessment which can be summarized as follows:

- the elements of competence define the performance requirements
- the performance criteria describe competent performance
- range statements specify the contexts of competent performance
- statements of knowledge and supporting evidence define the underpinning knowledge and understanding required
- levels specify the nature of work activities for competent performance, ranging from the routine and predictable to the complex and unpredictable.

A contentious issue about what is to be assessed concerns the optimum level of specificity. Storey et al (1995:382) say that 'if there is too little specificity, the result may be a lack of clarity, poor communication and diminished credibility'. This is the criticism directed at the Rule 18 competencies and the Rule 18a and Rule 33 outcomes. On the other hand, too much specificity can lead to assessment criteria which take too long to read and are cumbersome to use by busy practitioners. This criticism has been directed at the NVQ system. However, you may agree that the NVQ approach has the attraction of precision and clarity as to *what* is to be assessed to achieve competence. Advocates of this approach also emphasize its potential contribution to effective training and learning. Storey et al (1995) and Fletcher (1991), for example, argue that specific criteria for assessing competence are provided, thereby giving the much desired guidance for assessees and assessors. Individuals know exactly what they have to achieve and assessors can provide specific guidance and feedback. Educational provisions and employment needs can be brought together.

The appropriateness of the NVQ approach for assessing professionals such as in nursing and midwifery has been criticized (Le Var 1996, Norris 1991). What could be the trouble with an approach where the assessment of competence is grounded in performance in the workplace? The NVQ model is seen by Norris (1991:334) to be 'highly reductive, providing atomised lists of tasks and functions'. He elaborates further:

> the sum of the parts rarely if ever represents the totality of good practice . . . in their tidiness and precision, far from preserving the essential features of expertise, they distort and understate the very things they are trying to represent.

Competence is conceived of in terms of the discrete behaviours associated with the ability to complete individual tasks. This approach is unconcerned with the connections between tasks and ignores the possibility that the coming together of tasks could lead to their transformation (Hager and Gonczi 1996). Le Var (1996) fears that the care activities in nursing, midwifery and health visiting will become fragmented if students are trained within this approach. If holistic care is to be valued and provided, care activities need to be designed and integrated around the needs of the client at that particular time. Unless professionals are involved in the planning and evaluation of total care, they cannot engage in the processes of critical analysis and synthesis which lead to the development of theories and principles of practice. If this 'atomised' approach of the NVQ system is used by professionals, qualifications could be in danger of being reduced to a list of technical skills (Storey et al 1995). Hager and Gonczi (1996) and Le Var (1996) echo this concern when they point out that this approach ignores the complexity of performance in the real world and the role of professional judgement. Furthermore, the practice and assessment of 'components of care' do not engender the development of problem-solving skills.

A number of general concerns have been raised about the use of a competency-based approach to nursing and midwifery education. The degree to which competencies can be used to describe professional practice is questionable (Sutton and Arbon 1994, Benner 1982). The practice of health care professionals is undeniably complex and competency-based statements can only provide a limited view of this practice – they cannot be used to reflect the complexities of practice with accuracy. They must, by their very nature, provide a reductive analysis of practice (Sutton and Arbon 1994), which excludes learning derived from a whole performance (Benner 1982). Although competency statements purport to describe the attributes, including knowledge and skills necessary for effective and/or superior performance, the testing of intangible attributes such as attitudes is still subjective (Ashworth and Morrison 1991, Benner 1982). Benner pointed out the difficulties of testing some attributes and abilities such as empathy and the ability to relate to others as learning the behaviour does not guarantee the possession of the accompanying attitude and/or values.

If we return to the definition of a competent professional offered by Gonczi et al (1993) above, you will notice that the competent professional should also possess the appropriate underlying personal attitudes and traits. The assessment of these aspects of competence is not given due consideration in the NVQ system. The Training Agency (1988) states that competence should take into account the 'qualities of personal effectiveness that are required in the workplace to deal with co-workers, managers and customers'. Underlying attributes and qualities may include interpersonal and social skills; attitudes; perceptiveness, receptivity, creativity and maturity as well as knowledge, understanding and critical thinking capacity (Ashworth and Morrison 1991). These underlying attributes of the practitioner are crucial to effective performance (Hager and Gonczi 1996) and are fundamental to excellence in clinical practice (Novak 1988).

If the NVQ system for assessing professional practice is used, the reader is left to ponder the answers to the following questions:

- The UKCC is concerned about 'fitness for practice': Will the student who is assessed using this system be 'fit for practice' and be allowed to register?
- Employers are concerned about 'fitness for purpose': Will the newly-qualified nurse or midwife be able to function competently in clinical practice? Can the new practitioner fulfil the UKCC's definition of competence – i.e. have the 'skills and ability to practise safely and effectively without the need for direct supervision'? Due to the speed of change in the context and content of health care, fitness for purpose is an evolving entity: it is not fixed, and depends on the 'commitment of employers and employees to constant updating' (UKCC 1999:34). Having trained and been assessed using the NVQ system during clinical practice, how likely is the new practitioner in making this commitment?

The case for an integrated competency-based approach for assessing nursing and midwifery practice

The UKCC Education Commission (UKCC 1999) recommended refocusing pre-registration education on 'outcomes-based competency principles to ensure

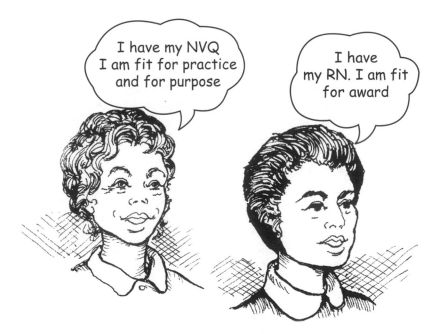

The NVQ represents a very particular application of competency-based assessment

that students develop not only higher order intellectual skills and abilities but also the practice knowledge and skills essential to the art and science of nursing and midwifery' (UKCC 1999:4).

In refocusing pre-registration education on outcomes-based competency principles, the UKCC believed that the needs of the three key stakeholders of pre-registration education – the UKCC, the prospective employers and the HEIs – are more likely to be met. This belief reinforces Hager and Gonczi's (1996) views that a competency-based approach to education and training potentially provides a framework for bringing together professional policies for training and employment requirements. Competencies provide consumers and professionals with some common understanding of standards expected of professionals, and may thereby enable both parties to relate to each other more successfully.

The nursing profession of Australia (Sutton and Arbon 1994) views competency development as one means by which the profession can monitor and maintain its own professional standards and thus enhance its accountability to the public. Hager and Gonczi (1996), however, recommend that any assessment strategy that utilizes the outcomes-based competency model should be 'holistically orientated' – a holistic/integrated competency-based model is more valid and reliable than current ways of assessing professionals. It enables us to come closer than we have in the past to assessing what we want to assess, i.e. the capacity of the professional to integrate knowledge, values, attitudes, skills and other attributes in the real world of practice.

It is clear that any holistic/integrated model of assessment that utilizes the outcomes-based competency approach to the assessment of professional practice needs to take into account the following:

- effective performance of work activities in a range of contexts
- the exercising of cognitive skills such as integration of theory with practice, critical analysis, problem solving and synthesis
- the ability to provide holistic care
- the underlying attitudes and traits of the learner
- that practice is up-to-date.

A holistic/integrated competency-based approach considers the complex combinations of attributes (knowledge, understanding, skills, personal traits, attitudes and values) that are used to understand and function within the particular situations in which professionals find themselves. The abilities of practitioners are considered in relationship to the tasks that need to be performed in particular situations. The notion of competence is relational – it is conceived of as the complex structuring of attributes needed for intelligent performance in specific situations. It incorporates the idea of professional judgement. Many authors (e.g. Jessup 1991, McGaghie 1991, Black and Wolf 1990) also consider that, other than practical skills and knowledge, cognitive skills are important underpinnings of competence. Jessup (1991:127) describe it this way:

An analysis of the knowledge which people actually draw upon, and need to draw upon, to perform competently, may not appear in what is taught as the body of knowledge underpinning a profession or occupation, or if it is covered, may not be accorded the priority it deserves. Competent professionals tend to acquire a set of guiding principles, of which they are often partially conscious, derived largely from their experience. These may build upon 'academic' theories and knowledge or be only loosely related. While this is recognised in areas such as management, it also appears to be true in well established professions such as medicine.

The holistic/integrated approach is to conceive of competent nursing and midwifery care as the capacity of the practitioner to employ a complex interaction of attributes in a range of contexts. Thus, a knowledge base and possession of a repertoire of practical skills will need to mesh with, amongst other things, ethical values and interpersonal skills. Practitioners may then be able to 'perform the task with desirable outcomes under the varied circumstances of the real world' (Benner 1982:304).

The real world of health care is dynamic, complex and unpredictable. Health care professionals face challenging and unique situations within practice and need flexible ways of responding to, and learning from, these situations. It follows then that competence is also developmental in orientation – never a total accomplishment, always looking forward to better performance, improved decision making and greater quantity of outcome (Bedford et al 1993). The holistic/integrated competency-based approach allows us to incorporate ethics and values as elements in competent performance, the need for reflective practice, the importance of context and the fact that there is more than one way of conceptualizing competence. In the nursing context, the holistic/integrated approach views that competence is (Percival et al 1994:139):

> The ability of a person to fulfil the nursing role effectively and/or expertly. It is an inner, highly differentiated characteristic of a person which is applicable to the very demanding and very specific context of nursing. It is an ability that effectively encompasses the entire demands of the nursing role; and therefore nursing competence itself possesses a complexity that increases with experience, and as responsibilities become more intricate.

The qualities expected by practising nurses and midwives of the competent professional nurse or midwife (see Figure 3.1) have many similarities to the holistic/integrated way of conceptualizing competence. Another inference which can be drawn from the information in Figure 3.1 is what Gonczi et al (1993:13) said of clinical competence, and that is: 'clinical competence is a complex phenomenon, which almost always requires the practitioner to use a combination of attributes simultaneously and, in addition, that the practitioners need to adapt their practices to different contexts'. It seems that if we are to use a competency-based model for assessing nursing and midwifery practice, adopting the concepts of competence inherent in the holistic/integrated approach is the way forward. In her critique of the use of the competency-based model for the nursing profession, Le Var (1996) came to the conclusion that the holistic/-integrated approach is in keeping with, and will also help fulfil, the current assessment philosophy and practice in professional nursing.

The components of the holistic/integrated competency-based model can be summarized as:

- a complex combination of attributes – knowledge, attitudes, personal traits, values, skills and understanding

- exercising cognitive skills, e.g. using professional judgement in specific situations
- effective performance on different occasions in different contexts
- developmental in orientation to emphasize the need for reflective practice.

Utilizing these components, an integrated competency-based model for assessing nursing and midwifery practice can be constructed, as shown in Figure 3.3.

Unifying assessment by using the holistic/integrated model of assessment is more likely to help nurses and midwives develop the technical competence and scientific rationality, as well as fulfil the paradoxical expectation of meeting the holistic care needs of patients and clients (Department of Health 1999). For the purposes of the discussion on assessment methodology (see Chapter 4) these components are grouped into the category of reflective practice and the three domains of learning classified by Bloom et al (1956):

- *cognitive domain*: knowledge, understanding, problem solving, decision making, professional code
- *affective domain*: attitude, ethics, professional code
- *psychomotor domain*: technical skills.

Using the holistic/integrated approach for competency-based assessment of clinical practice

The holistic/integrated approach to competency-based assessment used by the professions in Australia seeks to identify attributes as well as key functions and

| FIGURE 3.3 | *The components of a holistic/integrated competency-based model of assessment.* |

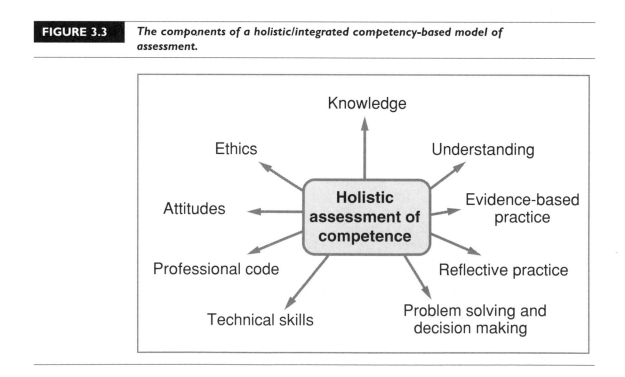

activities, and to combine these in an integrated set of competency statements (Gonczi et al 1993). This has meant that analysis into tasks has ceased at the level of relatively complex and demanding professional activities – typically, a profession does not develop more than 30–40 competencies. In the nursing and midwifery professions, the nurses' registration boards of Australia did not wish the competencies to drive a competency-based curriculum. The competencies were not designed to reflect the narrow behaviourist approach typical of the NVQ system: rather, they were designed to reflect the holistic nature of nursing and to represent the practice repertoire of the newly qualified nurse (Hager and Gonczi 1996).

A similar strategy has been used by the UKCC in developing the competencies for both the pre-registration midwifery and nursing programmes (UKCC 2000a, 2000b – Appendices 1 and 2). The primacy of practice underpins the competencies. The Department of Health (1999) calls for an increase in practical skills within training programmes. Additionally, the UKCC provided the following guiding principles that should be reflected in pre-registration nursing and midwifery programmes:

- nursing and midwifery are practice-based professions which recognize the primacy of patient and client well-being and respect for individuals
- the *Code of Professional Conduct* (UKCC 1992) applies to all practice interventions
- the importance of lifelong learning and continuing professional development are recognized
- skills and knowledge are transferable
- practice is based on the best available evidence.

The need for an integrated competency-based approach to the assessment of clinical practice has been highlighted. Within an integrated assessment framework, assessment approaches can assess a range of elements and performance criteria, rather than collect evidence for each element and performance criterion (Gonczi et al 1993). For example, in the case of a student midwife on a community placement, home visits of women and their babies can be used to assess elements such as the practical skills of examination of the woman and/or baby, conducting interviews, monitoring progress and compiling case records and reports. The performance on these visits can also be used to measure a number of attributes at the same time, such as communication and interpersonal skills, underpinning knowledge, understanding, problem solving and so on.

In Chapter 4, there is a consideration of the assessment methods available and how these may be used to generate the assessment evidence required to infer, and confer, competence. In Chapter 6, there is a discussion of how the components of the holistic/integrated competency-based model of the assessment of clinical practice can be incorporated and used within a learning contract.

A 'clinical skills checklist'

Currently, there is concern and unease about the lack of essential practical nursing skills of newly qualified nurses (UKCC 1999). Although concerns about the practical skills of newly qualified midwives were not as marked as those for nursing, they remain significant because of the requirement of midwives to practise autonomously on registration. Both the UKCC (1999) and the Department of Health (1999) call for an increase in the level of practical skills during pre-registration training. While the holistic/integrated competency-based approach to the assessment of clinical practice will concomitantly assess practical skills, it may not identify the nature and repertoire of the skills in which the student has become competent. Hilton (1996) found that there were reduced opportunities for students to acquire what many believe to be key psychomotor skills in some areas of clinical practice. Furthermore, with the rapidly changing nature of clinical learning environments and the increasing complexity of nursing practice, students were finding it increasingly difficult to identify what clinical skills they really needed to acquire to function as a newly registered nurse to help them negotiate appropriate learning opportunities.

Using a 'clinical skills checklist' will help both the student and the mentor/assessor keep track of clinical experiences and caregiving situations that the student needs to engage in to acquire these skills. It is emphasized that the checklist should not fragment the clinical experience and assessment of the student – rather, it should be used as a guide to planning clinical experiences so that the student has the opportunity to engage in those clinical activities to enable the acquisition of these skills and the statutory competencies of the UKCC (2000a, 2000b). The checklist should be seen as a formative tool used towards the achievement of the statutory competencies as the 'assessment of competence cannot be reduced solely to an assessment of a student's ability to carry out certain tasks' (UKCC 1999:38).

Following an extensive review of the literature and consultation with mentors/assessors, students and newly qualifying staff nurses, Hilton (2000) developed several checklists termed the *Clinical Skills Maps*. These checklists are intended to help students map their own clinical skills acquisition. The clinical skills are framed around the 12 'Activities of Living' model of Aggleton and Chalmers (2000 in Hilton 2000) and are to be achieved at five levels:

- *Level 1* – Have observed the procedure in the practice setting
- *Level 2* – Have participated in the skill under direct supervision
- *Level 3* – Have performed the skill on a number of occasions and required minimal supervision
- *Level 4* – Can perform the skill safely and competently giving the rationale for their actions
- *Level 5* – Have taught the skill to others.

The first 'map' lists the core skills that all student nurses are encouraged to achieve during the first year to a minimum of *Level 3*. The second 'map' lists the skills to be achieved by the end of the programme to a minimum of *Level 4*. There are separate skills 'maps' for students in all branches of the pre-registration programmes in order to take account of the differing nature of the mental health, learning disability and paediatric environments. Hilton (2000) states that the lists of skills are not exhaustive. Blank spaces allow students to add any skills acquired which are unique to their personal learning experiences. An example of some of the clinical skills related to the 'activity of breathing' from the first 'map' is shown in Table 3.1.

The 'record of practical instruction and experience for the certificate of general nursing' (GNC 1969) may also be useful in compiling a 'skills checklist'. A sub-section of this document can be found in Appendix 7.

| TABLE 3.1 | Skills related to the activity of breathing (reproduced from Hilton 2000 with the permission of The University of Sheffield, School of Nursing and Midwifery). |

Position client experiencing difficulty breathing							
Monitor and record expectorant							
Disposal of sputum secretions							
Obtain sputum specimen							
Maintain safe administration of oxygen as prescribed via:							
Mask							
Nasal cannulae							
Humidifier							

Levels of performance

Hilton (2000) requires students to achieve the skills at five levels – Level 4 is competent performance and is not expected to be achieved until the end of the course. The NCVQ (1991) approach requires performance to be judged as either competent or not yet competent only against pre-specified standards of the five NVQ levels (see above). The condition(s) of competent practice are not specified by the NCVQ or Hilton (2000). As can be seen in the NCVQ framework, each level specifies the tasks and nature of the tasks that is expected of the person to achieve competent performance. What seems to be the notion of 'levels' in the NCVQ framework is the ability of the person to achieve competent performance in an increasing range of work activities, commensurate with the routine and predictable to the complex and unpredictable, and the exercising of personal autonomy and responsibility for the work of others. There does not seem to be any doubt about what constitutes a 'level of practice performance' in the NCVQ framework. Neither is there any doubt about the purpose of levels: i.e. to cover the progression of individuals from being able to perform routine activities through to the complex activities.

The assessment of *levels of clinical practice* in pre- and post-registration nursing and midwifery education is not as clear-cut. In their review of the assessment of practice in nursing and midwifery education, Gerrish et al (1997) said that one consequence of the integration of pre- and post-registration nursing and midwifery education into higher education is the highlighting of some of the problems associated with the assessment of practice at different levels. There are difficulties agreeing a level of performance commensurate with an academic level. Phillips et al (2000) question the relationship between particular constructs of academic level and practice concepts such as safe, good, excellent and outstanding. Both Phillips et al (2000) and Gerrish et al (1997) discuss attempts which have been made to develop assessment tools that incorporate criteria of levels to assess diploma, degree and postgraduate levels of practice.

Phillips et al (2000) and Gerrish et al (1997) raise many issues surrounding the assessment of levels of clinical practice. Some of these are framed in the following questions:

- Is there any purpose in attributing levels to practice in nursing and midwifery education?
- If we accept the viability of the use of levels criteria to differentiate practice, what constitutes evidence of movement from one level of practice to another?
- Does learning in the practice setting progress in a linear fashion, as implied by assessment tools which apply Steinaker and Bell's (1979) taxonomy of experiential learning?
- If practice is assessed only in relation to a competent/incompetent distinction, as in the NVQ system, what are the criteria which constitute competent versus incompetent performance?

Pre-registration nursing and midwifery curricula generally prescribe the expected level of competent performance at pre-specified points of the programme (Phillips et al 2000, Gerrish et al 1997). Within a consideration of *what to assess* in clinical practice of a pre-registration programme is the necessity to determine whether a student is achieving competent practice as the training progresses. Bradshaw (1998) is concerned that we are able to state that the nurse or midwife has reached certain minimum standards of competence in the practical knowledge and skills needed to care for patients. We have to decide whether the student is learning, and therefore achieving, the competencies within the student's expected capability: this is generally determined by the stage of training the student is at. This assessment necessarily involves the use of criteria to decide how a competent/incompetent distinction can be made, and whether the student has made the requisite progress at the level specified at a particular stage of the course. These aspects of assessment are seen as part and parcel of the monitoring of progress of students and are discussed in detail in Chapter 7.

CONCLUSION

Everyone agrees that, on qualification, nurses and midwives should be competent to give both physical and psychological/emotional care. Evidence shows that new nurses, and to a lesser extent midwives, are not as clinically skilled as their predecessors (Castledine 2000). The Department of Health's agenda is that qualified practitioners should be 'fit for purpose' (Department of Health 1999): Is the nurse or midwife clinically competent and fit to be employed? Has the nurse or midwife maintained clinical competence? The UKCC, endorsed by the NMC, is primarily concerned about 'fitness for practice': Should the student's name be added to the professional register? Registration endorses an individual's fitness for practice: Does the individual maintain this right to practise?

To achieve these key aims we need to be clear about *what* we want to assess in the clinical setting. The UKCC (2000a, 2000b) specified statutory competencies for pre-registration nursing and midwifery education. These are to be achieved through the principles of a competency-based model of assessment.

Two particular applications of this model have been described in this chapter. First, the NVQ system, which is seen to focus almost exclusively on the performance of discrete tasks and is therefore reductionist in nature. This application of the competency-based model is therefore not entirely appropriate for assessing professional education such as nursing and midwifery. Secondly, the other application of the competency-based model utilizes the holistic/integrated approach as used by the professions in Australia (Gonczi et al 1993). This approach conceives of competent nursing and midwifery care as the capacity of the practitioner to employ a complex interaction of attributes needed for intelligent performance in a range of contexts. Thus, a knowledge base and the possession of a repertoire of practical skills will need to mesh with, amongst other things, ethical values and interpersonal skills. Clinically, the assessment can be integrated by using those methods which assess a number of elements and all their performance criteria simultaneously, so that evidence towards the achievement of one or several competencies can be generated.

All existing methods of clinical assessment are potentially appropriate for use in the holistic/integrated competency-based approach. This is because it is not the methods which are competency-based but the way they are used, the emphasis given to each method and the way in which the results are interpreted which are important. The following chapter examines the range of methods available and how these can be used in competency-based assessment.

REFERENCES

Abel-Smith B (1960) *A History of the Nursing Profession*. London: Heinemann.

Aggleton P and Chalmers H (2000) *Nursing Models and Nursing Practice*, 2nd edn. London: Macmillan Press.

Ashworth P and Morrison P (1991) Problems of competence-based nurse education. *Nurse Education Today*, 11, 256–260.

Baly ME (1995) *Nursing and Social Change*, 3rd edn. London: Routledge.

Bedford H, Phillips T, Robinson J and Schostak J (1993) *Assessing Competencies in Nursing and Midwifery Education: Final Report*. London: The English National Board for Nursing, Midwifery and Health Visiting.

Benner P (1982) Issues in competency-based testing. *Nursing Outlook*, **May 30**, 303–309.

Black H and Wolf A (1990) *Knowledge and Competence: Current Issues in Training and Education*. Sheffield: Employment Department.

Bloom BS, Engelhort MD, Furst EJ et al (1956) *Taxonomy of Educational Objectives, Handbook 1: Cognitive Domains*. London: Longman.

Bradshaw A (2000a) Editorial. *Journal of Clinical Nursing*, 9, 319–320.

Bradshaw A (2000b) Competence and British nursing: a view from history. *Journal of Clinical Nursing*, 9, 321–329.

Bradshaw A (1998) Defining competency in nursing (part II): an analytical review. *Journal of Clinical Nursing*, 7, 103–111.

Bradshaw A (1997) Defining competency in nursing (part I): a policy review. *Journal of Clinical Nursing*, 6, 347–354.

Castledine G (2000) New nurse competencies: are they adequate? *British Journal of Nursing*, 9(5), 314–315.

City and Guilds (1992) *3033: Care – NVQ Level 2*. London: City and Guilds of London Institute.

Davis M (1991) Professional development module: P4 – nursing competency. *Nursing Times* (Open Learning Programme), 87(43), i–viii.

Department of Health (1999) *Making a Difference*. London: Department of Health.

Department of Health and Social Security (1979) *Nurses, Midwives and Health Visitors Act*. London: HMSO.

Donnison J (1988) *Midwives and Medical Men – a History of the Struggle for the Control of Childbirth*. London: Historical Publications.

Fletcher S (1991) *NVQs Standards and Competence. A Practical Guide for Employers, Managers and Trainers*. London: Kogan Page.

Fraser D, Murphy R and Worth-Butler M (1997) *An Outcome Evaluation of the Effectiveness of Pre-registration Midwifery Programmes of Education*. London: The English National Board for Nursing, Midwifery and Health Visiting.

Gerrish K, McManus M and Ashworth P (1997) *Levels of Achievement: A Review of the Assessment of Practice*. London: The English National Board for Nursing, Midwifery and Health Visiting.

GNC (1969) *Syllabus of Subjects for Examination and Record of Practical Instruction and Experience for the Certificate of General Nursing*. London: the GNC for England and Wales.

Gonczi A, Hager P and Athanasou J (1993) *The Development of Competency-Based Assessment Strategies for the Professions*. National Office of Overseas Skills Recognition, Research Paper No. 8. Canberra: Australian Government Publishing Service.

Hager P and Gonczi A (1996) Professions and competencies. In Edwards R, Hanson A, Raggatt P (eds) *Boundaries of Adult Learning*, pp. 246–260. London: Routledge.

Hilton P (2000) Mapping clinical skills acquisition. *The Assessor* [online]. Sheffield: The University of Sheffield. Available from: http://www.snm.shef.ac.uk/news/assessor.htm

Hilton P (1996) Clinical skills laboratories: teaching practical nursing. *Nursing Standard*, **10**(37), 44–47.

Jessup G (1991) *Outcomes: NVQs and the Emerging Model of Education and Training*. London: The Falmer Press.

Kent J (2000) *Social Perspectives on Pregnancy and Childbirth for Midwives, Nurses and the Caring Professions*. Buckingham: Open University Press.

Le Var R (1996) NVQs in nursing, midwifery and health visiting: a question of assessment and learning? *Nurse Education Today*, **16**, 85–93.

McGaghie WC (1991) Professional competence evaluation. *Educational Researcher*, **20**(1), 3.

Manpower Services Commission (1985) *Guidance Notes for Two-Year Youth Training Schemes*. Sheffield: Manpower Services Commission.

NCVQ (1991) *Guide to National Vocational Qualifications*. London: National Council for Vocational Qualifications.

Norris N (1991) The trouble with competence. *Cambridge Journal of Education*, **21**(3), 331–341.

Novak S (1988) An effective clinical evaluation tool. *Journal of Nursing Education*, **27**(2), 83–84.

Nursing and Midwifery Council (2002a) *Code of Professional Conduct*. London: Nursing and Midwifery Council.

Nursing and Midwifery Council (2002b) *Complaints about Professional Conduct*. London: Nursing and Midwifery Council.

Percival E, Anderson M and Lawson D (1994) Assessing beginning level competencies: the first step in continuing education. *Journal of Continuing Education in Nursing*, **25**(3), 139–142.

Phillips T, Schostak J and Tyler J (2000) *Practice and Assessment in Nursing and Midwifery: Doing it for Real*. London: The English National Board for Nursing, Midwifery and Health Visiting.

Steinaker N and Bell M (1979) *The Experiential Taxonomy: A New Approach to Teaching and Learning*. New York: Academic Press.

Storey L, O'Kell S and Day M (1995) *Utilising National Occupational Standards as a Complement to Nursing Curricula*. London: Department of Health.

Sutton FA and Arbon PA (1994) Australian nursing – moving forward? Competencies and the nursing profession. *Nurse Education Today*, **14**, 388–393.

Training Agency (1988) *Development of Assessable Standards for National Certification. Guidance Note 1: A Code of Practice and a Development Model*. Sheffield: Training Agency.

UKCC (2000a) *Requirements for Pre-registration Midwifery Programmes/Registrar's Letter 25/2000*. London: United Kingdom Central Council for Nursing, Midwifery and Health Visiting.

UKCC (2000b) *Requirements for Pre-registration Nursing Programmes*. London: United Kingdom Central Council for Nursing, Midwifery and Health Visiting.

UKCC (1999) *Fitness for Practice*. London: United Kingdom Central Council for Nursing, Midwifery and Health Visiting.

UKCC (1998) *Midwives Rules and Code of Practice*. London: United Kingdom Central Council for Nursing, Midwifery and Health Visiting.

UKCC (1996a) *Issues Arising from Professional Conduct Complaints*. London: United Kingdom Central Council for Nursing, Midwifery and Health Visiting.

UKCC (1996b) *Guidelines for Professional Practice*. London: United Kingdom Central Council for Nursing, Midwifery and Health Visiting.

UKCC (1994) *The Future of Professional Practice – The Council's Standards for Education and Practice Following Registration*. London: United Kingdom Central Council for Nursing, Midwifery and Health Visiting.

UKCC (1992) *Code of Professional Conduct*, 3rd edn. London: United Kingdom Central Council for Nursing, Midwifery and Health Visiting.

UKCC (1990a) *Statutory Instrument 1990 No. 1624. The Nurses, Midwives and Health Visitors (Midwives Training) Amendment Rules Approval Order 1990*. London: United Kingdom Central Council for Nursing, Midwifery and Health Visiting.

UKCC (1990b) *The Report of the Post-Registration Education and Practice Project*. London: United Kingdom Central Council for Nursing, Midwifery and Health Visiting.

UKCC (1989) *Statutory Instrument 1989 No. 1456. The Nurses, Midwives and Health Visitors (Registered Fever Nurse Amendment Rules and Training Amendment Rules) Approval Order 1989*. London: United Kingdom Central Council for Nursing, Midwifery and Health Visiting.

UKCC (1986) *Project 2000: A New Preparation for Practice*. London: United Kingdom Central Council for Nursing, Midwifery and Health Visiting.

UKCC (1983) *Statutory Instrument 1983 No. 873. The Nurses, Midwives and Health Visitors Rules Approval Order 1983*. London: United Kingdom Central Council for Nursing, Midwifery and Health Visiting.

Wolf A (1995) *Competence-Based Assessment*. Buckingham: Open University Press.

4

How do we assess?

INTRODUCTION

It is discussed in Chapter 3 that competence is a construct which is not directly observable, but rather is inferred from performance. Assessing performance will therefore be important to infer clinical competence. Equally important will be the requirement to gather sufficient evidence to justify the inference, and in particular, that a safe inference has been made (Gonczi et al 1993). Clinical competence is a complex entity and it almost always requires the practitioner to use a combination of attributes simultaneously and adapt practices to different contexts. Thus, the assessment of clinical competence is not straightforward and no one method can hope to assess overall competence. Moreover, some competencies are less easily assessed through performance than others. Hager and Gonczi (1996) state that it is not enough merely to observe performance in the complex world of professional work – a breadth of evidence is required to enable assessors to make a sound inference that professionals can perform competently in the variety of clinical situations in which they can find themselves.

What is therefore needed is a 'range of forms of evidence' (Bedford et al 1993) to provide this breadth so that assessors can make valid and reliable inferences. Consequently, it is necessary to use planned combinations of a variety of methods of assessment to obtain this 'breadth of evidence' to evaluate overall clinical competence, so that assessors of clinical practice know with confidence that the student has the necessary knowledge, skills and attributes to ensure public safety and protection. Bedford et al (1993) suggest that the strategy of *triangulation* is utilized to obtain this breadth of evidence.

There is one key similarity between the processes of clinical assessment and research – simplistically, both seek to obtain data or evidence to add to the knowledge base and/or prove or disprove the case under investigation. In clinical assessment we seek data by which we obtain clearer perspectives of our learners, and evidence to confirm the achievement of competence for safe practice. When conducting clinical assessment there is much to be learnt from the rigour with which research studies are generally conducted in order to achieve validity and reliability of results. One rigorous research strategy is the use of triangulation.

In this chapter the importance of using the strategy of triangulation to achieve validity and reliability of assessment is explored. In research, the technique of triangulation is used to obtain more valid and reliable research data. The principles guiding the use of this technique will be extrapolated for use in assessment so that assessments can also be conducted with the same degrees of validity and reliability as in research. The uses, merits and limitations of a range of methods that can be used in the competency-based approach for the assessment of clinical practice are also explored and debated. To reflect the principle of integration through the use of the holistic/integrated competency-based model of assessment (see Figure 3.3), integrated assessment approaches that use a combination of methods are put forward so that a number of elements and their performance criteria can be assessed simultaneously.

TRIANGULATION

The theoretical perspectives of the term 'triangulation' are drawn from the literature on research, as literature which relates this term to the conduct of assessment is perfunctory and indirect (see, for example, Bedford et al 1993). Triangulation is a term borrowed by the social sciences from surveying and navigation. It refers to the principle of geometry that the third point of a triangle can be plotted using the two known points as the vertices (Fielding and Fielding 1986, in Redfern 1994). This concept of triangulation was first applied to research methodology by Campbell and Fiske (1959, in Redfern 1994) in psychological research as a metaphor to describe the use of several methods to measure a single construct in order to confirm a hypotheses. Triangulation in this context then does not mean three. Later researchers such as Denzin (1989) argue that triangulation is more than the use of several methods – it is the combination of 'methodologies' used to investigate the same phenomenon. These 'methodologies' are referred to as 'types of triangulation': four of them are described by Denzin (1989). From the work of Denzin, three types of triangulation are selected for exploration here, as these are seen to be relevant and applicable for the conduct of integrated assessments: they are therefore discussed, and extrapolated, to our discussion on assessment in this chapter. The types of triangulation are:

- method triangulation
- data triangulation
- investigator triangulation.

Method triangulation

There are two kinds of method triangulation: *within-methods* and *between-methods*. *Within-methods* triangulation is the application of different types of the same method to measure a phenomenon. An example is that of using different scales to measure pain, such as a visual analogue scale, a Likert-type scale and a semantic differential scale. All these scales are different in the way they assess the amount and/or the quality of pain but they are all examples of the same kind of method, that is, *scales*. As a test of validity, the issue is whether they come up with the same answer when applied to the same patients at the same time.

When a student is assessed caring for patients experiencing pain, the student can be observed by the assessor during clinical practice when caring for these patients. Arrangements can also be made for the student to be observed by a second assessor, thus generating evidence of performance using the 'testimony of others'. Both assessors are using the same assessment method, i.e. *observation*. As a test of validity, the issue is whether they come up with the same or similar answers of what the student is able to perform.

Between-methods triangulation uses different methods to measure the same phenomenon. The important point about using between-methods triangulation is that it is much more than the mere combination of several methods. Rather, the methods should be selected as a combined strategy so that the strengths of each are maximized and their limitations are minimized. Linking the data in a coherent and systematic way is essential. In the case of the student assessment above, an example of using between-methods triangulation is to ask questions about care you have observed the student giving. Questioning will establish, for example, whether there is a sound understanding of the needs of the patients who are experiencing the pain, which in turn should influence the care given. It may also reveal the attitudes of the student on this aspect of care or her attitudes towards the patients. The strengths and weaknesses of observation in determining performance evidence are complemented by the strengths and weaknesses of questioning in determining knowledge and understanding. As a test of validity, the answers of the student will augment the assessor's observation of performance.

Data triangulation

Data triangulation refers to the use of multiple data sources, with each source focused upon the phenomenon of interest (Denzin 1989). These data sources can differ by person, time or place. For example, data can be collected from different people or during different times or at different locations. The aim is that the data sources provide unique and diverse views about the same topic to contribute to validity and reliability: this enables the researcher to discover the dimensions of a phenomenon which are similar and dissimilar. As shown below, it is appropriate to make use of the three data sources as described by Denzin (1989) for the purposes of clinical assessment:

- *person* – assessment evidence is collected from other assessors and/or student self-evaluation

- *time* – assessment evidence is collected on different clinical shifts over a period of time
- *place* – assessment evidence is collected from the different instances of practice provided within the range of context in the learning contract (see Chapter 6).

If we return to the example of assessing the student caring for patients who are experiencing pain, we can see how evidence from the three data sources can provide the assessor with diverse views about the student when caring for patients experiencing pain. Evidence provided by the testimony of the second assessor and student self-assessment will contribute to the validity and reliability of assessments of the student. If all sources agree that the student has achieved the performance criteria and is able to care for this category of patients, the assessment is likely to have validity. Conversely, if there is disagreement, the assessment could lack validity and/or reliability. The use of continuous assessment of practice will help ensure that evidence collected on different clinical shifts reflects a wide a range of conditions – such as different patients, working at different times of the day, environmental stresses such as noise and busyness of the ward – as these factors may influence the student's practice positively or adversely. The evidence collected from a range of occasions when the student cared for patients experiencing pain will provide information about the quantity and quality of learning. It will also serve to identify the strengths and weaknesses of the student in this aspect of care. For instance, does the student provide better care for the younger than the older patient? How well does the student cope when caring for these patients? Is the student able to assess the patient's need for pain relief with accuracy?

Investigator triangulation

Investigator triangulation occurs when the different knowledge and expertise held by members of the research team are used in the analysis of raw data. When several investigators are involved in a study, this type of triangulation helps reduce the potential bias that occurs when only a single investigator is involved. In clinical assessment, investigator triangulation takes place when the range of evidence contributed by different assessors is used in the analysis of student competence. This will help reduce the potential bias of a single assessor. In their research report on the assessment of competence, Bedford et al (1993) recommend that:

> Assessment documentation should be broadened to include evidence contributed by more than one accredited witness . . .

These 'witnesses' could be the assessor, other clinical colleagues and the clinical link lecturer. Each person is likely to 'know' the student in slightly different ways and be able to contribute to identification of the range of learning that has taken place, what the strengths and weaknesses of the student are and so on. Investigator triangulation may be particularly valuable when attempting to evaluate the student's attitudes. Several people's views are likely to have been collected after independent assessment of the student, thus reducing biases and adding to the reliability of the assessment (Phillips et al 2000).

So far, then, triangulation is about:

- the use of different assessment methods or ways of collecting assessment evidence
- ensuring that different assessment methods and ways complement each other.

The main aim of using triangulation in clinical assessment is to obtain as complete a picture as possible of the student's achievement of competence, so that the assessment is valid and reliable. It is therefore important to remember that triangulation is more than just obtaining three (or more) sources or types of evidence: the evidence needs to be linked so that an integrated and comprehensive assessment of the student is made.

Advantages and limitations of triangulation

Practically, triangulation may be quite straightforward to arrange when we are arranging the supervision and assessment of our students. Using triangulation to the extent that an integrated and comprehensive assessment of the student is made can prove to be challenging, which may be construed to be a limitation by some. However, the use of triangulation carries many advantages. We will now consider what these advantages and limitations are.

You may wish to try Activity 4.1.

Advantages

1. *It allows confirmation of assessment evidence and increases our confidence in the assessment decision we make*: By combining the types of triangulation – i.e. method, data and investigator triangulation – we obtain a fuller and more complete picture of the student's achievement or non-achievement. Having a richer and deeper understanding of the student's learning, be it performance or knowledge and understanding or the development of some attitude or a set of values, confirms our assessment of the student and therefore increases our confidence when we are making the assessment decision. Consider this scenario: you have a student who is not achieving several competencies. You have come to this decision over several weeks of observing the student in practice and asking her questions about her practice. You wonder whether your decision is influenced by the fact that you do not like the student's green and red hair! Another assessor provides assessment evidence which confirms your decision. You probably breathe a sigh of relief and say: 'I'm not biased after all'. The testimony provided by another assessor increases your confidence in your assessment decision. *Does this enhance the validity, or reliability, or both, of your assessment?* (see discussion in Chapter 5).

ACTIVITY 4.1

From our discussion so far on triangulation, what advantages and limitations can you elicit? Make a list of them. Compare your list with the feedback in the text.

2. *It guards against a blinkered perspective*: The use of triangulation can potentially help us overcome the bias of 'single-method, single-observer' assessments (Redfern 1994). However, Redfern warns that the use of several methods and assessors may not compensate for assessor bias. It can be difficult to overcome strong likes and dislikes.

3. *It is more likely to portray a 'whole picture' of the student*: Rowntree's (1987) book has this question as the title: *Assessing Students: How Shall We Know Them?* Attempting to 'know' students so that we are fair in our assessments of them requires us to understand a complex and multidimensional being. Furthermore, competencies are generally complex, which requires the student to learn and develop several attributes concurrently (see Chapter 3 for a discussion of the holistic/integrated competency-based model). A range of assessment evidence will give us a richer and deeper understanding of the student's strengths and weaknesses and what has and has not been achieved, so that we obtain a fuller picture of the student's achievement. We will then be in a better position to provide the guidance and support that the student requires in order to learn and achieve some more.

4. *It allows divergent evidence to enrich explanation*: When we use triangulation we are more likely to obtain or be given unexpected and divergent assessment evidence about the student. This should be regarded as a bonus (Redfern 1994), as such evidence may explain some aspect of the student or the student's performance that has been eluding us. For example, a colleague who was working with your student may report to you that your student was observed to have been in tears when caring for a patient with terminal cancer. The student subsequently revealed that a close friend had recently died of cancer. For several weeks you have been attempting to involve the student in this aspect of care but had been unsuccessful as the student was always reluctant. You were getting concerned that the student is not learning about care of patients with terminal cancer. The evidence from your colleague has served as a source of divergent evidence.

Limitations

1. *It is expensive on resources*: When using triangulation, arrangements need to be made for the student to learn and practise over a range of contexts over time. Several assessment methods, including other assessors, need to be used: more resources, such as time and extra assessors, are required. In today's climate of health care, where such resources are in scarce supply, the need for student supervision and assessment competes with the need to deliver care. It would be tempting, and certainly easier, to ignore the use of triangulation when assessing students! As was practised by the General Nursing Council for England and Wales in the 1970s, the use of 'one-off' assessment when a student nurse was assessed on one occasion, for a stated period of time, for one aspect of learning, was much more economical on resources: *Did you experience this form of assessment? And how valid and reliable were the assessments?*

2. *It cannot compensate for assessor bias*: If we cannot overcome our biases, the use of triangulation will not help us achieve the validity and reliability we desire in our assessment.

3. *It may compound sources of error*: This point relates to Point 2 above. If we hold some biases and the other assessor also holds some biases which are different from ours, our assessment evidence will not be as objective as we perceive. In fact, the student could be more disadvantaged than if we had not used the evidence from the other assessor.

4. *Methods selected may be inappropriate*. As discussed earlier, the assessment methods we select should complement each other so that a 'rich' range of evidence is provided to allow us to assess fully the development of professional competence. This means we have to assess the development of knowledge, attitudes, skills and attributes. The selection of methods should allow us to assess those areas of learning, performance and development equally, and not focus on the assessment of one or two domains of learning. For example, if we use observation to assess the student's performance, the testimony of another assessor was also based on observation of practice and simulation as our assessment methods, we have assessed very well the student's abilities to perform but may not have assessed attributes such as understanding and attitudes well, if at all.

5. *Triangulation is no use with the 'wrong' research question*: This limitation is equally relevant to assessment. If we are not clear about *what* we want to assess, then triangulation is not going to enhance the validity and reliability of our assessment. It is therefore important to define, and describe, clearly the competency statement, the knowledge and performance outcomes we wish our student to achieve.

If you wish to try Activity 4.2, find some colleagues who experienced the 'one-off' assessments conducted by the GNC.

Despite the challenges and difficulties associated with the use of triangulation, the advantages of using this strategy indicate that it gives us better opportunities to achieve validity and reliability of assessment. What this means when using the holistic/integrated competency-based approach to assessment is that both the *attributes* of the learner and the *performance* of key professional tasks are assessed. The discussion of competence in Chapter 3 stated that the attributes of individuals do not in themselves constitute competence. Nor is competence the mere performance of a series of tasks. Rather, the notion of competence integrates attributes with performance. Another point about competence to be reiterated is that competence is a construct which is not directly observable but is inferred from successful performance. Therefore, combinations of assessment methods need to be considered and used so that a range of evidence is provided to enable a safe judgement of competence to be made (Gonczi et al 1993).

ACTIVITY 4.2

Debate the following with your colleagues:
- the limitations of the different types of triangulation are real and daunting
- we should return to the use of the traditional 'one-off' assessments practised by the General Nursing Council!

ACTIVITY 4.3

What methods do you frequently use to assess students you work with?
Can you give reasons for your selection?

ASSESSMENT METHODS

This section starts with Activity 4.3.

In my experience, the following methods are the most commonly used by assessors:

- working with the students and observing their practice
- asking questions leading to reflective discussions on contextualized practice
- obtaining the opinion (testimony) of other assessors
- checking nursing care records made by the students.

Gonczi et al (1993) say that all existing methods of assessment used by a profession could potentially be appropriate for use in the competency-based approach to assessment. They go on to explain that it is not the methods themselves which are competency-based but the *way* they are used, the *emphasis* given to the methods and *how results* are interpreted that are important in competency-based assessment. The uses, merits and limitations of a range of methods which can be used for the assessment of the different components of professional competence are now explored.

Observation of practice

Observation simply means watching and noting what you see (Stoker 1994). Stoker (1994:iv) says that 'observation is an essential tool in assessment – it is one of the most effective ways of finding out whether learning has taken place'. There is a better chance of making more accurate assessments if observation is part of a continuous process of working with the learner. Learners can be assessed on a number of occasions in their everyday working environment while they are performing in their 'natural' surroundings to give us a picture of their ability to perform a variety of real tasks so that direct evidence of competence can be collected. As we watch the learner in action, we obtain direct evidence of behaviours and behavioural patterns. Much more reliable judgements about professional competence are therefore possible than with assessments conducted in limited time periods on limited ranges of context. Assessments are also more likely to have predictive validity.

There are two ways we can observe the learner's performance: by participant and non-participant observation. Working directly with the learner is known as *participant observation*. In research, during participant observation, researchers join the group, often keeping their identities a secret to try to minimize any changes in behaviour which participants may be inclined to make as a result of being observed (Swanwick 1994). In clinical assessment, however, we cannot make our identity a secret! Therefore, the effects of being observed – the *observer* effect – may affect the learner's performance. Observer effect is discussed in

ACTIVITY 4.4

If you were being directly observed, how may your performance be affected?

Chapter 5. Another important point to bear in mind when observing practice is that of *observer bias* and how this may affect our assessment. This is also discussed in Chapter 5.

Try Activity 4.4.

The fact that someone is looking at us may make us nervous. Our actions may not be as smooth as usual or we may have lapses of memory. I can recall an instance when I was observed during teaching practice – I dropped all my papers and acetates during the middle of the teaching session and I felt that I stuttered for the whole hour! *Have you had similar experiences?* On the other hand, we may exercise more attention to the task than we normally would. Again, I can recall many instances of teaching practice when I knew in advance that I would be observed and assessed. I have never since prepared my lectures, audiovisual aids, hand-outs and so on as meticulously and lost so many nights of sleep!

In the above instances, we are obviously not giving a true picture of the way we practise. *Is the validity, or reliability, or both, affected?*

- Observing the learner 'from a distance' is known as *non-participant observation*. In research, the researcher does not interact with the participants unless approached. If this happens, interaction is kept to a minimum (Swanwick

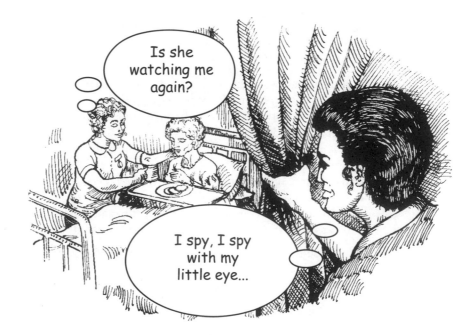

Nerve wracking – or an opportunity to outshine?

1994). During clinical assessment, we may observe the learner caring for a patient while we are performing another activity, such as dispensing medications, talking to someone else and so on. *What strategies have you used for observing a learner 'from a distance'?*

■ There are occasions when evidence of ability to perform may be inferred from an examination of the product of the learner's work – items which the learner produces or has worked on, e.g. a made bed and the surrounds, the bandaged stump of a below-knee amputation and so on. The level of achievement is judged by assessing the quality of the piece of work.

Using the standards and performance criteria in a checklist

Fletcher (1991:66) stated that in competence-based assessment 'it is individual performance which is judged – and judged against explicit standards which reflect . . . the expected outcomes of that individual's competent performance . . .'. When assessing for the development and achievement of a professional competency, we look for pre-specified behaviours, like the ways a skill is performed or the ways the learner interacts with a patient. We use these criteria to determine whether learning has taken place. When using observation to assess performance, noting these criteria in the form of a mental or written checklist (Stoker 1994) will guide our observation. Dawson (1992) says that:

> The use of observation schedules in assessment is quite acceptable, and accurate, when the observer is seeking to identify pre-specified behaviours concerned with a given operation.

Ewan and White (1996) recommend the use of written checklists, as they have a high inter-observer agreement. They also have the advantages of ensuring *validity, discriminating power* and *feasibility* (Stoker 1994), concepts that are discussed in Chapter 5. As checklists are generally detailed, they provide a useful profile of performance that can be discussed with the learner.

When using written checklists, the following points may be useful to remember (Ewan and White 1996):

■ longer checklists tend to be more reliable than shorter ones
■ as checklists require the observer to judge whether certain behaviours have taken place, they are most effective where components of performance are specified in detail
■ it is possible to include behaviours which may underpin aspects of attitudes and interpersonal relationships
■ have three options for recording, i.e. *observed, not observed, not applicable*
■ important errors should also be noted
■ if any essential component of the performance is omitted, the learner is assessed as *not yet competent* and is re-assessed

In particular instances it becomes necessary to assess the process of performance (Gonczi et al 1993). When observing these instances of practice, the ways of performing a task can also be included in a checklist, such as:

■ accuracy or lack of error
■ speed of performance
■ choice of the correct techniques

- the proper sequence of techniques
- adherence to regulatory and policy requirements.

Although the use of checklists has advantages, Ewan and White (1996) warn that if the criteria in the checklist emphasize the performance of a specific skill, beginning students may become fixated on specifics rather than learning the perspectives of care as a whole. Conversely, Benner (1984) thinks it necessary to break a psychomotor skill down into sequenced elements that the student can grasp in order to become technically competent as a beginning practitioner in the real world of clinical practice. One key facilitation skill of the mentor/assessor is to be able to coach the student through the necessary paces to learn the psychomotor skill and, at the same time, learn about how to care for the patient.

Allow enough time for observation

Assessments, in general, sample only a fraction of what a learner is expected to know. This is inevitable as it is not feasible or desirable to attempt to assess every aspect of learning, e.g. it would be impractical to attempt to assess a pharmacist's knowledge of every drug that could be encountered in everyday practice. Likewise, when assessing the competent clinical practice of nursing and midwifery practitioners, inference of competence is inevitably based on a sampling of performance. Fish and Twinn (1997:114) made this important point about observing practice: 'all seeing is selective, and all reporting of what is seen is interpretive; there is no such thing as purely objective factual observation'. We should also bear in mind that competence is a construct that is not directly observable but is inferred from successful performance. There must therefore be enough evidence so that we are confident that it is safe to make the inference that the learner is competent. The assessor must therefore allow enough time to observe the learner on a number of occasions so that it is possible for sufficient evidence of learning to be demonstrated. Guidelines from the English National Board (1997) state that the assessor should directly observe and support the pre-registration student for a minimum period equivalent to 2 days per working week for full-time students and pro rata for part-time students. This working arrangement will give the assessor more time to work with the student so that learning and progression can be monitored with accuracy.

How does the assessor know when there is enough evidence? Making an assessment decision based on concrete evidence is one of the key principles of competency-based assessment. This important aspect of competency-based assessment is developed in Chapter 7.

So far, there has been a consideration of how to use observation as an assessment method, its usefulness or otherwise in ascertaining a true picture of the learner's ability in 'natural' surroundings and some of the difficulties associated with its use. To summarize, effective observation (Stoker 1994) requires you to:

- use a checklist
- allow enough time for observation
- be aware of observer bias
- be aware of observer effect.

ACTIVITY 4.5

Make a list of the uses/merits of observation and another of the limits of observation.

Which components of competence can be assessed with any accuracy using observation? When we observe a learner's performance, we can only see overt behaviours and behavioural patterns as the learner performs care. Although behavioural patterns may indicate the underlying attitude (Andrusyszyn 1989) we cannot see inwardly held beliefs, values or feelings (Dawson 1992), nor can we determine knowledge and understanding of the care or task. As an observer we can only say that the observable performance is mainly a reflection of the possession of skills. Observation is therefore only useful for the assessment of the skills developed which are contributing to effective performance at the time. Gonczi et al (1993), however, claim that observation allows assessment of attitudes and interpersonal skills.

Try this next activity (Activity 4.5) on the use of observation as an assessment method.

Advantages of observation of practice

- *Can provide a high level of integrated assessments*: As the learner is observed performing care and tasks, it is possible to use evidence of performance to assess several competencies and several components of competence simultaneously.

- *Allows assessment of attitudes and interpersonal skills*: Attitudes can be inferred from behaviours and behavioural patterns. Interpersonal skills can be directly observed.

- *Offers realistic evidence of competence*: Competence-based assessment uses explicit standards of occupational performance as its foundation. The logical way to assess whether someone is meeting those standards is to watch them working in that occupation (Fletcher 1991).

- *Allows evaluation of problem solving*: As the learner is observed managing a situation, it is possible to assess how well the learner has managed the situation. From this, it can be inferred that the learner has been able to solve the problem.

- *Mistakes in performance can be corrected*: Direct observation and supervision of practice will enable the assessor to identify and correct any mistakes at the time or immediately afterwards.

Disadvantages of observation of practice

- *Circumstances of observation may be too specific*: Evidence obtained about the ability to perform in care situations that occur rarely generally cannot be used with any degree of validity towards the assessment of many competencies.

- *Requires lengthy and costly assessments for reliability*: The learner needs to be observed on more than one occasion to ensure reliability. This means that the period of assessment is longer rather than shorter and is therefore costly in terms of time and effort required.

■ *Gives indirect evidence of knowledge/understanding only*: If a learner is able to perform the care or task it can only be inferred that knowledge/understanding underpins that performance.

■ *Does not assess ability to learn through practice*: Even if a learner is able to perform a task, or care for a patient, it cannot be assumed that the learner can transfer this performance to another situation and perform to the same standards another time.

■ *Subject to observer bias and observer effect*: Polit and Hungler (1989:212, 231) state that one of the most pervasive problems with observation is the vulnerability of observational data to distortions and biases – human perceptual judgemental errors can pose a serious threat to the validity and accuracy of observational information.

In summary, direct observation of clinical practice is used primarily to obtain evidence of ability to perform when we assess the learning of practical skills and behaviours and behavioural patterns, which may indicate the underlying attitudes and value systems held by the learner.

An ability to perform is only one component of competence. Evidence of achievement of the other components of competence needs to be obtained using other assessment methods. Questioning frequently complements observation in that we are obtaining the 'indirect evidence' of competence which is 'hidden' and not open to observation (Stoker 1994).

Questioning

It is discussed in Chapter 1 that one of the purposes of assessment is to maximize learning. Gipps (1994:15) made the point that 'assessment alone will not develop higher-order skills in the absence of clearly delineated teaching strategies that foster the development of higher order thinking in pupils'. Asking questions is an integral part of teaching and learning, and places students in the role of active learners (De Young 1990). It is one teaching/learning strategy to help students develop higher-level cognitive skills. Questioning can also serve as positive reinforcement for students when we indicate that answers are correct and/or insightful. This gives feedback to the student that material has been understood and higher-level thought processes were used.

Try Activity 4.6.

In clinical assessment, questioning can be used for the following purposes:

■ To assess baseline knowledge, e.g. knowledge of the stages of the grieving process.

ACTIVITY 4.6

For what purposes have you used questioning?

- To assess ability to form links between previously isolated information, e.g. if a student midwife is learning how to support women in labour, questions could be asked about the support strategies used for the individual woman and how well these worked for that woman. Further questioning could then lead the student to explore those common strategies that work, or do not work, for the majority of women.

- To assess application of theory to practice, e.g. using the policy on infection control you had discussed, ask your learner to go over the actions she would take when preparing for the admission of the next patient who requires to be barrier nursed.

- To assess understanding of care given, e.g. the rationale for using certain communication skills when comforting the dying patient; if the learner understands the *why* behind the care, it indicates that theory underpins practice.

- To assess problem solving skills, e.g. by posing: . . . *What other information do you need before you can solve this problem . . . How else could you . . . Give reasons for . . . What would happen if you tried . . . What other options do you have . . . .*

- To assess decision making skills, e.g. by posing: . . . *What action would you take if . . . Give reasons . . .*

- It is possible to obtain an indication of underlying attitudes, values and beliefs, e.g. by posing: . . . *What do you think of euthanasia? . . . detaining psychiatric patients under the mental health act? Do you agree with Jenny's opinions? Why?*

- It is possible to assess verbal communication skills by the ability of the student in verbalizing responses.

From the above discussion of the uses of questioning it can be seen that learning in the cognitive domain and affective domain (Bloom et al 1956) – thus, several attributes of competence – can be assessed using this assessment method. When we assess learning in the cognitive domain, it is important to assess not only the knowledge base but also higher-level thinking, so that the range of cognitive skills are assessed. The kinds of questions asked will reveal to the learner the kind of thinking expected and the stimulation of different kinds of thinking (Perrott 1982). Formulating questions to assess higher-level thinking can be tricky. An understanding of how questions can be classified may assist in the framing of those questions which are necessary to elicit the level of thinking we require of the learner.

The most popular classification system is based on Bloom's taxonomy of educational objectives (Bloom et al 1956). Although the taxonomy was developed to classify educational objectives, questions can be related to each level of the taxonomy. Table 4.1, adapted from De Young 1990, lists the cognitive activity at each level, as well as some sample questions.

- With the assistance of the information in Table 4.1, try Activity 4.7.

ACTIVITY 4.7

Examine one learning outcome that a learner of yours needs to achieve.
Formulate one question at each level of Bloom's taxonomy so that you can assist your learner to develop the range of higher-level cognitive skills.

TABLE 4.1 Question classification according to Bloom's taxonomy (adapted from Craig & Page 1981)

Category	Cognitive activity required	Sample question words		Examples of questions
1. Knowledge	*Recall* Questions, regardless of complexity, can be answered by simple recall of previously learnt material	What When Which	Identify Describe Who	Define List	What is the definition of glaucoma? At what age do infants begin to crawl?
2. Comprehension	*Understanding* Questions can be answered by merely restating and reorganizing material in a rather literal manner to show that there is understanding of the essential meaning	Compare Contrast Differentiate Explain Extrapolate			What does the nursing process have in common with the scientific method? Why does intravenous tubing have to be free of air?
3. Application	*Solving* Questions involve problem solving in new situations with minimal identification or prompting of the appropriate rules, principles or concepts	Apply Consider How would Checkout			Given these arterial blood gas results, what nursing interventions are needed? How would you get a blood pressure reading on a person with third-degree burns of all extremities?
4. Analysis	*Exploration of reasoning* Questions require the student to break an idea into its component parts for logical analysis, facts, opinions, logical conclusions, etc	Support your What assumptions What reasons			What is the major premise behind Kubler-Ross's theory of death and dying? What data would you need to support this nursing diagnosis?
5. Synthesis	*Creating* Questions require students to combine ideas into a statement, plan, product, etc., that is new for them	Think of a way Create Propose Plan Suggest			Given all of the data in this case study, what nursing diagnoses can be developed? Think of a way that we could research the relationship between those variables.
6. Evaluation	*Judging* Questions require students to make a judgement about something using some criteria or standard by making their judgement, principles, or concepts	Judge Which would Consider Defend What is the most appropriate			Of the two possible nursing interventions in this situation, which would be more appropriate?

The aim is to structure questions so that they define a linking path, as these are more valuable in assessing the quality of learning and helping the learner to develop higher-level thinking (Minton 1997). Do not be too concerned if you have had difficulties formulating the questions. Many trained teachers only manage to ask questions predominantly at the lower cognitive levels (De Young 1990). In view of the high-level thinking required of health professionals, however, it is beneficial to assess students at the application through to evaluation levels (see Table 4.1). Stoker (1994) says that using questions effectively is an essential skill in assessment. This skill should be, and can be, developed. The reader is referred to the chapter on questioning in De Young (1990) for a further discussion of how to frame and ask questions.

It is important to remember that when we use questioning in clinical assessment, our main aim is to gain evidence about how much learning has taken place, i.e. how much of the competency the student has achieved. Questions asked should therefore be related to the competency and be based on the context of the practice event. The following checklist (Stoker 1994) on the use of questioning may be helpful:

- Are the questions relevant to the learner? Do they relate to things the learner needs to know and should know rather than focusing on unusual aspects of the subject?
- Is the wording clear? Does it indicate what sort of answer you require?
- Have you provided some sort of feedback at the time? Be especially aware of how you deal with incorrect or incomplete answers. Try not to let your reaction have the effect of demotivating the learner.
- Be careful not to make learners feel that you are trying to catch them out.

The limitations of using questioning for assessing clinical practice are:

- Questions cannot assess attitudes, values and beliefs with accuracy, as what the learner says may not be a reflection of inwardly held beliefs.
- The learner may feel threatened. This may affect the responses, and an inaccurate picture is formed of the student's ability.
- Inappropriately framed questions may not elicit the correct responses.
- Questioning can be time consuming.
- It may not have predictive validity. Correct responses to questions may not reflect the ability to perform.

As the use of questioning in the clinical setting is frequently related directly to the caregiving experiences of the learner, questioning sessions may lead to a discussion of these instances of practice. It is generally believed that *reflection on practice* – where the thinking done in one situation is made explicit and built on to be used in another – should be developed through discussion that takes place away from the arena of care activity (Bedford et al 1993). The use of discussions in clinical assessment is now examined.

Discussion around care and care activities

De Young (1990) says that topics that are most suitable for discussion are controversial issues, clinical or professional problems, and emotionally laden topics such as death and dying. After deciding on which clinical event you wish to explore further with the student through discussion, you need to provide some structure for the discussion. De Young (1990:87) made this important point about the use of discussion: 'Good discussions do not just happen spontaneously; they require careful planning'. She suggests making the following arrangements before you start:

- be clear about what you want the student to learn – set some objectives
- plan the physical environment – use a room where you will not be interrupted; ensure that the seating is adequate.

During the discussion, take on the role of the facilitator (Rogers 1983). As we work with students during discussions, we can assess their development of those attributes desirable of a competent practitioner. Depending on the topic and the skills of the facilitator (Ewan and White 1996, Oliver and Endersby 1994, De Young 1990), students may have the following learning opportunities:

- Consider and explore the principles, concepts and theories used in that particular practice situation and transfer such learning to new and different situations.
- Clarify information and concepts.
- Develop critical thinking skills, leading to the development of problem-solving and decision-making skills. Bedford et al (1993) emphasize the importance of post-event discussion in fostering the development of high-quality decision-making and problem-solving skills
- Develop and evaluate their beliefs, values and attitudes, leading to attitude change. The use of discussion to bring about attitude change is well documented (De Young 1990). As students are facilitated to give and take during the discussions, they learn whether the stance they take on a particular issue is clear, logical and defensible.

Bedford et al (1993:139) advocate that discussions should be critical and take place *before*, *during* and *after* an activity 'through which the activity is reviewed and analysed'. They say that these critical discussions move the assessment activity from being mere surveys of 'activities "done" and skills "covered" to a collaborative, analytical discussion about practice' and divorce criticism from personal attack. Bedford et al (1993:136) emphasized that it is 'assessment discussion' rather than simple discussion that complements observational data in the assessment of competent practice:

> Through discussion about a particular event, students can demonstrate
> the knowledge, understanding and values that have informed their actions
> in the clinical area on a given occasion, enabling assessors to test their
> own observation-based judgements about the quality of those actions.
> The great advantage of assessment dialogue, as opposed to simple
> discussion, is that it facilitates learning as part of the assessment process.

Assessment discussions can help students develop 'situational understanding' that will help them live with, and negotiate a way through the competing and contradictory values they encounter as they perform care (Phillips et al 2000). Elliott (1991) and Schon (1987) postulated that professional practice is learned and developed through 'doing' and 'reflection on doing'. During the course of assessment discussions then, as we allow students to voice their understanding, views and opinions, disagreements and doubts, we can assess the student's *range of cognitive skills* and *attitudes, values and beliefs.*

Assessment discussions around practice can then be held:

- *Before* an activity – when we prepare the student for taking part in the care. As we question and discuss, we can assess the student's knowledge, understanding and perhaps attitude, values and beliefs.
- *During* an activity – when we discuss and check understanding, as the student performs.
- *After* an activity – when we review and analyse care. During the analysis, we can assess the range of cognitive skills, such as knowledge, understanding and problem solving and attitudes, values and beliefs developed or altered as a result of the experience. Post-activity discussion should be held as soon as possible after the experience, while events are still fresh in the mind, to allow more accurate recall of details and for any feedback to have more impact.

Learning diary

Assessment discussions can also be conducted using the student's learning diary entries as the basis. In proposing that reflective understanding should be developed around written evidence of practice, Bedford et al (1993) call for assessment documentation to require:

> . . . written accounts of analytical reflection on the relationship between particular clinical events and general nursing and midwifery principles.

They believe that documentation – in this instance the student's learning diary – that requires discussion between assessor and student is more likely to promote assessment discussion on practice. Learning diaries can offer insight into how students make sense of and feel about their practice. It is possible that students may choose to write only that which they want us to read (Phillips et al 2000). Nonetheless, it provides an evidence base and focus for dialogue (Phillips et al 2000) and gives us a starting point from which to begin an assessment discussion with the student. As a source of evidence of practice, learning diaries can be considered by more than one assessor. The creation of a databank of sharable evidence was advocated by Bedford et al (1993). The views of another assessor would enrich the assessment evidence base on the student and is one way of achieving investigator triangulation.

Facilitating and assessing learning through reflective assessment discussions using the student's diary is not straightforward (Stuart 1997). Flexibility and abilities to deal with the unexpected are required. When 'working' with a student's diary entry, the following framework may assist in carrying out the reflective assessment discussion with intent:

1. *Consider the level of detail in the student's account of the incident.*
   - Is there any description/discussion of the incident in relationship to personal involvement?
   - Have the actions taken by the student been discussed in terms of the negotiation undertaken within the situation (Phillips et al 2000)?

- Is there any description/discussion of the incident in relationship to the involvement of others?
- What suggestions would you make so that the quality of the account could be enhanced?

2. *Consider the ways in which the student has explored personal behaviours, feelings and thoughts and those of others involved.*
   - Is there a constructive exploration of behaviours and actions, thoughts and feelings?
   - How perceptive is the student?
   - Was there an objective appreciation of how and why self and others behaved, felt and thought as they did?
   - Was there any indication of how these affected the incident?
   - What suggestions would you make to help the student explore these further?

3. *Consider the ways in which the student has used or referred to relevant theory and literature.*
   - Is relevant underpinning knowledge identified?
   - Is there any indication of application of theory to practice?
   - Has the student critically analysed theory and current literature and their relationship to practice?
   - What broad theoretical areas may be included in order to explore the incident further?
   - What broad professional issues may be brought into this incident?

4. *Consider the amount of learning the student has extracted through the incident.*
   - Has the student identified any implications for future practice?
   - Does the student specify how own practice can develop?
   - Does the student integrate any 'new' learning with previous knowledge to reach different/new perspectives about care?
   - Have any assumptions about current practice been critically appraised?
   - Has the student suggested alternative ways for practice?
   - What influenced the choices made about the way care was done (Phillips et al 2000)?
   - What constraints affected any decisions made (Phillips et al 2000)?
   - What suggestions would you make to help the student develop the above issues further?

Try Activity 4.8. Do not rush it.

Diaries are considered to be an effective way of encouraging active reflection on experience, particularly where a review takes place with the mentor at some point in the future (Boud et al 1985). As the basis for reflective assessment discussion, it will allow the student opportunities to justify personal actions by

ACTIVITY 4.8

Obtain a learning diary entry of a student. Using the above framework, work through the diary entry with a colleague.

giving the rationale for choices in different circumstances. The student is likely to feel valued as the incident under discussion has been personally identified as important. To an extent, the student is taking control of personal learning by identifying what is important. By an inclusion of the requirement to record not only behaviours and actions but also feelings and thoughts, the student may indicate attitudes, values and beliefs held about particular situations. Although diaries can be used to assess attitudes, values and beliefs, Dawson (1992) says that any such assessment should be formative, as attitude is dynamic and changes over time.

What aspects of learning can be assessed through the reflective assessment discussion of a student's diary? Assessing learning through this process is complex (Boud et al 1985). In using the above suggested framework to facilitate the reflective discussion, the following aspects of learning may be assessed:

- the perceptiveness of the student in the situation
- the self-awareness of the student
- communication and interactive skills
- unobserved practical skills
- underpinning knowledge
- ability to apply theory to practice
- higher-level cognitive skills such as problem solving and decision making
- attitudes, values and beliefs.

Every assessment method has disadvantages and limitations! The limitations of using the student's learning diary for assessment may be listed as:

- does not assess ability to perform in the practical setting
- can be time consuming
- may not have predictive validity
- may not have reliability, as each incident is different
- may not elicit the appropriate responses if the assessor is unskilled in facilitating reflective assessment discussions.

Harlen (1994:3) observed that 'all forms of assessment are subject to human judgement and thus require some form of moderation'. In the section on triangulation the use of investigator triangulation was suggested as a means of reducing the potential biases of a single assessor. The potential diversity of views from more than one assessor would also enrich and strengthen the assessment database on the learner. The next section will consider the use of testimony of others as an assessment method.

Testimony of others

As the student's key assessor, you need to take into account the several perspectives about the achievement of the student and, during that process, draw out both commonalities and points of disagreement (Bedford et al 1993). In practice, explicit arrangements are made for the student to work with other assessors – nursing or midwifery colleagues – who may assess the student by observing the student's practice and complementing this form of evidence by evidence from other assessment methods. When students spend time working with members of the multidisciplinary team, these professional colleagues may also be called upon to provide assessment evidence. Making arrangements for the student to work with, and be assessed by others, has the advantage of making the assessment more feasible, as the student will have more opportunities to practise. As the key assessor you are responsible for coordinating learning and assessment activities so that they are purposeful – the student will then have a fair chance of achieving learning outcomes and competencies. The arrangements you make with other assessors should include:

- briefing them about the learning experiences that the student needs
- the learning outcomes and competencies to be achieved
- the level of performance expected of the student.

Bedford et al (1993) and Ewan and White (1996) caution that we have different standards of practice which may lead to inconsistent expectations and judgements of our student. In their literature review of the assessment of practice, Gerrish et al (1997) found that there is much unease about the expertise of assessors on two counts: first, the concern that there are insufficient practitioners with academic qualifications equivalent to those sought by the students they are assessing; secondly, the concern that a number of clinical assessors are inadequately prepared and do not keep up-to-date with developments in the assessment process. In these instances, the reliability of assessments will be reduced and validity may be compromised.

Try Activity 4.9.

Some suggestions you and your team of assessors may wish to consider are:

- Regular assessor meetings to confer on criteria for high standards of practice.
- Regular assessor meetings to confer on the expected levels of performance in comparison with an ideal standard. Having a common standard amongst assessors will help assessors rate a student's performance at the level expected of students for that stage of the training, which has the advantage of ensuring that assessments have discriminating power.
- Using a checklist for observation.
- Discussing the criteria in the checklist with the other assessors to avoid multiple interpretation.
- Appropriate training and regular updating of assessors.
- Openly discussing personal biases with each other so as to deal with them objectively.

Assessment evidence from others – termed 'witness testimonies' – should be collated by the key assessor. This could be in the form of verbal discussions between assessors or in a written format. Written witness testimonies are a requirement of the national vocational qualification (NVQ) system (City and Guilds 1992). Testimonies should:

- be specific to the clinical activity

ACTIVITY 4.9

Make some suggestions to reduce inconsistencies amongst assessors and thus increase the validity and reliability of your assessment.

- give a brief description of the background and circumstances of practice
- identify the aspects of competence demonstrated.

Box 4.1 is an example of a witness testimony.

Another group of people who could potentially provide testimonies about student performance are the patients and clients. As recipients of care given by students, patients and clients are a legitimate source of assessment data. Who can say with more accuracy whether the nurse was kind or gentle or explained and reassured before giving the injection. Neary (2001:9) found that patients and clients do assess students informally, as illustrated by this statement from a patient: 'Nurse [name] took me for a bath today, I feel safe with her, the way she encouraged me into the bath, ... I was frightened I'd fall . . .. Nurse [name] never left my side, gave me confidence, she did, good lass that she is'.

However, formalizing and gaining access to this source of assessment evidence is fraught with ethical, and even legal problems. Lankshear and Nicklin (2000) suggest developing the many quality audit documents currently in use as a source of information about the performance of individual staff. Patient and client comments and complaints could, and should, feed into the assessment of individual students.

Another group of possible assessors are the student's peers. Peer reviews are becoming an increasingly important feature of professional practice (Lankshear and Nicklin 2000). Peer assessment during training provides opportunities for students to learn to rate the work of other students, helping students to develop collaborative skills; it builds on communication skills of giving feedback and develops professional responsibility (Gomez et al 1998), thereby preparing these aspiring professionals for evaluating the work of

BOX 4.1	Witness testimony on student nurse Mary

During an afternoon shift Mary was assisting in the care of clients on the short-term area of the unit. When sitting with a client called Joseph during tea time, Mary observed him having an epileptic seizure. I was away from the area at the time, so Mary immediately called for help. On entering the dining room I observed that Mary had moved Joseph's food and drink away from him and was supporting his upper body and head while offering reassurance. It was obvious to me that Joseph was experiencing a series of seizures as he appeared to regain consciousness for a short time and then enter into another seizure. Both of us continued to support him until he had fully recovered.

During discussion which followed this incident, I praised Mary for acting quickly by calling for help and ensuring a safe environment by removing the food and drink which may have harmed Joseph. Although Mary could not name the specific type of seizure, she was able to describe the client's behaviour, which allowed me to assess the type of seizure. More important, Mary had remembered the importance of maintaining the safety of the client by supporting his upper body and head to ensure a clear airway. Mary also reported that she had made a note of the time and duration of the seizure and was able to explain the reasons for recording such information in the client's care file.

Mary acted in a competent and professional manner during this incident and followed the correct procedure when administering first aid.

others. Stengelhofen (1993) says that peer feedback is important in laying down the concept that it is part of professional work to be observed and evaluated by one's own colleagues.

The student's peers have a useful contribution to make in the overall assessment process of both theory and practice. Peers frequently work for sustained periods in close proximity; they therefore have the opportunity to make assessments that may be inaccessible to others. Burke (1969 in Rowntree 1987) found that students are realistic when assigning grades to their peers. However, Gomez et al (1998) report that peers may be biased in providing only favourable information because of not wanting to cause trouble for someone or having unrealistic expectations of their peer. A criticism of student peer assessment is that students are not experts – so this is a case of the 'blind leading the blind' (Jarvis and Gibson 1997). If students are to be expected to perform peer assessment, training should be provided.

In some situations it may not be possible to assess learners' performance in the real situation as exemplified in Box 4.1. Reasons may be a shortfall of learning opportunities, e.g. dealing with emergency situations, or it may not be desirable to assess learners' performance with real patients or in real situations because of risks or discomfort to patients or the learner. In midwifery education, student midwives could qualify without having had experience in dealing with obstetric emergencies (Westwood-Timms 1995). In these instances, the same simulation exercises used for teaching can be used to assess learning (De Young 1990). The next section discusses the use of simulation to provide another source of assessment evidence.

Simulation

A simulation is a resemblance of a social or physical reality that corresponds to a real-life situation that a student or client might encounter. It aims to put learners in a position where they can experience some aspect of the real situation by becoming involved in activities that are closely related to it. Gibbs (1988) maintains that simulation is an invaluable substitute for experience. When using simulations, the aim is to create a scenario that resembles the real-life situation as closely as possible so that the learner's responses and behaviours can be assessed with some degree of validity and reliability (De Young 1990). Such learning is more likely to be transferred to the real setting.

All simulated activities cannot take account of the complexities of the 'real' clinical environment. The amount of learning that can be transferred to the real-life setting is debatable (Quinn 2000). Rethans et al (1991 cited in While 1994) claim that such assessments have predictive validity for performance in actual practice. Research on the use of simulations as an assessment activity has shown that achieving reliability is generally not a problem (De Young 1990). What is questionable is the validity of this testing procedure. At the very least, students will have had the opportunity to experience, and perhaps internalize, the actions and reactions required of a given situation.

Simulated activities give us more control over what happens in the assessment. For example, if we use the same scenario to assess the achievement of several students, the conditions of performance and the criteria for assessment will remain the same. The assessment is more likely to be reliable. The validity of the assessment can be increased by close representations of simulations to actual practice situations (Forker and McDonald 1996).

Simulations can take the following formats:

- enacting a simulated clinical situation
- analysing a simulated clinical problem
- using educational models
- using computer-based simulation
- staging objective structured clinical examinations.

Enacting a simulated clinical situation

This format can be used for many social and emergency situations. It closely resembles the use of role play, except that the learner will 'play' the part of the health professional and someone else will 'play' the part of the patient or relatives or some other role. In simulating the clinical situation, we should remember that we are assessing the learner's development into the health professional – this, therefore, requires the learner to play that role. Quinn (2000) states that one of the hallmarks of simulating the clinical situation is that the learner is not expected to act out any kind of script but, rather, is expected to behave and react in a way that is thought and felt to be appropriate. It therefore involves learners to be themselves and to deal with situations using their repertoire of normal everyday behaviour.

Hoban and Casbergue (1978 cited in DeTornyay and Thompson 1987) put forward four principles to consider when using simulations:

- the responses and behaviours – knowledge, attitude, skills – that are expected at the end of training should be specified, as well as the minimal acceptable level of performance the learner is required to demonstrate
- the simulation should represent reality, with enough fidelity to ensure face validity of the test of the learner's performance
- the simulation being used to assess performance should be standardized for all learners to achieve validity and reliability of assessment
- decisions regarding the purpose of the assessment should be made before a simulation is used.

An activity is now used to illustrate how a simulated exercise of a clinical situation can be carried out (Activity 4.10).

There are several key steps to follow:

1. Thoroughly prepare the scenario, including setting learning outcomes for enacting the simulated clinical situation. In Activity 4.10, we will need to collect information about the patient and any problems the patient may encounter at home, the illness of the patient, the home and surrounding envi-

ACTIVITY 4.10

We are planning to involve our learner in a simulated exercise to give her practice in explaining aftercare and home visits to a patient following discharge from the ward. How should we plan for, and conduct the simulation?

ronment, any social support and so on. Creating a simulation as near as possible to the real-life situation that the learner will encounter enhances retention so that the established behaviours can be transferred more easily to the real setting (Quinn 2000).

2. Brief the learner, and the person who is playing the part of the patient. The learner and the 'patient' need to be prepared, particularly if they have not been involved in a simulated exercise before. This involves thorough briefing about the roles they will be playing, the intended learning outcomes to be achieved and agreeing any ground rules. Briefing ensures that the learner is more likely to benefit from the activity.

3. Allow sufficient time to carry out the activity. The learner is expected to behave and react in any way she/he feels is appropriate, as the simulation is not scripted. As discussed above, a simulation involves the learner in 'being herself/himself' and dealing with the situation using her/his natural reactions and behaviours. The success of the exercise therefore depends to a large extent on the selection of the simulated 'patient' (Ewan and White 1996). A 'patient' who is a good role player will put the student through her/his paces!

4. Debriefing and processing the learner's responses and behaviours to give feedback is an important final step. The following points may be used to guide the debriefing:

- allow the student to self-evaluate
- identify the concepts learned
- relate learning to the outcomes of the exercise
- discuss any problems encountered
- discuss application to clinical practice
- give feedback, e.g. discuss if the student needs to do it differently.

What aspects of learning can be assessed using enactment of a simulated clinical situation?

What we can assess will depend on the simulated activity. In the example above we will be able to assess the following:

- knowledge of how the illness has affected the patient
- knowledge of resources and social and support services for the patient
- knowledge of the arrangements to be made prior to discharge of a patient
- communication and interpersonal skills
- decision-making and problem-solving skills
- attitude about discharge planning.

If a scenario requires the performance of physical activities such as enacting the drill for an emergency situation as in a cardiac arrest, responses and reactions during an emergency can be assessed. In these simulated clinical situations the use of the 'thinking aloud' technique is helpful in developing knowledge and clinical reasoning processes (Corcoran-Perry and Narayan 2000). The 'thinking aloud' technique requires the learner to think aloud while making decisions: this makes the reasoning process of the learner explicit and transparent. In their study, Corcoran-Perry and Narayan tape-recorded the thinking aloud verbalizations for later transcription. Analysis of the transcripts revealed the cues attended to, the inferences generated and the actions proposed.

Analysing a simulated clinical problem

This format can be used for many social and emergency situations. A written simulated clinical problem, as close to life as possible, is presented to the learner, who analyses the problem and discusses how the problem would be managed. De Young (1990) recommends that written simulated clinical problems have these features:

- Use real cases as far as possible – these are better because of the wealth of information from which to draw; fabricated cases too often become just summaries of what supposedly happened. The more complex simulations should be based on real cases with all the variables that were involved. Phillips et al (2000:161) recommend that 'assessees should be enabled to work with accounts of practice that tell it like it is and thereby map real practice problems with richly described contextual details'. The assessment is more likely to be valid by focusing on the reality of practice rather than idealized versions.
- The cases that you choose should not be esoteric or unique – the purpose of simulations is to teach and assess learners to solve typical problems and confront commonplace information that they can transfer to their clinical practice.
- The case should be appropriate for the learner's level of knowledge and experience. Cases that are too easy are boring. Those that are too difficult may defeat the objectives – the emphasis in simulations is on the learning process; the learning of content should be a by-product (Ewan and White 1996, De Young 1990)

De Young suggests that simulations can be taken home for the learner to work on for subsequent presentation or they can be used for 'on-the-spot' assessment. Westwood-Timms (1995) reports the use of written simulations in midwifery education to assess student midwives' ability to manage obstetric emergencies. These were used for 'on-the-spot' assessment; these assessments were reported to have reliability. The validity of these assessments was not reported. Box 4.2 gives an example of a clinical problem used by Westwood-Timms.

What aspects of learning can be assessed using analysis of a simulated clinical problem? To analyse a simulated clinical problem successfully, the student requires prior knowledge and, perhaps, practical experience of similar situations. During the analysis, and subsequently solving the problem, the student

BOX 4.2	*Undiagnosed twin delivery*

It is fairly busy on the labour ward in a consultant obstetric unit. There are three midwives on duty including you and two student midwives. One of the student midwives is with you for the shift.

You admit a 30-year-old multigravida at 36 weeks pregnant in advanced labour. She is accompanied by her husband. A female baby is delivered soon after admission. The baby appears smaller than you expect for the gestation. On palpation of the mother's abdomen a second fetus is detected. Fortunately, the oxytocic drug has not been administered.

How would you manage this situation?

has to exercise higher-level cognitive skills. Westwood-Timms (1995) devised assessment criteria to assess the full range of cognitive skills, including the higher cognitive skills of analysis, evaluation and synthesis. In the scenario given in Box 4.2 it is possible to assess the following aspects of learning:

1. *Underpinning knowledge, ability to assess the situation and planing the care*:
   - analysis of the facts presented
   - formulation of action plan
   - rationale for the choices and strategies in the action plan.

2. *Problem-solving and decision-making skills:*
   - ability to predict potential problems and/or complications
   - ability to select relevant cues and to discriminate in order to reach an appropriate decision
   - ability to prioritize actions and the rationale for the decisions
   - ability to delegate care.

It is possible to assess attitudes and values held by the student. Practical skills cannot be assessed. Gipps (1994) warns us that intentions to measure higher-order thinking can be subverted by repeated practice on the task. Intended higher-order tasks such as analysis of a simulated problem can be turned into rote tasks. If many opportunities are provided to practise a task so that the criteria for its assessment are learnt – e.g. how to resuscitate a person – that task is learnt through rote learning.

Try Activity 4.11 with your colleagues.

Using educational models

Educational models may be used to assess skills such as cardiopulmonary resuscitation, suctioning, catheterization, dressing change, administration of injections and so on. In midwifery education, models may be used to assess a learner's ability to perform complex skills and manoeuvres such as performing a breech delivery or managing a shoulder dystocia. Aspects of learning which can be assessed are:

- ability to perform the practical skill correctly in the right sequence
- other aspects of performing the procedure correctly, such as maintaining cleanliness or asepsis, using the right equipment, preparation of the environment, disposal of used equipment and so on
- attitudes towards the performance of the skill, e.g. the importance attached to the observation of maintaining asepsis

ACTIVITY 4.11

Compile a list of problems that you and your colleagues have dealt with that can be used for simulated problem solving and management. Include details of each problem. This set of teaching/learning resource can be kept in a file and be added to.

- if the 'thinking aloud' technique is used (see above), the 'thinking' of the learner can be assessed while the procedure or skill is being performed
- if observation is supplemented by the use of questioning, it is possible to assess knowledge and understanding of performing that skill.

What are the advantages and disadvantages of learning to perform a skill using a model?

- patient safety is not compromised
- patient rights are protected
- learner anxiety is reduced, as practice is in a protected environment
- 'unlimited' opportunities for practise until 'perfection' is achieved!
- may not have predictive validity, as the complexities of the real world are absent
- communication skills and interpersonal skills cannot be assessed.

Using computer-based simulation

Computers are used increasingly to provide sophisticated simulations of clinical events, both for training and assessment purposes. Students' understanding of the systems and concepts upon which the simulations are based are then usually assessed in a conventional way such as using a written test. There are, however, a variety of ways of designing assessment directly around the use of computer simulations. Using computer graphics, realistic patient care situations similar to those likely to be encountered in clinical practice are presented which closely represent actual reality. Learners are assessed managing that simulated situation by their responses to a series of cues and changes in variables of the patient condition. Responses are recorded and a print-out is then handed in for assessment.

An example of a computer simulation is MACPUFF, which was developed by Manchester University Medical School for learning about and assessing the management of patients with respiratory problems (Brown et al 1996). The simulated patient can be set up with a chosen set of respiratory variables in a particular atmospheric environment. The patient is then 'run' for several minutes to see what happens to various vital indicators of physiological functioning. Biochemical measures are calculated, listed every 3 seconds and plotted on graphs. The complex chemical interactions involved in maintaining a stable and healthy respiratory state can thus be observed. Students' understanding of these interactions which inform the management of the patient can be assessed by setting up the patient using different variables. The student is then required to manipulate conditions such as the amount of oxygen required to stabilize the patient's condition. The assessment of the student could include the requirement to stabilize the patient's condition within certain parameters and within a certain time limit. Such a goal cannot be achieved by trial and error but only through an understanding of the biochemistry of respiration.

Aspects of learning which can be assessed using computer-based simulations are discussed in 'Analysing a simulated clinical problem' above. It needs to be acknowledged that to implement computer-based simulation, students and assessors must be 'computer literate' and adequate computing facilities should be available.

Staging objective structured clinical examinations (OSCEs)

This form of assessment requires students to rotate through a series of standardized simulated professional tasks set up at testing points called 'stations'. During an OSCE, students are tested at several stations by spending a fixed period of time at each station. As the students have to be tested at each station in turn, it means that several students can be tested during each OSCE – in practice, the number of stations set up will determine the number of students going round during the OSCE.

OSCEs have been used predominantly by teaching staff in university laboratory settings to assess competence in performing psychomotor skills, ability to analyse and interpret data, take a patient's history, identify problems, make clinical decisions and the use of interpersonal and communication skills (see, for example, Govaerts et al 2001, Phillips et al 2000, Ladyshewsky 1999, Fahy and Lumby 1988). The assessment evidence of competence from this source can supplement other sources of evidence. It should, however, be noted that evidence of its reliability and validity as an assessment method is conflicting. Govaerts et al (2001) and Ladyshewsky (1999) report high reliability and validity of this test procedure, whereas Phillips et al (2000) report that as a form of assessment it is seriously flawed, having neither inter- or intra-assessor reliability.

The next three methods of assessment to be considered will focus on the use of written evidence of competence. These methods are:

- care records made by the learner
- case study presentation by the learner
- project or assignment compiled by the learner.

Care records made by the learner

We will start by considering a scenario: try Activity 4.12.

The learner has to demonstrate the ability to obtain the history in the first instance, and subsequently to record the history, assessment and plan of care in writing. The most appropriate way to assess this is to observe the student taking the history and then examine the written records made by the learner. The activity of interviewing a client to obtain a history followed by the formulation and documentation of a care plan is one way of integrating assessment so that several competencies can be assessed concurrently.

What can we learn about the learner?

The observation will tell us how the student attempted to establish rapport and develop a relationship with the patient, how and what type of communication

ACTIVITY 4.12

We wish to assess our learner's ability to record an accurate history, assess, plan and document the nursing/midwifery care needs of a client admitted to the unit. How can the learner be assessed?

skills were used, the accuracy of the questioning and so on The nursing/midwifery care plan and records made by the learner will tell us whether:

- all the relevant information has been obtained
- the student is able to analyse and synthesize the information in a meaningful way, resulting in an accurate assessment of care needs
- the student is able to plan care using the above information
- the student has achieved the standards of record keeping required; in the case of nurses and midwives these standards are laid down by the United Kingdom Central Council (UKCC 1998).

Subsequently, as the learner cares for the client and is able to maintain a continual review of care needs, this should be reflected in the changes made to the care plan. In this instance, we will be able to assess the learner's ability to:

- evaluate the effectiveness of care given
- solve any problems
- make decisions about client needs
- manage change.

Most of these are higher-level cognitive skills which the beginning student may not have acquired. It would therefore be inappropriate to assign such a task to a junior student. There are other areas of learning which can be assessed through a student obtaining a client history with the subsequent development of a care plan:

- knowledge of the history to be taken and effective communication skills in order to obtain an accurate and comprehensive history
- underpinning knowledge of the illness, an understanding of the information obtained, the ability to apply theory to practice and the ability to analyse the information in order to synthesize information meaningfully
- problem-solving and decision-making skills and the ability to apply theory to practice in order to evaluate and make changes to care as required
- effective written communication skills in order to maintain standards of record keeping
- the standards of the records may tell us about how important the student views record keeping.

Examination of care records, however, may not tell us about the student's attitudes towards the task. Rowntree (1987) gives the example of the ability of a medical student in eliciting information from the case histories compiled but the fact that he antagonized each and every one of the patients by his arrogant and insensitive manner was concealed.

Case study presentation by the learner

Case studies provide students with the opportunity to carry out an in-depth study of one particular patient in their care over a period of time. In the written format this method of assessing learning is more frequently used for the assessment of theory. However, the evidence of learning provided by a case study can be used as one source of evidence for the assessment of competence in the clinical setting. This evidence can be in the written format or be presented verbally by the student. Some elements guiding the compilation of a case study are:

- an orientation to the patient
- the socioeconomic background of the patient and the influence of this on the development of the illness
- draw on and integrate theory from a range of subjects to explain the nature and cause of the disease condition
- the problems/difficulties encountered by the patient and the care required
- the rationale for the care, management and treatment
- contributions made by other members of the multidisciplinary team and their importance
- identify services available
- evaluate the effectiveness of care.

What aspects of competence can be assessed using a case study?

- knowledge base surrounding the case study
- an understanding of that knowledge
- application of theory to practice
- ability to assess, plan, implement appropriate care and evaluate care
- possible to assess attitudes.

Practical skills cannot be assessed. A difficulty when assessing the case study is that it may reflect idealized standards of care rather than actual care given (Lankshear and Nicklin 2000). This will then reduce the validity and reliability of that assessment.

Project or assignment compiled by the learner

It is possible to arrange for the learner to carry out a small-scale project or assignment. On completion of the work it is usual to provide a written record for examination. Rowntree (1987) suggests that if students are allowed to set their own objectives and how to achieve them, we can assess not only the product but, more importantly, the process of learning. Like the case study, a project or assignment is more frequently used for the assessment of theory. The evidence of learning, however, can be used as one source of evidence for the assessment of competence in the clinical setting to give us a more holistic measurement of competence. Through examination of a project or assignment, it is possible to assess the following (Quinn 2000, Rowntree 1987):

- knowledge and understanding of the subject under investigation
- application of theory to practice
- creativity
- independence and resourcefulness
- how the situation was managed, e.g. coming up with solutions to problems will be indicative of problem-solving and decision-making skills.

The above qualities and attributes are some of the hallmarks of a competent practitioner and are therefore important for the student to develop. Practical skills and attitudes cannot be assessed with accuracy.

SELECTING AND COMBINING METHODS OF ASSESSMENT

Gonczi et al (1993) say that in competency-based assessment we should always try to select the methods that are most direct and relevant to the nature of the competency being assessed. Some methods of assessment are simply inappropriate to the assessment of certain aspects of competence. For example, interpersonal communication skills cannot be assessed using written assessment methods; manual dexterity and psychomotor skills cannot be assessed through verbal assessment methods. Attitudes, the most difficult aspect of competence of all to assess, may elude assessment altogether if special care is not exercised. The careful selection of method is thus required so that the assessment method matches the type of attribute being assessed. An examination of the uses, advantages and limitations of the assessment methods discussed in this chapter will help you consider which combination of methods will be most suitable to assess the attributes of competence.

When selecting methods for use in the holistic/integrated competency-based assessment system, Gonczi et al (1993:20) provide two guiding principles:

1. The assessment should be as integrated and holistic as possible, i.e. combinations of attributes should be assessed simultaneously. For example, when a student is observed when admitting a patient, attributes such as knowledge of the admission procedure, communication and interpersonal skills, record keeping skills and so on can be assessed simultaneously.

2. The assessment should be as direct as possible, i.e. as close as possible to the real-work situations in which these combinations of attributes are employed.

The key question arising is this: How well will the methods assess the capacity to function appropriately across the uncertain situations of professional practice? Inevitably, not all the professional attributes needed to function thus can be assessed holistically and directly. Therefore, combinations of methods need to be considered which will provide the range of evidence on which a judgement of competence can be made. The principles underpinning the use of the strategy of triangulation should also be taken into account when selecting and combining methods.

Other factors to be considered when selecting methods are:

- The time available to assessors – busy practitioners are generally hard-pushed for time to be mentors and assessors to learners who end up competing for the practitioner's time (Phillips et al 2000, Bedford et al 1993)

- The confidential nature of some aspects of work limits the capacity to undertake assessment in the real situation, e.g. when learning counselling skills in the mental health setting, it may not be desirable to learn the skills and be assessed when working directly with these clients. Simulated activities may be required.

- The methods are not biased against particular groups of learners. Rowntree (1987:60) made the point that 'to treat people equally is not necessarily to treat them fairly. Indeed, people being so different, equal treatment probably means injustice for most'.

- The methods should be acceptable to the learners, e.g. not all learners feel comfortable taking part in enacting simulated clinical situations.

The following combinations of methods are suggested for assessing the components of competence, as discussed in Chapter 3.

1. To assess the components of competence in the cognitive domain use:
   - questioning
   - assessment discussion
   - analysis of simulated clinical problems
   - computer-based simulation
   - OSCE
   - care records
   - testimony of others
   - project or assignment
   - case study.

2. To assess technical skills and performance use:
   - direct observation of practice
   - examination of work products
   - testimony of others
   - simulation of clinical situations
   - OSCE.

3. To assess reflective practice use:
   - questioning
   - assessment discussion
   - testimony of others
   - care records
   - case study
   - project or assignment.

4. To assess attitudes and ethics of care use:
   - questioning
   - assessment discussion
   - observation
   - testimony of others
   - simulation of clinical situations.

It is difficult to assess and measure attitudes, beliefs and values directly. Assessment of the affective domain of learning abounds with difficulties (Dawson 1992, Andrusyszyn 1989), and frequently poses a 'gap' in assessment strategies (Fraser 2000). We can, however, observe behaviours and behavioural patterns which may be reflective of the underlying attitudes and values held by the student (Andrusyszyn 1989). Recent research by Fraser et al (1997) and Hart et al (2001) identify some key attributes that professional midwives should possess. Using the empirical evidence provided by the above research and the behaviours identified by midwives as 'essential' behaviours that a student midwife should demonstrate, a tool termed the 'Professional Behaviours Inventory' has been developed by one higher education institution to assess pre-specified behaviours expected of a professional exhibiting the accepted conduct of a midwife. These professional behaviours consist of highly specified descriptors against which the student will be assessed. These descriptors are observable and can be readily used by the assessor and other members of the team working with the student. Each descriptor is graded along a continuum, as shown by the numbers along the first row – the continuum follows the banding consistent with the university's marking grid. Appendix 12 contains one 'professional behaviour' with its descriptors.

CONCLUSION

In a system of competency-based assessment, any of the assessment methods described in this chapter can be used. From the discussion on the uses and limitations of the range of assessment methods, it can be seen that no one method will enable us to assess all the components of competence. It is of course not desirable or economical to use all the assessment methods. It is, however, important to select and combine methods so that their strengths and weaknesses complement each other and methods are relevant to the nature of the competency being assessed. In choosing the methods to be used there will always be a need to balance competing demands and the necessity to obtain the range of evidence required to make a judgement of competence.

In general, a move in the direction of competency-based assessment requires the greater use of more direct methods of assessment that more closely match the kinds of day-to-day tasks that professionals undertake. This emphasizes the importance of the use of methods that directly assess performance and the other attributes of competence and requires clinical assessors to make professional judgements in interpreting what the minimum acceptable levels of competence are in respect to professional standards. Assessment methods which are 'subjectively scored', such as observation and simulation of practice, need to be managed to ensure reasonable reliability to accompany greater validity. A high level of professional expertise is required to assess the work of others (Phillips et al 2000, Gerrish et al 1997, Bedford et al 1993). Being an expert in a profession is essential but is not enough. It is important to have some level of expertise in the assessment process. The next chapter addresses issues relating to the management of the assessment process, in particular the competency-based assessment system, so that assessments can be made with validity and reliability.

REFERENCES

Andrusyszyn MA (1989) Clinical evaluation of the affective domain. *Nurse Education Today*, 9, 75–81.

Bedford H, Phillips T, Robinson J and Schostak J (1993) *Assessment of Competencies in Nursing and Midwifery Education and Training*. London: The English National Board for Nursing, Midwifery and Health Visiting.

Benner P (1984) *From Novice to Expert: Excellence and Power in Clinical Practice*. Menlo Park, CA: Addison-Wesley.

Bloom BS, Engelhart MD, Furst EJ et al (1956) *Taxonomy of Educational Objectives, Handbook I: Cognitive Domain*. London: Longman.

Boud D, Keogh R and Walker D (1985) What is reflection in learning? In Boud D, Keogh R and Walker D (eds) *Reflection: Turning Experience into Learning*, pp 7–17. London: Kogan Page.

Brown S, Race P and Smith B (1996) *500 Tips on Assessment*. London: Kogan Page.

Burke RJ (1969) Some preliminary data on the use of self-evaluation and peer-ratings in assigning university course grades. *Journal of Educational Research*, **62**(10), 444–448.

Campbell DT and Fiske DW (1959) Convergent and discriminant validity by the multi-trait, multi-method matrix. *Psychological Bulletin*, **56**, 81–105.

City and Guilds (1992) *3033: Care – NVQ Level 2*. London: City and Guilds of London Institute.

Corcoran-Perry S and Narayan S (2000) Teaching clinical reasoning in nursing education. In Higgs J and Jones M (eds) *Clinical Reasoning in the Health Professions*, pp 249–254. Oxford: Butterworth-Heinemann.

Craig JL and Page G (1981) The questioning skills of nursing instructors. *Journal of Nursing Eduction*, **20**, 20.

Dawson KP (1992) Attitude and assessment in nurse education. *Journal of Advanced Nursing*, **17**, 473–479.

Denzin N (1989) *The Research Act,* 3rd edn. New York: McGraw Hill.

DeTornyay R and Thompson MA (1987) *Strategies for Teaching Nursing*, 3rd edn. New York: John Wiley and Sons.

De Young S (1990) *Teaching Nursing*. Menlo Park, CA: Addison-Wesley.

Elliott J (1991) *Action Research for Educational Change*. Milton Keynes: Open University Press.

English National Board (1997) *Standards for Approval of Higher Education Institutions and Programmes*. London: English National Board for Nursing, Midwifery and Health Visiting.

Ewan C and White R (1996) *Teaching Nursing: A Self-instructional Handbook*, 2nd edn. London: Chapman and Hall.

Fahy K and Lumby T (1988) Clinical assessment in a college program. *Australian Journal of Advanced Nursing*, **5**(4), 5–9.

Fielding NG and Fielding JL (1986) *Linking Data*. Beverly Hills, CA: Sage.

Fish D and Twinn S (1997) *Quality Clinical Supervision in the Health Care Professions*. Oxford: Butterworth-Heinemann.

Fletcher S (1991) *NVQs Standards and Competence. A Practical Guide for Employers, Managers and Trainers*. London: Kogan Page.

Forker JE and McDonald ME (1996) Methodologic trends in the healthcare professions: computer adaptive and computer simulation testing. *Nurse Educator*, **21**(4), 13–14.

Fraser D (2000) Action research to improve the pre-registration midwifery curriculum. Part 3: can fitness for practice be guaranteed? *Midwifery*, **16**, 287–294.

Fraser D, Murphy R and Worth-Butler M (1997) *An Outcome Evaluation of the Effectiveness of Pre-registration Midwifery Programmes of Education*. London: The English National Board for Nursing, Midwifery and Health Visiting.

Gerrish K, McManus M and Ashworth P (1997) *Levels of Achievement: A Review of the Assessment of Practice*. London: The English National Board for Nursing, Midwifery and Health Visiting.

Gibbs G (1988) *Learning by Doing: A Guide to Teaching Learning Methods*. London: Further Education Unit.

Gipps CV (1994) *Beyond Testing: Towards a Theory of Educational Assessment*. London: The Falmer Press.

Gomez DA, Lobodzinski S and Hartwell West CD (1998) Evaluating clinical performance. In Billings DM and Halstead JA (eds) *Teaching in Nursing: A Guide for Faculty*, pp 407–422. Philadelphia: WB Saunders.

Gonczi A, Hager P and Athanasou J (1993) *The Development of Competency-Based Assessment Strategies for the Professions*. National Office of Overseas Skills Recognition, Research Paper No. 8. Canberra: Australian Government Publishing Service.

Govaerts MJB, Schuwirth LWT, Pin A et al (2001) Objective assessment is needed to ensure competence. *British Journal of Midwifery*, **9**(3), 156–161.

Hager P and Gonczi A (1996) Professions and competencies. In Edwards R, Hanson A and Raggatt P (eds) *Boundaries of Adult Learning*, pp 246–260. London: Routledge.

Harlen W (ed) (1994) *Enhancing Quality in Assessment*. BERA Policy Task Group on Assessment. London: Paul Chapman Publishers.

Hart A, Lockley R, Henwood F et al (2001) *Evaluation of the Effectiveness of Midwifery Education in Preparing Midwives to Meet the Needs of Women from Disadvantaged Groups*. London: The English National Board for Nursing, Midwifery and Health Visiting.

Hoban JD and Casbergue JP (1978) Simulation: a technique for instruction and evaluation. In Ford CW (ed) *Clinical Education for the Allied Health Professions*, pp 145–157. St Louis: Mosby.

Jarvis P and Gibson S (1997) *The Teacher Practitioner and Mentor in Nursing, Midwifery and Health Visiting,* 2nd edn. Cheltenham: Stanley Thornes (Publishers).

Ladyshewsky R (1999) Simulated patients and assessment. *Medical Teacher,* **21**(3), 266–269.

Lankshear A and Nicklin P (2000) Methods of assessment. In Nicklin P, Kenworthy N (eds) *Teaching and Assessing in Nursing Practice,* 3rd edn, pp 119–138. London: Baillière Tindall.

Minton D (1997) *Teaching Skills in Further and Adult Education*, rev. edn. Basingstoke: Macmillan.

Neary M (2001) Responsive assessment: assessing student nurses' clinical competence. *Nurse Education Today,* **21**, 3–17.

Oliver R and Endersby C (1994) *Teaching and Assessing Nurses: A Handbook for Preceptors.* London: Baillière Tindall.

Perrott E (1982) *Effective Teaching.* London: Longman.

Phillips T, Schostak J and Tyler J (2000) *Practice and Assessment in Nursing and Midwifery: Doing it for Real.* London: The English National Board for Nursing, Midwifery and Health Visiting.

Polit DF and Hungler BP (1989) *Essentials of Nursing Research*, 2nd edn. Philadelphia: JB Lippincott.

Quinn FM (2000) *The Principles and Practice of Nurse Education*, 4th edn. London: Chapman and Hall.

Redfern SJ (1994) Validity through triangulation. *Nurse Researcher,* **2**(2), 41–56.

Rethans JJ, Sturmans F, Drop R, van der Vleuten C and Hubbs P (1991) Does competence of general practitioners predict their performance? Comparisons between examination settings and actual practice. *British Medical Journal,* **303**, 1377–1380.

Rogers C (1983) *Freedom to Learn for the 80's.* Columbus, Ohio: Charles E. Merrill.

Rowntree D (1987) *Assessing Students: How Shall We Know Them?* 2nd edn. London: Kogan Page.

Schon D (1987) *Educating the Reflective Practitioner.* San Francisco: Jossey-Bass.

Stengelhofen J (1993) *Teaching Students in Clinical Settings.* London: Chapman and Hall.

Stoker D (1994) Assessment in learning: (iii) methods of assessment. *Nursing Times,* **90**(13), Section 7 (iii), i–viii.

Stuart CC (1997) Reflective journals as a teaching/learning strategy. *British Journal of Midwifery,* **5**(7), 434–438.

Swanwick M (1994) Observation as a research method. *Nurse Researcher,* **2**(2) 5–12.

United Kingdom Central Council (1998) *Guidelines for Records and Record Keeping.* London: United Kingdom Central Council for Nursing, Midwifery and Health Visiting.

Westwood-Timms J (1995) Critical incident scenarios. *MIDIRS Midwifery Digest,* **5**(3), 268–270.

While AE (1994) Competence versus performance: which is more important? *Journal of Advanced Nursing,* **20**, 525–531.

5 Conducting fair assessments

INTRODUCTION

Learners' lived experience in authentic practice contexts and their competence in dealing with the dilemmas they face should form the basis of assessment (Phillips et al 2000). Competency-based assessment in the professions therefore needs to be based on realistic, complex workplace problems to generate the range of evidence of competence required to make valid and reliable assessments (Masters and McCurry 1990). This can be done by the careful selection and combination of methods of assessment which will best assess the particular component of competence, e.g. using observation to assess psychomotor skills and questioning to assess cognitive skills.

It is not possible or desirable to assess everything a person might need to know or be able to do. Assessment of clinical practice is inevitably based on a sample of the student's performance on assessment tasks perceived to be relevant. An inference of competence is then made from the student's performance on the set of arranged tasks. Competence is a construct that is not directly observable: rather, it is inferred from performance. Most typical assessments involve making inferences, e.g. tests of knowledge usually sample only a fraction of the required knowledge. On the basis of that score, an inference is made as to whether or not a student knows enough to be assessed as satisfactory (Rowntree 1987). Grades and degree classifications are made on that basis: hence, assessment of clinical practice, in common with other types of assessment, involves inference – and inferences are subject to error (Gonczi et al 1993). This is perhaps one major weakness of most, if not all, of our assessment systems.

As I see it, two major expectations are made of clinical assessors. First, they are required to make professional judgements in interpreting what the minimum acceptable levels of competence are in respect to professional standards. These judgements are frequently made within the role relationship of that of a mentor cum assessor to a student – this role relationship may very well influence assessment judgements. The reader is directed to a discussion of the issues and dilemma of the mentor–assessor interface in Chapter 2. Secondly, assessment evidence obtained through the methods used requires to be 'subjectively scored'. Reliability, and perhaps even validity, may be compromised. Students may then be assessed unfairly; and what could be worse than passing a student who has not achieved the goal of professional nursing and midwifery education, and that is, to be 'fit for purpose' and 'fit for practice' (UKCC 1999).

We rely on assessments to make some quite specific but also far-ranging judgements about our students' future behaviour as registered practitioners. In deciding whether the assessments are sufficiently satisfactory to enable us to make such judgements soundly, we need to use quite clear criteria for deciding if the assessments are satisfactory. A question we need to ask is this: Do our assessments enable us to make such judgements soundly? Deciding whether or not an assessment lives up to this task is not straightforward.

There is now an examination of those factors we need to consider in order to make sound judgements in assessments. Measures to attain objective assessments and avoid subjective assessments are suggested.

THE KEY CONCEPTS OF CONDUCTING FAIR ASSESSMENTS

Justice is a basic part of the functioning of a civilized society: we believe in justice not only for the accuser and the accused in criminal trials but also for parties in any dispute. When we are involved with any situation when a decision about fair play has to be made, as a person with a sense of justice, we generally like to think that the decision we have made to carry out a certain action is just and fair, and the other person has had fair treatment. As an assessor you have to make assessment decisions continually and these decisions about student performance must be just and fair. How can you ensure that this is so? Furthermore, assessment for certification, as in nursing and midwifery education, should offer sufficient reliability and validity for public scrutiny. Assessments at national levels, which is the case with pre-registration nursing and midwifery education, must offer comparability (Gipps 1994). In its document *Making a Difference*, the Department of Health (1999) stated that the health service of the country needs to know that nurses and midwives are trained to broadly the same standards and have the same skills. How can we achieve these 'orders' through our assessment activities? Or are these orders too tall?

What does the word 'fair' mean to you? According to the *Collins Pocket Dictionary and Thesaurus* (1993), to be fair is to act 'according to rules'. The next question then may be: *What are the rules of fair assessment?* Stoker and Hull (1994) state that four attributes need to be fulfilled to make assessment fair to all parties – these attributes may thus form the rules of fair assessment. Quinn (2000) refers to these as the four cardinal criteria of every effective test. The four cardinal criteria or attributes are:

- validity
- reliability
- feasibility
- discriminating power.

Validity

Gonczi et al (1993) maintain that the most important issue in competency-based assessment is that of validity. The traditional definition of validity is the extent to which a test measures what it was designed to measure. If it does not measure what it purports to measure, then its use is misleading (Gipps 1994). There are two key issues here which are important to the assessment of clinical practice: *how* we measure and *what* we measure. The use of the strategy of triangulation will help ensure that a more complete picture of the student's competence is obtained, thereby enhancing validity. The reader is referred to Chapter 4 for a discussion of the use of appropriate methods of assessment and the strategy of triangulation to achieve validity of assessment. Valid assessment in clinical practice depends on methods of assessment used which are appropriate to the attribute of the competence being assessed, e.g. valid assessments of psychomotor skills are unlikely to be provided by the use of questioning. In nursing and midwifery education, what we purport to measure must be that of 'the ability to actually care for patients' (Gerrish et al 1997:70). Assessment for accountability purposes, as in the nursing and midwifery professions, should aim for high validity, as nurses and midwives must be fit for the purpose of caring for patients and clients. We therefore have to be clear about *what* we want to measure. Rowntree (1987) tells us to 'articulate as clearly as possible the criteria by which we assess, the aims and objectives we espouse, what qualities we look for in students'.

When assessing in clinical practice we infer validity. It is difficult to measure validity (Gonczi et al. 1993). The way to infer validity is to collect evidence of the different types of validity which matter to us in clinical practice. The types of validity to be discussed here are:

- face validity
- content validity
- predictive validity
- construct validity
- concurrent validity.

Face validity

This is the extent to which an assessment appears to be testing what we want students to be able to do. Gerrish et al (1997) point out that many pre-registration nursing programmes require students to produce written evidence of the achievement in practice but that this did not necessarily indicate their ability to actually care for patients: i.e. this form of testing for clinical competence lacks face validity. Another example of a test lacking in face validity comes from Wolf (1995), who gives the example of the use of multiple-choice tests of the type often used to license professionals in the United States. For example, in the case of a physician after qualification, the multiple-choice questions that have to be taken do not test the physician's competence to practise (McGaghie 1991 in Wolf 1995). Masters and McCurry (1990) believe that face validity is likely to be enhanced by making set tasks resemble those encountered in day-to-day practice in a profession.

Content validity

This concerns the coverage of appropriate and necessary content (Gipps 1994). The following questions can be asked in association with this concept:

- Has the assessment sampled adequately the content of the course? In the case of pre-registration nursing and midwifery students, has the assessment sampled adequately the UKCC competencies?
- Has the assessment covered the skills necessary for good performance?
- Is the item being assessed within the content of the course?
- Does the item being assessed require to be assessed at this stage of the student's training?

It is of course necessary to have knowledge of the content and structure of the course of students being assessed in order to achieve content validity.

Predictive validity

This relates to whether the assessment predicts accurately or well some future performance (Gipps 1994). Rowntree (1987:189) gives us this warning about predictive validity:

> Predicting how a person will turn out in the future, on the basis of what we know about him now, is hazardous. Even if he retains the ability, he may no longer have the disposition.

In the health care profession, it is important to try to predict our students' competence in the future so that, as a minimum, at the point of qualification, they are competent to practise. Whether they remain competent in the future is of course beyond our control. What can be done in attempts to achieve predictive validity? The use of continuous assessment may help here. The constant and regular supervision, guidance and feedback we give our students will reinforce learning and hence their development and achievements. Ensuring that students have a range of clinical experiences, with repetitions if necessary, will help them acquire the skills to practise with confidence and perhaps predictability. Stoker (1994:v) says that:

> If a learner can do it once, it's an event; twice may be a coincidence; three times may show that a consistent pattern is emerging.

If there is consistency of performance, there is a higher chance of predictive validity in our assessment as 'the best indicator of future performance is past performance' (Wolf 1995:44). Correspondingly, the best predictor measure will be to incorporate and assess those future behaviours which are of interest.

Construct validity

Constructs are the qualities, abilities and traits we look for to explain aspects of human behaviour that cannot be observed directly (Rowntree 1987). Honesty, maturity, kindness and intelligence are some examples of constructs. Construct validity is the extent to which our assessment reveals the construct we are measuring. We are required to make value judgements about certain aspects of the student's behaviour or personality. Rowntree (1987:84) asks whether we are deluding ourselves when we make those judgements. 'Is what we see (or not see) in students a figment of our imagination – a fabrication of the mind of the beholder to some extent?' To what extent do our personal constructs influence construct validity? Abstract concepts such as attitudes and values are notoriously difficult to measure (Nolan and Behi 1995, Ashworth and Morrison 1991). Again, the use of continuous assessment may be helpful here. Working with and assessing the student over a period of time, in conjunction with other assessors, and utilizing a range of caregiving situations, will give us more opportunities to assess the student's attitudes and values, thus making our assessment in this area of learning more accurate. It will also allow students more opportunities to demonstrate the attitudes and values they hold. For example, imagine you are trying to assess a student's attitudes to the elderly and you work with her on one occasion with one elderly person. Your student appears to have difficulty demonstrating sensitivity to the needs of the patient, even though questioning reveals that she is theoretically well aware of those needs. Do you then assume that her attitudes towards the elderly are not good? No, of course not. Your student's performance on that occasion might be due to a number of factors: e.g. she may find it particularly difficult to relate to that individual patient or she may simply be very tired or have some other pressing problems.

Concurrent validity

This is concerned with whether an assessment in an aspect of performance correlates with, or gives substantially the same results as another assessment in a related area of performance (Gipps 1994, Davis 1986). In other words, does the assessment predict performance in related areas? How far can we generalize from the ability to perform one task to an ability to perform other tasks in the same domain? For example, if you are working with a student who is able to assess and give the immediate nursing care to asthmatic patients in relation to their dyspnoea – that of nursing them at rest in a comfortably supported and upright position – can you conclude from the student's care of these patients that the student is able to assess and give the necessary immediate nursing care to patients with dyspnoea from other causes? I would suggest that you could, because the principle of care is the same for all patients with dyspnoea. Your assessment has concurrent validity. Let us use another example: there is assessment evidence to say that the student is able to give intramuscular injections safely into the gluteus muscle. Can you assume that the student is able to give intramuscular injections safely into other sites of the body? I would suggest that you could not make this assumption because even though the principles of giving an intramuscular injection remain the same, there are different dangers associated with the use of these alternative sites.

To achieve concurrent validity the assessor needs to be aware of the range of context of practice (see Chapter 6) to achieve competence in an area of care so that the student has the necessary experiences. Specifying the range in the assessment plan is therefore necessary to achieve concurrent validity. In other words, we should increase the number of tasks and ensure comprehensive coverage of the domain to improve generalizability (Linn 1993).

The final point to make about validity in relationship to the assessment of competence comes from Gonczi et al (1993), who state that a general principle underlying validity in competency-based assessment is that the narrower the base of evidence for the inference of competence, the less generalizable it will be to the performance of other tasks. Generalizability is a particular problem for performance assessment, as direct assessments of complex performance do not generalize well from one task to another (Gipps 1994). This is because performance is heavily task-dependent.

Reliability

Reliability is concerned with the accuracy with which the test measures the performance or attainment it is designed to measure (Gipps 1994). A test or assessment is said to be reliable if it gives similar results when used on separate occasions and with different assessors. There are two underlying reliability questions: Would an assessment produce the same or similar results on more than one occasion? Or if done by other assessors? There are three key issues here:

- consistency of student performance
- consistency of interpretation
- consistency, and therefore agreement of interpretation, between assessors.

The core of any assessment is the judgement of the assessor – any form of assessment involves activity and judgement on the part of the assessor (Wolf 1995). For judgement to be valid and reliable, all assessors are presumed to be able to 'feel, understand and judge in much the same way when confronted with the work of a particular student. It is [also] presumed that they would notice and value the same skills and qualities and would broadly agree in their assessments' (Rowntree 1987:191). There is abundant evidence which attests to the falsity of these assumptions (see, for example, Gipps 1994 and Rowntree 1987). The unreliability of assessment first became an issue when it was noticed that the mark awarded for a student essay depended on who marked it. The following excerpt is rather amusing and illustrates the unreliability of assessment. Ben Wood (1921, cited in Rowntree, 1987) tells how one of the six college professors grading a set of history papers wrote out, for his own satisfaction, what he considered to be a model paper for the set of questions. By some mischance this paper got amongst those being marked. It was unsuspectingly graded and deemed unworthy of a pass mark! According to standard precautions, this paper was duly marked by the other professors to double-check its grade and was given marks ranging from 40 to 90.

Factors which can affect the reliability of assessment in the clinical setting can be grouped under the three headings of *student factors*, *environmental factors* and *assessor factors* (Stoker and Hull 1994). Each set of factors is now considered in turn.

Student factors

As stated above, to achieve reliability, student performance has to be consistent. Can students perform with consistency all the time? Obviously not. There are many human factors which militate against being the 'perfect all-singing all-dancing' student. Those physical and emotional factors which may affect performance could be poor health; fatigue; lack of interest in the placement and therefore motivation to learn; anxiety and lack of confidence about giving

ACTIVITY 5.1

Make a list of those student factors that you have encountered, either personally or from a colleague's experience, that have affected assessments either positively or negatively.

patient care; and personal problems affecting concentration at work. Physical disabilities such as mobility problems and any speech impediments may affect learning. The presence of other students in the clinical area may be supportive and positive for each other, thereby enhancing learning, or it may be detract from learning if students are negative.

That group of factors that students have no control over such as their gender and racial background may also affect the way they are assessed. In mainstream education it has been shown that when markers can infer gender or racial group from the pupil's name, stereotypes come into play which affect marks awarded. For example, both male and female markers rated the same paper more highly when it was attributed to John T McKay than to Joan T McKay (Gipps 1994). Even when names are not attached to scripts, surface effects such as neatness can affect marking. Now, try Activity 5.1.

A group of clinical assessors came up with the following list of factors which they thought might have affected the way they view the students and potentially their assessment of the students:

- Physical appearance, such as dress code, body piercing, tattoos and dyed hair
- Age of the student in relationship to themselves – the younger mentor/assessor may feel threatened by the older student and the mature mentor/assessor wishing to 'mother' a younger student
- Social class of the student – more may be expected of the student from a higher socioeconomic background as these students are 'associated with higher intelligence'. Conversely, less may be expected from the student from a lower socioeconomic background
- Accent of the student – students speaking with the 'Queen's English' accent are accorded a higher intelligence and assessed accordingly.

Environmental factors

There are particular problems which are the direct consequences of assessing in the clinical setting. These problems will contribute to assessments being unreliable if they are not recognized and managed:

- There is an inherently high variability in the context of clinical assessment: we cannot standardize patients/clients or situations and therefore cannot produce identical situations in which students can be assessed. The conditions for learning and practice can be highly inconsistent, which will directly impact on the consistency of performance of the student and the assessment.
- The work environment is often very busy. Phillips et al (2000) found that there are a large number of clinical environments where the level of staffing is such that all available time is given to coping with the demands of patient

care. Assessors are simply too busy as carers. There is, therefore, insufficient time for reliable evidence collection. In the United Kingdom, the government is taking measures to improve levels of staffing (Department of Health 1999) so that students can be better supported by clinical assessors during placements.

■ There are many distractions which may interfere with the student's and the assessor's concentration. A preoccupation with something which has happened, concern with jobs still to be done and the busyness and noise on a ward are examples of distractions which will affect learning and assessment activities.

■ The learning climate of the working environment should also be considered. The support and encouragement given to learners contribute to their confidence, which will enable them to participate more effectively in the learning and assessment process (Neary 2000).

As can be seen, there are many environmental factors which may contribute to the unreliability of assessments. Phillips et al (2000) recommend that time should be prioritized for assessment-only activity, so that there is more time for reliable evidence collection. The length of time spent on each clinical placement should also be sufficiently long to enable continuity of assessor/student contact. Longer placements will also provide more opportunities for the student to engage in a range of care situations, thereby giving the student more opportunities to achieve consistent performance.

Assessor factors

As with factors attributed to the student and the environment, there are many factors attributed to the assessor which can detract from the reliability of assessment. The research evidence that we have on assessors' behaviour emphasizes the very active role that their own concepts and interpretations play when making judgements and final assessment decisions (Wolf 1995). These concepts and interpretations are likely to be influenced by the assessors' own competence and standards of practice. Wolf explains that assessors do not simply 'match' students' performance to assessment criteria in a mechanistic fashion. On the contrary, they draw on an internalized, holistic set of concepts about how and how far they can take account of the context of the situation, what students should 'get out' of an assessment and how much allowance they can make by offsetting lapses and weaknesses with strengths from other areas of performance and so on. Making allowances is particularly apparent when assessing students performing difficult and complex tasks. In short, assessors make what Wolf describes as judgemental aggregation which is to 'compensate, make allowances, interpret, explain away' (Wolf 1995:71). The more experienced the assessor, the more they will have internalized a model of competence which in turn affects the degrees of judgemental aggregation. People are often unaware of the degree to which they are operating in this way. Conversely, the inexperienced practitioner/assessor does not make as much compensation or as many allowances – there is a tendency to expect every performance criterion to be achieved.

One claim made with competency-based assessment is that because the assessment criteria are so clearly defined in such detail, assessors are required to

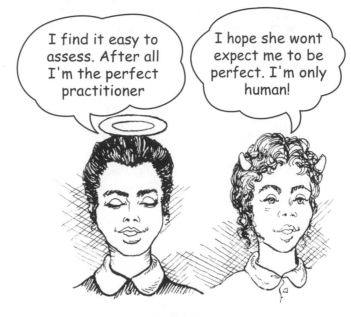

Reliability

make far less in the way of complex judgements. Fletcher (1991:66) stated that 'individual performance . . . is judged against explicit standards . . . and individuals know exactly what they are aiming to achieve'. There is evidence to say that this is far from the truth (Wolf 1995). The inherent variability of the contexts and complexity of clinical practice in which competence is displayed and assessed means that assessors have to make complex judgements and constant major decisions. They must also determine how to take account of the conditions of practice when judging whether a piece of evidence fits a defined criterion. It is not clear that judgements, in particular complex judgements, are derived from specified assessment criteria. Wolf (1995:69) states:

> The key judgements have far more to do with whether someone has actually performed up the *assessor's* standards than with the individual performance criteria at all. And whether or not one assessor applies standards which are the same as another's will also, in a case like this, have rather little to do with the focus on competence and outcomes.

An example of the above situation comes from a study by Hayter (1973) where 31 nurse educators viewed a film of students in three clinical situations. The educators were instructed to assess only the students' ability to care for a patient in shock. They were required to assign and justify the letter grade awarded (A for best performance to F for worst performance). Only 27 of the 155 reasons for the grades related to the care of the patient in shock. Some reasons for below-average grades were: 'seemed very cold and distant', 'did not seem sure of herself' and 'she was clumsy when taking the pulse'. The grades awarded in one clinical situation were: A – 1 student; B – 10 students; C – 16 students; D – 3 students; and F – 1 student. These grades were also typical of the grades awarded in the other two situations.

Up to now the discussion has been on how the assessor's judgement is influenced by personal concepts and expectations which are likely to be based on the person's standards and model of competence. Another set of factors which can influence the assessor's judgement and detract from reliability of assessment even more is our personal biases. We all carry prejudices of some kind, many of which we are not even aware of. If we are biased either in favour of or against the student – based on prior knowledge of the student's work or prejudices or stereotypes we might hold about the student – our assessment of the student is likely to be influenced. If this prior knowledge of the student or some personal aspect about the student which we like influences us to make a more favourable assessment, it is known as the *halo* effect. If the student's performance is underrated because our knowledge of that student's poor past performance has influenced that judgement, it is known as the *horn* effect (Philp 1983). I once knew a student who shaved his head bald, chewed gum frequently, had nose and ear rings and several visible tattoos. Coincidentally, he failed the placement but that is another story! I'm sure you have other similar stories.

Assessors should also consider the influence which their presence may have over students. A student who is being observed may become nervous. Conversely, the student may become much more attentive to the task and attend to detail more than she normally would. If the latter situation is the result of a positive and constructive relationship between the assessor and the student, it is known as the *Hawthorne effect* – 'the tendency for persons to perform as expected because of special attention' (Sullivan and Decker 1988). This inconsistent performance on the part of the student may affect reliability of assessment if the assessor overlooks the student's usual lower standards when the student is working with others.

The point is not that assessors cannot assess to an acceptably common standard: they can, but the process is complex and judgemental. Furthermore, each set of factors influencing reliability – student, environmental, assessor – does not operate on its own to affect reliability; rather, they all have an impact on each other. The conclusion to be drawn from this is that the reliability of assessment is threatened even more. An awareness of those factors which may influence the reliability of assessment will help the assessor in overcoming difficulties contributing to unreliable assessments. Problems of reliability reinforce one recommended aspect of assessment practice that comes from Bedford et al (1993): summative assessment should consider a broad range of evidence of competence from several sources.

There is much call (see, for example, Phillips et al 2000, Gerrish et al 1997, Bedford et al 1993) for the training of assessors to include developing their competence in collecting evidence and analysing data. These authors also recommend that issues of validity and reliability with full regard to making

ACTIVITY 5.2

During your next spell of duty, identify an item you assess in others, e.g. feeding a patient or a similar simple item. Complete the following:

■ I assessed the following item: . . . .
■ the assessment of this item was/was not reliable because: . . . .

judgements and assessment decisions in a busy work environment should also be looked at.

Try Activity 5.2. This activity is to help you consider those factors in your work environment which may contribute to unreliable assessments.

Remember to ask the following questions about reliability:

- Would I interpret the student's performance in the same way if I saw it again?
- Would other assessors agree with my interpretations of the student's performance?
- How consistent is the student's performance?

Feasibility

If we are given a task to do but have not been given the time or resources to complete the task, we would say that it is unfair because it had not been feasible to complete the task, and perhaps even complain bitterly! Likewise, in assessment, it is a fair assessment if it is feasible in terms of:

- allowing sufficient time for the student to practise and demonstrate competence
- there are sufficient resources in terms of, for example, learning opportunities for students to learn and demonstrate that they have developed the abilities and skills
- assessors have had enough time and opportunities to work with and assess the student.

Try Activity 5.3.

Time constraint is likely to be one major restriction – the result of the student's perceived 'short' placement or your workload or differing shifts with your student. All these factors could result in students not having enough time to practise or you are not able to spend enough time with the student to perform a fair assessment.

Generally, a student's length of placement in a clinical area cannot be altered, as these periods have already been determined in the curriculum. Prior planning of clinical experiences – e.g. by agreeing a learning contract with the student – will maximize the potential of clinical time. The use of alternative assessment methods and strategies other than observing the student in practice by yourself can make the assessment fairer. These strategies are discussed in Chapter 4.

Remember to ask the following questions about feasibility:

- Has the student been given enough time to practise?
- Has the student been given enough learning opportunities?

ACTIVITY 5.3

Make a list of any restrictions that you think your clinical environment may place on what is feasible in terms of assessment. Can anything be done to reduce/remove these restrictions?

- Has enough time been spent assessing the student, either by yourself or another assessor?

Discriminating power

An assessment that has discriminating power is one which:

- reflects the different levels of ability in those for whom it is used (Stoker and Hull 1994)
- decides clearly between those students who are of a certain standard and those who are not (Davis 1986).

Most of us do not possess the same level of ability nor do we learn at the same rate. During formative assessments, it is important to identify areas that require improvement. During summative assessments we need to be able to identify whether the student has attained the required level of competence and thus achieved the standard of training required at that stage of the course.

As far as the health care professions are concerned, we have a basic level of measure for many professional activities – that of *safety* (Davis 1986). For example, where asepsis is concerned we cannot have a standard which is 'fairly safe'! An aseptic technique is either safe or not safe. On the other hand, some professional activities do not come into this category – empathy is an example. Attempting to decide what is and what is not acceptable behaviour over a wide range of variables such as can be encountered with measuring the ability to show empathy is difficult.

Remember to ask the following questions about discriminating power:

- Has my assessment identified the correct level of ability of the student?
- Has my assessment identified the correct standard to be achieved?

CONCLUSION

Validity is traditionally considered to be more important than reliability: a highly reliable test is of little use if it is not valid. However, according to classical test theory a test cannot be valid if it does not have a basic level of reliability (Gipps 1994). Validity and reliability are in constant tension – what is needed is an appropriate balance between the two. Gipps goes on to say that generalizability bridges validity and reliability – inferences of competence are based on a sample of performance and we have to generalize from this sample in conferring fitness for purpose and fitness for practice. In order to generalize with any confidence, we need to ensure that what we want to assess is carefully defined to achieve validity and the assessment itself is reliable. To generalize without achieving validity and reliability would be unsafe.

The situation surrounding conducting and achieving fair assessments is complex. Gipps and Murphy (1994) say that the notion of a fair test is simplistic. The biggest challenge to fairness faced by assessors and students during clinical practice is the context: we cannot assume identical clinical experiences for all.

However, by paying attention to what we know about factors that affect the fairness of assessment we can begin to work towards assessments that are more fair to all students.

REFERENCES

Ashworth P and Morrison P (1991) Problems of competence-based education. *Nurse Education Today*, **11**, 256–260.

Bedford H, Phillips T, Robinson J and Schostak J (1993) *Assessment of Competencies in Nursing and Midwifery Education and Training*. London: The English National Board for Nursing, Midwifery and Health Visiting.

Collins Pocket Dictionary and Thesaurus (1993, reprinted 1995). Glasgow: Harper Collins.

Davis M (1986) *Managing Care (Pack 11): Assessing Nurses*. London: South Bank Polytechnic, Distance Learning Centre.

Department of Health (1999) *Making a Difference*. London: Department of Health.

Fletcher S (1991) *NVQs Standards and Competence. A Practical Guide for Employers, Managers and Trainers*. London: Kogan Page.

Gerrish K, McManus M and Ashworth P (1997) *Levels of Achievement: A Review of the Assessment of Practice*. London: The English National Board for Nursing, Midwifery and Health Visiting.

Gipps CV (1994) *Beyond Testing: Towards a Theory of Educational Assessment*. London: The Falmer Press.

Gipps C and Murphy P (1994) *Assessment, Achievement and Equity*. Buckingham: Open University Press.

Gonczi A, Hager P and Athanasou J (1993) *The Development of Competency-Based Assessment Strategies for the Professions*. National Office of Overseas Skills Recognition, Research Paper No. 8. Canberra: Australian Government Publishing Service.

Hayter J (1973) An approach to laboratory evaluation. *The Journal of Nursing Education*, **12**, 17–22.

Linn RL (1993) Educational assessment: expanded expectations and challenges. *Educational Evaluation and Policy Analysis*, **15**, 1.

McGaghie WC (1991) Professional competence evaluation. *Educational Researcher*, **20**(1), 3.

Masters GN and McCurry D (1990) *Competency-Based Assessment in the Professions*. National Office of Overseas Skills Recognition, Research Paper No. 2. Canberra: Australian Government Publishing Service.

Neary M (2000) *Teaching, Assessing and Evaluation for Clinical Competence*. Cheltenham: Stanley Thornes (Publishers).

Nolan M and Behi R (1995) Validity: a concept at the heart of research. *British Journal of Nursing*, **4**(9), 530–533.

Phillips T, Schostak J and Tyler J (2000) *Practice and Assessment in Nursing and Midwifery: Doing it for Real*. London: The English National Board for Nursing, Midwifery and Health Visiting.

Philp T (1983) *Making Performance Appraisal Work*. Maidenhead: McGraw-Hill.

Quinn F (2000) *Principles and Practice of Nurse Education*, 4th edn. Cheltenham: Stanley Thornes (Publishers).

Rowntree D (1987) *Assessing Students: How Shall We Know Them*, 2nd edn. London: Kogan Page.

Stoker D (1994) Assessment in learning: (i) Understanding assessment issues. *Nursing Times*, **90**(11), Section 7(i), i–viii.

Stoker D and Hull C (1994) Assessment in learning: (ii) Assessment and learning outcomes. *Nursing Times*, **90**(12), Section 7 (ii), i–viii.

Sullivan EJ and Decker PJ (1988) *Effective Management in Nursing*, 2nd edn. Menlo Park, California: Addison-Wesley.

UKCC (1999) *Fitness for Practice*. London: United Kingdom Central Council for Nursing, Midwifery and Health Visiting.

Wolf A (1995) *Competence-Based Assessment*. Buckingham: Open University Press.

Wood BD (1921) Measurement of college work. In *Educational Administration and Supervision*. Vol. VII.

6

Assessment as a learning process: using learning contracts

INTRODUCTION

It is discussed in Chapter 2 that assessors of professional practice have both professional responsibility and accountability to ensure that students they assess achieve safe and competent standards of clinical practice. These onerous tasks of assessing and conferring safety and competence are based on inferences made on a sample of the student's performance. Such inferences are subject to error (Gonczi et al 1993). Procedures need to be in place to make sure that the kind and amount of evidence gathered are sufficient to make a safe inference and the assessment is managed to ensure reasonable reliability to accompany greater validity. In other words, a carefully planned and managed assessment strategy is required so that through our assessment processes we achieve the goal of professional nursing and midwifery education which is to achieve fitness for purpose and practice. It would perhaps be a truism to say that students do not just achieve this 'fitness' – their learning requires to be facilitated as they work alongside us during clinical placements. This implies that assessment has another key function other than that of obtaining evidence of competence – that of having a constructive focus where the aim is to help rather than sentence the individual (Gipps 1994). An important message from Crooks (1988) is that assessment appears to be one of the most potent forces influencing education: it can have positive as well as negative effects. It is therefore necessary to plan and manage clinical assessment so that the positive impact on learning can be realized.

The continuous assessment process will be explored as the key assessment strategy to facilitate assessment as a learning process. Integral to the continuous assessment of clinical practice are the strategies of using the learning contract, with its concomitant assessment plan, formative assessment and summative assessment. These are examined with respect to the successful management of the continuous assessment of practice in order to realize the positive impact of assessment.

CONTINUOUS ASSESSMENT OF CLINICAL PRACTICE

This section starts with an activity (Activity 6.1). The assumption made here is that not all of our experiences of being assessed are positive ones!

You may have thought that the assessment was unfair because:

- you were not given sufficient opportunities to develop and prove yourself
- you were unaware of incorrect practices
- your assessor did not know you well enough to make the assessment decision
- you did not have enough time to practise.

Nicklin and Kenworthy (1995) believe that assessments give students opportunities to demonstrate the learning that has taken place. Assessments should thus have a constructive focus (Gipps 1994) whereby students are given the support, supervision and opportunities to demonstrate learning. Glaser (1990:480) emphasizes the importance of placing assessment in the service of learning, saying that assessments should:

> display to the learner models of performance that can be emulated and also indicate the assistance, experiences, and forms of practice required by learners as they move toward more competent performance.

In health care, practical assessments of a student's learning are context bound. Each patient or client we care for has different health care needs, which means that the student has to learn different aspects of care constantly. An 'accurate estimate' of total learning can only be made fairly over a period of time, after a student has had continuous supervision and sufficient learning opportunities to provide the range of clinical experiences required to develop competence. In the United Kingdom, the impetus for the use of continuous assessment of theory and practice in nursing and midwifery education can be directly attributed to the perceived injustices of the final 'one-off' assessment, where factors such as anxiety and ill health may adversely affect the competence demonstrated on the day of the assessment. The result may not be representative of the overall abilities demonstrated by the student. Within early guidelines for continuous

ACTIVITY 6.1

Recall an occasion as a learner when you felt you were assessed unfairly. What were the circumstances surrounding that assessment?

assessment, the English National Board for Nursing, Midwifery and Health Visiting (ENB 1986) stated that:

> Assessment should be a cumulative process, relating to learner *progress* as well as *achievement*, and be more closely integrated with learning (rather than separated from it) and with development of the individual student. (original emphases)

In later guidelines (ENB 1997) for continuous assessment the ENB stated:

> The assessment of learning of theory and practice is a continuous process culminating in a judgement of achievement. Formative processes guide student learning and summative assessment measures integration of subject disciplines and the application of theories in practice.

The position of the ENB in 1986 and 1997 on continuous assessment, then, calls for the use of formative and summative assessments, with the formative assessments feeding into, and informing, the summative assessment. The use of the continuous assessment of practice requires assessments to take place continually with periodic discussion, feedback, educational counselling and documentation throughout the student's placement. Good continuous assessment demands substantial time and effort. This allows students' performances to be monitored continuously during their day-to-day activities in clinical practice. Student efforts have to be steady and regular throughout (Rowntree 1987). Over the duration of the programme then, 'a series of progressively updated measurements of a student's achievement and progress' are formally maintained in the student's portfolio (ENB 1996). Such measurements are made against given learning outcomes. The reference by the ENB in 1986 that 'assessment should be a cumulative process' means that every effort made by the student is assessed, and these series of assessments obtained through the continuous assessment process contribute to the summative assessment (see below) – a final 'end-of-the placement' assessment is generally dispensed with (Rowntree 1987). The use of continuous assessment allows the quality and quantity of information about the student to be increased. The more we know about a student's abilities the more likely it is that our assessment will be accurate. Continuous assessment of clinical practice has the following advantages:

- Practitioners who are responsible for student learning can assess progress as it takes place.
- The context-bound nature of practical assessments is reduced as the learner is assessed over the varied circumstances of different patients/clients cared for.
- The learner receives continual and accurate feedback on performance and can identify areas where improvement is required. The assessor's personal knowledge of the learner and understanding of the context of the performance are significant advantages in providing valid feedback.
- Areas for development and improvement can be planned jointly by the assessor and the student.
- The student is likely to feel supported and encouraged, as any learning and achievement is seen as contributing to the summative assessment. Rowntree (1987) reports that students in higher education who have experienced

continuous assessment believe it to be less stressful than the 'all-or-nothing' final assessment. However, White et al (1994) found that student nurses in their study felt continuous assessment during clinical practice to be stressful, saying that they were under scrutiny at all times and consequently had to exhibit best behaviours always. And is that such an onerous requirement, remembering that the behaviours of health care professionals towards their patients and clients and colleagues should be of an acceptable standard at all times?

Most systems of continuous assessment allow for the concept of compensation (Nicklin and Kenworthy 1995, Rowntree 1987). This means that within a module or a year of study, a poor result in one assignment or examination may be balanced by a better result attained for a different piece of work. This, in theory, does not penalize students for one-off poor performance which may be attributed to unrelated contextual factors. In midwifery and nursing pre-registration education, the competencies to be achieved by the end of those programmes were statutorily defined by the United Kingdom Central Council for Nursing, Midwifery and Health Visiting (UKCC 2000a, 2000b). This means that all competencies must be achieved. Accordingly, regulations governing assessment published by the ENB (1996) state that compensation is only allowed in exceptional circumstances. The ENB does not state what those exceptional circumstances may be. In any case, the ENB states that compensation cannot be applied when the assessment/examination failed:

1. forms a substantial proportion of the total assessment process
2. is central to the fulfilment of the programme objectives
3. is testing an area of knowledge/competence, required to be tested under the Nurses, Midwives and Health Visitors Rules, and which has not and will not be sufficiently tested elsewhere in the programme.

Now, try Activity 6.2.

In your debate you may have considered the responsibilities and accountability of the professional practitioner in the clinical setting. You may also have considered the statutory competencies that must be achieved. The following question may have been raised: *If compensation is allowed, will the student still become safe and competent?* As I see it, in nursing and midwifery education, there is *no* room for compensation in the assessment of clinical practice in any circumstance. Of course, not everyone takes this position. Pre-registration nursing and midwifery education in the United Kingdom (UKCC 1999) and Australia (Sutton and Arbon 1994) now utilizes the competency-based assessment system. There is the contention that the use of the competency-based assessment system allows only two judgements of competence: competent or not yet competent (Wolf 1995:22). Wolf goes on to say:

ACTIVITY 6.2

Debate the following question:
In nursing and midwifery education would you allow compensation in the assessment of clinical practice in any circumstance?

. . . either the person has consistently demonstrated workplace performance which meets the specified standards or they are not yet able to do so – 'competent' or 'not yet competent'.

This has to be the position of the assessment of clinical practice in the professions, as the main purpose of assessment is for accountability purposes.

FORMATIVE ASSESSMENT

Formative assessment refers to assessment taking place during the learning activity and throughout the placement. It is conducted while the event to be assessed is occurring and focuses on identifying student learning and progress (Reilly and Oermann 1990). It focuses on parts of learning. Formative assessment is founded on the principle of maximizing learning – assessment information about the student's knowledge, understanding and skills are used to feed back into the teaching/learning process (Gipps 1994). The assessor determines whether to re-explain, arrange further practice or move to the next stage. The assertion is that formative assessment can, and will, aid learning (Torrance and Pryor 1998). For this to take place, it is crucial that formative assessment becomes a process whereby both 'feedback' and 'feedforward' occur. Within this, assessor–learner interaction becomes an important part of the process: it goes beyond the communication of assessment results, judgements of progress and provision of additional instructions. The assessor and learner collaborate actively to produce a best performance (Torrance and Pryor 1998). An important role for the assessor is to assist the learner in comprehending and engaging with new ideas and problems. The process of assessment itself is seen as having an impact on the learner as well as on the result of the assessment.

Student self-assessment in formative assessment

Involve the student in self-assessment. It is important to allow students to assess their own learning – their achievements and level of competency acquired on previous placements – so that learning can start from, and build on, what the student already knows and can already do. Some educationalists believe that assessment is only truly formative if it involves the student directly (Torrance and Pryor 1998, Sadler 1989). Self-assessment helps students feel that they own the learning and can thus control the way they meet their learning needs (Stoker 1994). It is linked with motivation, monitoring one's own learning and becoming an independent learner (Gipps 1994). Additionally, Chambers (1998) says that self-assessment is an efficient and effective learning tool in that students are required to identify their own strengths and weaknesses.

Students have an important role to play in planning their own learning and assessment. If they are to become competent assessors of their own work, they need sustained experience in ways of questioning and improving the quality of their work, and supported experience in assessing their work. They are often well placed to assess their own learning and to regulate their own work appropriately. They will thus be able to indicate the amount and nature of clinical experiences they have had and recognize what clinical experiences they need in order to achieve competence. Falchikov and Boud (1989:395) highlight the need for students to take more responsibility for their own learning: 'life-long learning requires that individuals be able not only to work independently, but also to assess their own performance and progress'. This ability will help students develop awareness of their own standards of practice. It is therefore important to handle student self-assessment well and in a positive, constructive way rather than in a negative norm-referenced way, as this can be demotivating (Gipps 1994). By listening to students the assessor will learn what students consider to be their own learning needs. What we know about how adults learn tells us that adults learn best when they can see the relevance of what they are learning (Jarvis and Gibson 1997, Knowles 1990). The assessor should therefore respond to the student's expressed learning needs. It may be necessary to probe more deeply so that the self-assessment helps students monitor their own learning to help them become independent learners (Gipps 1994). Finally, encourage students to consider what they want feedback on, as this will help them develop self-awareness of personal and professional development (Bailey 1998).

Opportunities and time should be created to engage in the essential process of formative assessment to provide learners with targeted and evidence-based feedback, so that action plans for further learning and development of competence can be made. In clinical practice, how does the formative assessment process discussed above fit into the teaching/learning and working cycles of the assessor and the learner? These issues will be taken up in subsequent sections.

FEEDBACK IN ASSESSMENT

Torrance and Pryor (1998) argue that it is important to identify not just what learners have achieved but also what they might achieve and what they are now ready to achieve. In his review, Crooks (1988) concluded that feedback assists learning unless the material is too difficult for the students, in which case feedback appears to become demoralizing. Sadler (1989) emphasizes the importance of both the content and the quality of the feedback. Sadler's views stemmed from the observation that even when teachers (in mainstream education) gave students valid and reliable judgements about their work, improvement did not necessarily follow. The mere provision of feedback is insufficient for optimal learning. What students need in order to make any improvement is to have knowledge of the desired standard or goal, to be able to compare their own performance with the desired performance and, subsequently, to take part in the appropriate activities to close the gaps: *they need to know in some detail what to do, and what they can do, in order to improve.*

Formative assessment processes, then, require feedback to be of the kind and detail which tells learners what to do in order to improve: detailed factual feedback is more effective, as students know explicitly and reliably what they are expected to do. The award of grades or simply confirming correct responses or performance has little effect on subsequent performance (Crooks 1988), as such feedback is very nonspecific. It does not tell the student what has been done to merit such a grade or response, or what could be done to earn a better grade or to improve performance. Rowntree (1987) considers that such nonspecific feedback becomes increasingly useless to the student as the size and diversity of performance being assessed increases. This factor is important for the clinical assessor to consider, as students are required to engage in, and learn, through a diverse range of clinical activities. Feedback is required on a myriad of activities and situations that the student will have taken part in.

Managing feedback sessions

The following framework is suggested for managing feedback sessions:

- timing of the feedback session
- format of the session
- involving the student in self-assessment
- using some 'rules of thumb' for managing constructive feedback.

Timing of the feedback session

For feedback to have maximal motivational impact on learning, it should take place while it is still relevant and points raised are therefore more meaningful and alive (Bailey 1998, Gipps 1994); furthermore, the event and its details are fresh and accessible to memory and not distorted with time (Jones 1995). In the clinical setting, if appropriate, this could take place as a running commentary, as the learner is performing, or as soon as possible after the event. This gives the learner the opportunity to act upon feedback as soon as possible to improve future performance. A quote from a first-year student nurse in Neary's (2001:8) study illustrates this point:

> I was nervous because [assessor] worked with me all week and right away she told me where I was going wrong. She responded quickly by helping me to understand what I needed to learn. [Assessor] did not waste any time in telling me how and what to do. I like that, I know where I need to improve . . . . I can respond to this level of feedback. I feel more confident now, I can get on with the job.

The assessor who works alongside the student should take advantage of the unique position in being able to offer accurate feedback on all aspects of learning.

Feedback sessions after the event will be more beneficial if the assessor takes the responsibility for making time available and arranging a suitable venue (Gomez et al 1998). It will not be conducive for engaging in constructive feedback if either the assessor or the student is still preoccupied with activities on the ward or after a busy clinical shift. The session could then prove to be counterproductive.

Format of the session

The format can be oral or written. Students usually look for both. Fish and Twinn (1997) believe that written notes are essential in providing continuity in the monitoring of progress. When written notes are kept, the valuable details of the situation are not forgotten, which increases the potential for learning (Bailey 1998). Within the continuous assessment process of pre-registration students' written records of sessions reviewing progress are generally required. Constructive feedback sessions may be used to review progress formally and written records kept of these sessions.

Involving the student in self-assessment

This is discussed in the sections on formative assessment above, and 'Discussion with the student' in Chapter 7.

Using some 'rules of thumb' for managing constructive feedback

It is essential that constructive feedback is management systematically and with discipline. The following rules of thumb for the management of constructive feedback are based upon and extended from the work of Bailey (1998) and Fish and Twinn (1997):

- Keep your appointment with the student and give your undivided time, attention and interest – do not look at your watch constantly.
- Maintain privacy and be careful not to be interrupted.
- Do not tackle too many things at once – try to foster a sense of progress. Gipps (1994) says that the most effective forms of feedback are those which focus students' attention on their progress in mastering the required performance. This emphasis tends to enhance self-efficacy and encourages effort attribution.
- Always try to make the session a learning situation for the student. Be positive as a first step. Temper negative comments with praise – the so-called praise sandwich (Hinchliff 1999). Rowntree (1987:45) quoted the pioneering chemist Sir Humphrey Davy, who wrote of 'the love of praise that never, never dies'. Students tend to remember the negative rather than the positive – good points therefore need reinforcing. Help the student to see negative comments as growing points.
- Use evidence from the episode of practice in as objective a way as possible. Stick to facts and present them in as neutral a way as possible. Use any written evidence from the student's portfolio to provoke discussion.
- Avoid generalizing and making subjective comments. A statement such as 'you were brilliant' may be pleasant to hear but does not give any detail to be useful as a source of learning. Try to pinpoint what the student did which led you to use the label 'brilliant'.
- Do not compare with other students.
- Above all, remember that criticism is usually counterproductive.
- Be clear about your role – that of being an assessor giving constructive feedback on practice. It is your responsibility to *establish communication*, *clarify any problems* and either *get a commitment for change* or *offer a solution* (Paul 1988).

Establish communication:

- Use positive and warm nonverbal communication. Smile. Make eye contact. Do not be confrontational.
- Listen to the student. Get the comments and ideas from the student. Asking makes the student feel valued and is better than telling.

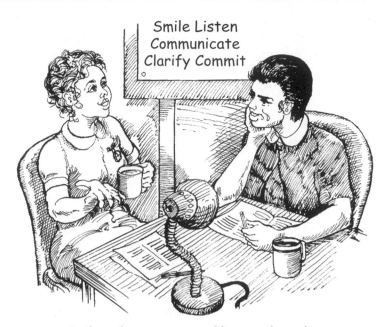

Smile Listen
Communicate
Clarify Commit

Smile, make eye contact and listen to the student

- Work *with* the student not *on* her or him. Avoid a power struggle. Do not take control of the situation.
- Giving negative feedback or leading the student to focus on the things that did not work is also important and should not be avoided. It is tempting to avoid unsatisfactory work but performance will not improve without knowledge of what was wrong. Remember that there will come a time when it may be too late to give negative feedback.
- Use open-ended questions and give reasons for your questions and comments.
- Encourage frankness and share worries and uncertainties – we are all learners.

Clarify any problems:

- Always take account of as many dimensions of the practice situation as possible. Try not to be biased by your own strong reaction or views about any individual part of the situation as this might colour the feedback session.
- If the student counterattacks, do not rise! Try to see it from the student's point of view – take account of the student's prior experiences, interpretations and perceptions of what has happened. Explore and clarify what the student is saying.
- Be prepared to see that your own and perhaps different value-base and skills are only of indirect importance. You are not trying to cast the student into a mould of you but, within professional parameters, to help the student be more fully herself or himself.

Get a commitment for change or offer a solution:

- Ask the student how performance can be improved.
- You may need to show how performance can be improved. Be specific: offer alternatives. Avoid suggesting that there are simple right answers. Suggest a small new target that will lead to success.

■ Make sure the student understands what is expected by asking the student to say what she or he will aim for and what first steps will be taken.

■ You may wish to make a written agreement with the student in the form of an action plan. Within this, set clear targets for the next period of supervised practice.

SUMMATIVE ASSESSMENT

Whereas formative assessments take place throughout the student's clinical placement, summative assessments usually take place at the end of the placement, where the aggregate of learning is represented. Summative assessment focuses on the whole and is used to provide information about how much students have learned and to what extent learning outcomes have been met. In the event of negative consequences, nothing can now be done to remedy the situation. The ENB (1997) clearly expected summative assessments to be made as it stated that 'the assessment of learning of theory and practice is a continuous process culminating in a judgement of achievement'. It further stated that in order to meet relevant statutory professional and academic requirements, the student is required to demonstrate competence within practice through the achievement of learning outcomes in both theory and practice. Within the competency-based assessment system a 'competent' or 'not yet competent' decision is made. The specified competencies for each clinical placement must be achieved at the summative assessment in order to progress in the training. Students who are not yet competent are generally not allowed to progress further in their training until they have successfully achieved competence.

Two positions are taken with formative assessment in this discussion: first, it is a facilitative process that aims to guide and maximize learning; secondly, it serves to provide a series of assessments so that a summative assessment can be compiled from them. Rowntree (1987) suggests that final 'end-of-the-placement' assessments may be dispensed with altogether if a satisfactory summative assessment can be compiled from the series of formative assessments. However, Harlen et al (1992) maintain that summative assessments should be separated into two types: 'summing-up' and 'checking-up'. In the former, information collected over a period of time is simply 'summed' every so often to assess how students are getting on. This collection of pieces of assessment evidence from formative assessments is kept in the student's portfolio of learning in order to preserve the richness of the data. The summing-up provides a picture of current achievements. 'Checking-up' is when summative assessment is done through the use of assessment tasks specifically devised for the purpose of assessing competence at a particular time. For example, at the end of the placement, on summing-up the evidence of competence of a learner in relationship to admitting a client to the ward, the assessor requires some more evidence of competence. Checking-up can be in the form of observing the learner admit a client or to simulate the activity. In your clinical area you may identify competencies which are crucial for the safe delivery of care and choose to use 'checking-up' as a matter of course when assessing the learner summatively.

Having examined formative and summative assessments, and the continuous assessment process in general, it is now appropriate to go on to examine how to engage in and use the process of continuous assessment.

ENGAGING IN THE PROCESS OF CONTINUOUS ASSESSMENT

The three little words 'assessment takes time' was probably written with much feeling and understanding by Phillips et al (2000:150) after their intensive investigation of the assessment of clinical practice in pre-registration nursing and midwifery education. Assessment does indeed take time. I would contend that good assessment takes even more time. Time has to be allocated for 'assessment-only' activity to enable assessors to engage in the process of continuous assessment so that assessments serve the intended purposes. The assessment activities to be undertaken within the continuous assessment process may be represented in Figure 6.1.

It can be seen from Figure 6.1 that one of the central assessment devices is that of student–assessor meetings. Bedford et al (1993) found that these valuable meetings do not function as effectively as they might because they are

FIGURE 6.1   *The process of continuous assessment of clinical practice.*

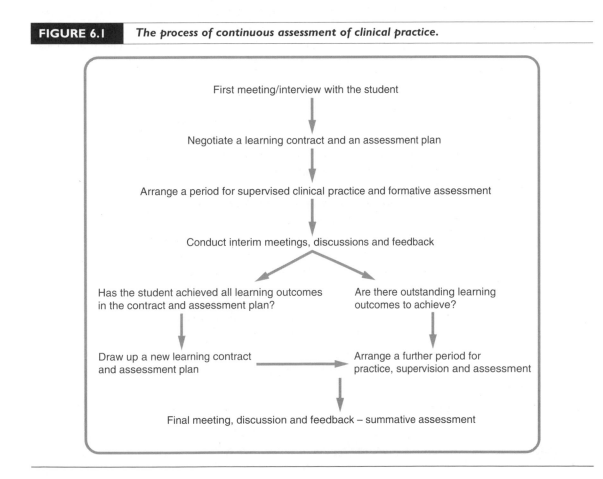

hurriedly carried out. If students feel that they pose an additional burden in a busy clinical area, the quality and quantity of learning is extremely negatively affected (Phillips et al 2000). Protected, that is timetabled, time should be prioritized and allocated for 'assessment-only activities' (Phillips et al 2000, Bedford et al 1993). Professional responsibility and accountability for learners require us to ensure that learning takes place, and allocating and spending time with learners is part of that contract we enter into with learners in our care.

The first meeting/interview

This first formalized meeting/interview is important for students: they will be feeling anxious in a new place of work (Phillips et al 2000) and unsure about what to expect from their mentor and assessor they may be meeting for the first time. When asked about their first day on clinical placement, most students in Phillips et al's study (2000:72), provided, as their first word descriptor, 'scary', 'frightening', 'terrified' and 'anxious'. Together with this anxiety, may be an uncertainty about how the ward functions and what they are going to learn, particularly if the student has never worked in that area of speciality. The student will thus be looking for support and guidance from the mentor/assessor. Anxiety can be a barrier to learning (Rogers 1983). The first meeting/interview gives the mentor/assessor an ideal opportunity to start forming a facilitative relationship with the student and introducing the student to the ward routine. What we know about what helps learners in a new clinical area tells us that 'beginners' feel more secure if their practice can be guided by the structure of a specified routine (Benner et al 1996).

The first meeting/interview with the student should be done as soon as possible – preferably within the first 2 days of the commencement of the placement. This is important to enable the mentor/assessor and the student to draw up a learning contract and an assessment plan using the information from the student self-assessment to identify learning needs. Phillips et al (2000) found that students on new placements often had to endure being treated as though they knew nothing – previous learning and accomplishments were ignored. Apart from this being disabling and demotivating, it can lead the mentor/assessor to shape learning experiences inappropriately. Phillips et al (2000), very rightly in my view, contend that all students know something and some know a great deal.

As soon as the contract and assessment plan are negotiated and agreed, the direction that both the mentor/assessor and the student require for the teaching/learning and assessment processes to commence is provided.

Try Activity 6.3.

In Chapter 2, we said that one of your responsibilities as an assessor is to be familiar with the structure, organization and content of the programme of students you are assessing. This will allow you to have cognizance of the learning outcomes that your student will be required to achieve during the placement. The first meeting/interview allows you to evaluate what prior learning has taken

ACTIVITY 6.3

Make a list of the points you would discuss with your student during the first meeting/interview. Why have you included these points?

FIGURE 6.2	*The outcomes of a first meeting/interview.*

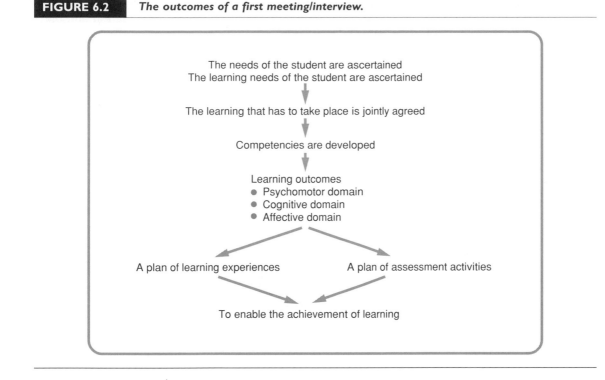

place to inform and guide subsequent plans for learning. The points to discuss with the student should include the following:

- find out and attempt to allay any anxieties
- confirm the student's stage of training and current module to ascertain course learning outcomes
- discuss any personal learning outcomes the student may have planned
- jointly examine and discuss the portfolio of learning
- ask about any written assignments or projects that have to be prepared
- discuss the learning opportunities the placement can provide to generate assessment evidence to enable achievement of competencies and learning outcomes
- discuss arrangements to supervise and support the student in your absence
- discuss the ward's routine and care philosophy.

The outcomes to aim for after the first meeting/interview may be represented in Figure 6.2. This meeting/interview should culminate in the mutual drawing up of the learning contract and assessment plan. The next section examines the learning contract, which also contains the assessment plan.

THE LEARNING CONTRACT AND THE ASSESSMENT PLAN

The use of learning contracts can be made integral to the continuous assessment process, as both the formative and summative assessment components of this process can be fulfilled. As discussed above, the intention of formative and summative assessment processes is to guide learning. Careful negotiation and planning of a learning contract will result in a framework to guide the teaching, learning and assessment requirements of the student. This framework will also provide the direction for teaching and assessing activities for the mentor/assessor. In the clinical setting, the learning contract approach involves an individual student negotiating with, and entering into an agreement with, a mentor/assessor to pursue certain goals of a proposed course of training. Commonly, in a pre-registration programme, these goals are to achieve the competencies of the training programme. Post-registered practitioners may enter into contracts with their preceptors or managers to develop further their competence, roles and expertise. As the purpose of these kinds of learning is to develop and/or improve one's competence to perform as a professional, the needs and expectations of the profession must be taken into account. How the learning is to be assessed is usually determined by the necessity to produce practitioners who are 'fit for purpose' and 'fit for practice' (UKCC 1999). Learners frequently have no choice in what they have to learn and how they are assessed. Furthermore, in the clinical setting, although there are many resources for learning, these are not unlimited. Constraints may also be imposed by timing of the availability of some resources. For example, certain clinical experiences such as rarely occurring clinical events do not manifest to order so that the student can learn and be assessed.

The above imposed structures on learning and assessment frequently conflict with an adult learner's need to be self-directing and having the 'freedom to learn' (Rogers 1983). They may also stifle a learner's creativity and motivation to learn and, according to Knowles (1986), may induce resistance, apathy or withdrawal. The use of learning contracts could be one way of reconciling the requirements imposed by the above structures and the learner's internal need of

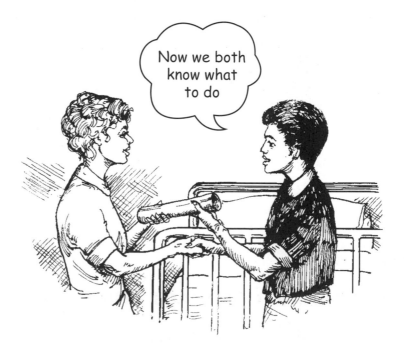

Have you contracted with your student?

having 'freedom to learn'. Chan and Chien (2000), Neary (1998) and Tompkins and McGraw (1988) found this reconciliation possible within the constraints of the curriculum – they used learning contracts in the clinical setting, which successfully increased individualized learning and student autonomy. Interactions for planning and feedback activities between the clinical instructor and the student also improved – this finding confirmed Knowles' (1986) belief that learning contracts provide the means through which the planning of learning experiences can become a mutual undertaking between the student and the mentor. In the nursing literature, Chan and Chien (2000), Neary (1998), McAllister (1996), Donaldson (1992) and Tompkins and McGraw (1988) for example, report other benefits of using the learning contract in the clinical setting. Knowles (1986) reported the disadvantages and benefits of contracting based on the experiences of a number of teachers in higher education. It is not the intention here to enter into a debate of the advantages and disadvantages of using learning contracts. The reader is therefore directed to the work of these authors for a further discussion of the advantages and disadvantages of using learning contracts.

The elements of a learning contract

The core that underpins any learning contract is made up of learning objectives, learning activities to be completed, strategies and resources for learning and both learner and mentor evaluation of outcomes. Specific elements can be developed from this core to suit individual and institutional practices as well as fulfil the learning needs of students in a complex and rich area of learning such as the clinical setting. For the purposes of competency-based assessment in the clinical setting, the elements given in Box 6.1 are suggested as the framework for the development of a learning contract. A discussion of these elements and how to develop them follows.

Planning a learning contract

An understanding of the format of the learning contract and the process of contract learning is important for the successful implementation and use of learning

BOX 6.1	The elements of a learning contract for competency-based assessment

1. Clear statements of the aim and learning outcomes
2. State the level of performance to be achieved
3. Define the range of context for clinical practice to enable the achievement of the aim and learning outcomes
4. Specify the resources and learning activities
5. Develop an assessment plan
6. Identify the roles and responsibilities of both the learner and the mentor/assessor
7. Decide a time frame – set review date(s) and a target date
8. Signatures

BOX 6.2	*The steps to the construction of a learning contract/assessment plan*

Step 1

At the initial interview/meeting:

- Facilitate student self-assessment
- Identify prior learning and clinical experiences the student has engaged in
- Examine student portfolio

Step 2

- Identify and jointly agree learning needs and competencies to be achieved
- For each competency, identify the knowledge outcomes, performance outcomes and attitudes and values to be developed

Step 3

- Identify the range of context of practice for each competency
- Identify resources and learning activities such as clinical experiences which are required to enable the student to achieve each competency

Step 4

- Consider how evidence of learning can be generated and evaluated
- Decide most appropriate assessment methods to assess learning
- Map methods against clinical activities and other learning activities

Step 5

- Agree the roles and responsibilities of both to achieve the learning contract/assessment plan

Step 6

- Set and agree review and target dates

contracts. Students must be well prepared for contract learning for this form of learning to succeed – preparation is crucial and should not be omitted (Knowles 1986). Personal discussion with students and mentors tell me that planning, developing and writing a learning contract is not a straightforward affair. Authors such as McAllister (1996) and Donaldson (1992) report that contract formats can be confusing to use.

Using the elements of a contract as shown in Box 6.1 as the basis for planning, the sequence of steps given in Box 6.2 are proposed for planning and developing a learning contract/assessment plan for competence-based assessment in the clinical setting.

There is now a discussion of the rationale underpinning each element of the contract and how each element can be developed and used for learning and assessment activities.

1. Statements of the aim and learning outcomes

Once the learning needs and expectations are outlined from the perspective of the student and the mentor, both will be in a position to define and describe what the student intends to achieve. These require to be translated into statements that can provide the direction for learning and assessment strategies. They can then act as the criteria against which student progress can be measured. In its document *Fitness for Practice*, the UKCC (1999:38) recommends that:

Students, assessors and mentors should know what is expected of them through specified practice outcomes which form part of a formal learning contract.

In a pre-registration programme, the learning, of necessity, requires to be related to the achievement of the statutory professional competencies. In the case of midwifery and nursing students in the UK, these competencies are laid down by the UKCC (UKCC 2000a, 2000b). In terms of statements of the aim and learning outcomes for competency-based assessment, the following aspects should be addressed:

- define the element of competency to be achieved
- define the attributes that underlie the successful performance of the competency.

For the purposes of this discussion, we use the example of a student nurse or student midwife who has identified the need to learn about caring for clients and others at times of loss and death. Elements of competence are the tasks within the wider function described by a 'unit of competence', which represents a wide work function. This element of competency may be written thus: *to be able to care for clients and others at times of imminent death, death and loss*. In the case of nursing students, it is suggested here that this element of competency may fall within the wider function of the UKCC competency *demonstrate sound clinical judgement across a range of differing professional and care delivery contexts* (UKCC 2000b). This UKCC competency may thus be the 'unit of competence'. The reader is directed to the discussion on competence and competencies in Chapter 3.

Professionals are competent as a result of the possession of a set of relevant attributes such as knowledge, understanding, skills, personal traits, attitudes and values. The attributes that underlie the successful performance of the element of competency *to be able to care for clients and others at times of imminent death, death and loss* require to be specified so that they serve as the criteria for the assessment of successful performance of this element of competency. These criteria are the standards in competency-based assessment. Performance is judged against these pre-specified standards. It is suggested here that these standards are specified under the three domains of learning:

- the cognitive domain – *knowledge outcomes*
- the psychomotor domain – *performance outcomes*
- the affective domain – *attitudes and values to be developed*.

Thus, the standards, which are not intended to be an exhaustive list, for the above element of competency may be grouped under these headings.

Knowledge outcomes

- Discuss the stages of the grieving process and the individual's needs during each stage
- Describe the policies and guidelines relating to care of clients and others at times of loss and death
- Discuss recent research in this area and recommendations for practice.

Performance outcomes

- Support clients, significant others and friends of clients during their initial adjustment to learning of the client's condition

- Support clients during the critical period before death
- Comfort and support significant others and friends of clients who have suffered loss
- Comfort and support significant others and friends of clients who have died
- Debrief and support colleagues as necessary
- Use the appropriate verbal and nonverbal communication skills
- Perform the necessary care of the dead person.

Attitudes and values

- Be empathetic towards grieving clients, significant others and friends of clients
- Be empathetic towards colleagues
- Possess the appropriate respect for clients from diverse cultural and religious backgrounds
- Show the appropriate respect for the dead person.

Bedford et al (1993) found that documentation of this nature is most likely to promote reflective discussion of practice and integrate theory and practice. This research team also found that defining and documenting the competency statement, knowledge and performance outcomes and the attitudes and values enabled the assessor to use them as measures against later analysis of student achievement of competence. This is perhaps the most persuasive argument for using standards in the assessment of clinical practice – standards define what we mean by quality care practices and quality practitioners. When standards and other requirements of good performance (see subsection 2 below) are made clear before tasks are attempted, misdirected efforts and undue anxiety are avoided.

2.   State the level of performance to be achieved

Work in psychology and learning tells us that for effective learning to take place, the task must be matched to the student's current level of understanding, and either pitched at that level to provide practice, or slightly higher in order to extend and develop the student's skills (Bigge 1982). If the new task is too easy, the student can become bored; if too difficult, the student can become demotivated. By matching the learning tasks to the student's level, the learning contract/assessment plan is individualized and the emphasis on assessment is placed on the student's progress and learning.

Stating the level of performance tries to make clear the degree of proficiency expected of the learner. The specified level of performance required is an important component of any learning contract because it is the measure used for the summative assessment of the element of competence. The specified level of performance also guides the development of the learner. Generally, in a 3-year pre-registration programme, there are three levels of performance to be achieved: Level 1 performance to be achieved by year-one students; Level 2 performance to be achieved by year-two students; and Level 3 performance to be achieved by year-three students. Standards of performance to be reached in assessment should be clearly specified to students – they should be high but attainable (Gipps 1994).

Bedford et al (1993) found that clinical assessors frequently experienced difficulty in ensuring that students were advised and assessed at the appropriate level. Specifying the criteria for a level of performance is a thorny issue (Phillips

TABLE 6.1   Matching the levels of performance to levels of supervision and practice and conditions of competent practice

Level of performance	Level of supervision/support	Level of practice	Conditions of practice for the achievement of clinical competencies	
			Competence achieved	Competence not achieved
Level 1	Direct to close supervision	Observes, participates, assists in	Performs with few prompts Can explain the rationale underpinning practice	Requires detailed and explicit instructions Cannot explain the rationale underpinning practice
Level 2	Close to minimal supervision	Active participation Planning most activities and leading some	Performance is smooth and complete Does not require prompting in practised activities Can explain the rationale underpinning practice and discuss pertinent research	Performance lacks completeness Requires prompting in practised activities Cannot explain the rationale underpinning practice
Level 3	Minimal to indirect supervision	Active participation Planning all activities and leading most	Does not require prompting Is organized and efficient Critiques evidence-based practice and its implementation	Requires prompting Unable to organize care Does not consider evidence-based practice

et al 2000, Gerrish et al 1997). The reader is directed to a discussion of this issue in Chapter 3. As I see it, one possible way around this problem is to specify the level of performance and then match this with the amount of supervision/support needed, the level of practice that can be expected of the student and the conditions of competent practice for the specified performance level. This eclectic framework to assess clinical practice is shown in Table 6.1. The reader is referred to Chapter 7, where there is a discussion of the theoretical basis of this format, and how to monitor and assess the progress of students using this framework.

3. Define the range of context for clinical practice to enable effective performance of the element of competence

The range of context for clinical practice identifies the various caregiving events that the student will require in order to carry out the element of competence in a specified clinical setting. These different caregiving events will provide the student with the opportunities to achieve the knowledge and performance outcomes and develop the appropriate attitudes and values specified in the learning contract. Here, there is room for negotiation and the exercise of autonomy by the student. If the student has already had particular clinical experiences that fulfil the requirements of any of the range statements (see Chapter 3), then these specific clinical experiences may not be required.

An example of the range statements for the element of competence – *to be able to care for clients and others at times of imminent death, death and loss* – is given below. The following range statements assume that the clinical setting is that of a medical unit:

- the imminent death of patients who have suffered a protracted illness
- the imminent death of patients with a sudden acute illness
- the imminent death of patients with different cultural and religious needs
- patients who have died.

In the midwifery setting, range statements may include:

- women who require the termination of their pregnancy for an abnormal fetus
- women who have experienced an intrauterine death
- women who have experienced a neonatal death
- women whose babies are in the special care baby unit
- women whose babies are acutely ill in the neonatal intensive care unit
- women who give up their babies for adoption.

It can be seen that the range statement serves to indicate the range of clinical situations to which the element of competence applies. It ensures that the element of competence has been learnt and can be demonstrated in a range of contexts. Jessup (1991) warns that although range statements can act to broaden the range of contexts in which mastery can be assumed, specifying the range can also be limiting.

Notwithstanding the possible disadvantage of specifying the range, there are sound educational reasons for doing so. What we know now of cognitive processes indicates that there is a close connection between skills and knowledge, and the context in which they are learnt and practised. Gipps (1994) suggests that we cannot teach a skill component in one setting and expect it to be applied automatically in another. This means, in turn, that we cannot validly assess a competence in a context very different from the context in which it has been practised. In mainstream education, Koretz et al (1991 in Gipps 1994) found that high performance on a regularly used test did not generalize to another test for which students had not been specifically prepared. The conclusion that can be drawn from this is that teaching to perform for a particular test invalidates the test results as indicators of more general learning.

In their work with young people in the Youth Training Scheme, Wolf et al (1990) found that the transferability of complex problem-solving skills was limited. Trainees were given training on problem-solving tasks either within their own occupational group only or in a range of occupational groups; a control group was given no training at all. Both groups that received training showed improved performance over the group that did not, and the group that had received training in a variety of contexts performed better outside their occupational area than did the group that had training within their own occupational area. The authors concluded that varied training encouraged generalized learning, i.e. generalized skills do not develop from context-specific learning. Experiences with performance-based licensure examinations in medicine confirm the need for a large number of tasks in order to achieve acceptable levels of generalizability (Linn 1993). In his review of the generalizability of performance from one task to another, Linn (1993:12–13) concluded that:

> . . . low levels of generalisability across tasks limit the validity of inferences about performance for a domain and pose serious problems regarding comparability and fairness to individuals which are judged against performance standards based on a small number, and perhaps different set, of tasks.

Generalizability is a particular problem in performance assessment because performance is heavily context-dependent – direct assessment of complex performance does not generalize well from one task to another. Linn (1993) recommends that, in performance assessment, increasing the number of tasks on the assessment is the most effective way of enhancing generalizability. Students must therefore be given new problems to solve or be asked to apply the concepts in different contexts of care to assess whether they can transfer and apply skills and knowledge. Increasing the number of tasks assessed clearly increases the resources required, such as time and expense. This is, however, justified by the need to achieve more valid assessment, so that health care professionals are the safe and competent practitioners we desire. Wolf (1995:43, 49) suggests the use of this guiding principle in assessment:

> . . . the best predictor of future performance is past performance . . . [therefore] . . . assessments should be as close as possible to the outcomes one is interested in . . . you will get the best results if you sample directly the item you are interested in.

The specification of a range of contexts will enable this important guiding principle to be put in place. Assessments will then have more validity.

4. Specify the resources, learning activities and learning opportunities

Resources required may be both material and human. These need to be identified and their use planned. Material resources, which should be available, up-to-date and directly relevant to the desired learning outcomes, include equipment, textbooks, journal articles, videos and self-directed learning programmes. There should be a discussion of how these resources can be best utilized to contribute to the achievement of learning outcomes. Learning activities around material resources may include reading text material, viewing a video and learning to use a piece of equipment. The mentor should arrange to provide the necessary instructions.

When identifying human resources, the name, designation, availability and contact details of the person, usually another professional, should be specified. There should be a discussion of how the person can contribute to the learning, so that the student is better prepared to utilize the expertise of that person. Learning activities here may include observing and working with the person, followed by discussions, or simply asking questions and talking to the person. In the example of the element of competence – *to be able to care for clients and others at times of imminent death, death and loss* – we have used so far, human resources and learning activities could include observing the hospital chaplain, observing and working with the bereavement counsellor, and so on.

Some learning opportunities, such as clinical experiences, may not be identified ahead of time. It should, however, be made clear to students those specific types of clients/patients whose care they need to participate in. The student will then be in a better position to negotiate with other team members to work with when they are looking after such clients/patients.

The reader is directed to the discussion on identifying and utilizing resources and learning opportunities in the clinical environment in Chapter 8.

5.   Develop a learning and assessment plan

There should be a clear plan of how the learning and assessment of the element of competence are to proceed over a specified period. Both the student and mentor should agree the following:

1. How learning and assessment will be managed, e.g. making firm arrangements:
   - to look after certain clients/patients
   - to work together on specified shifts
   - to spend time together to review progress on specified occasions.

2. What evidence needs to be collected.

3. How the evidence will be generated and collected.

4. What will be accepted as evidence that learning outcomes have been achieved.

Students should be allowed to exercise choice and autonomy, where feasible, when decisions are made about how evidence is to be generated and provided. The student may negotiate to do written pieces of work, or present information verbally to peers, to support the achievement of specific learning outcomes, in particular the knowledge outcomes. The student must know at the outset how the assessment will be done: e.g. if a written piece of work is used, a description of what must be included is identified. If an oral presentation is to be given, the student must know how long the presentation will last and how it will be evaluated.

Evidence of having taken part in care may be collected in a written format in the form of an evidence log. It is suggested that the student has the responsibility for maintaining this log. Within an evidence log, the student records details of clinical activities undertaken that will act as evidence of achievement of learning outcomes in the learning contract. Questioning and reflective discussions of these records will provide evidence of the underpinning knowledge and understanding of care delivered. The reader is directed to the section on *recording evidence* in Chapter 7 for a further discussion of the use of evidence logs.

Within a scheme of the continuous assessment of clinical practice, the student will generally work alongside the mentor so that the mentor is facilitating learning, at the same time assessing learning and progress as both work together. The mentor will be gathering evidence of learning that should be discussed with the student during feedback sessions. In the absence of the allocated mentor, firm arrangements should be made for the student to work with another practitioner. The learning contract should be explained to the other mentor so that continuity of supervision and support is maintained, and the validity and reliability of the assessment is enhanced.

6.   Identify the roles and responsibilities of both the learner and the mentor/assessor

A written learning contract signals a commitment from both the student and the mentor. In contract learning, the student and mentor work together to achieve the specified outcomes. Tompkins and McGraw (1988) emphasized the importance of recognizing that contracting does not mean that the student learns *independently*; rather, an *interdependent* relationship develops between the student and the mentor. Within this interdependent relationship, the roles and responsibilities of each party should be made clear.

While one key aim of using learning contracts is to promote student autonomy and responsibility by encouraging self-directed learning, this may be intimidating for some students. McAllister (1996) found that some students did not enjoy the freedom and control when they were working through their learning contracts. Both Chan and Chien (2000) and McAllister (1996) discussed the uncertainties and anxieties students felt when contract learning was an unfamiliar learning strategy. However, levels of anxiety diminished quickly as students learned how to manage their own learning. Students' active participation in the development of the contract and agreement to what work must be done for achievement are helpful in reducing anxiety.

The mentor needs to assess the level of readiness and ability of the student to deal with the demands of using learning contracts as advanced learning skills are required. These advanced learning skills include self-direction, critical self-appraisal, the ability to participate actively in the learning activities provided and in the management of their learning and to seek help, guidance and feedback when appropriate (Refshauge and Higgs 2000).

Knowles (1986:43) suggested that in contract learning, 'the role of the instructor shifts from that of a didactic transmitter of content and controller of learners to that of a facilitator of self-directed learning and content resource'. In the case of the mentor in the clinical setting, it is suggested here that the role shifts from someone who has the responsibility for making sure that learning experiences take place, and indeed controls the clinical experiences that students have, to that of someone whom students approach to negotiate the types of clinical, and other learning, experiences they require to achieve the outcomes in the contract. McAllister (1996) observed that mentors still need to be aware that, even though power is more evenly distributed, they should not abrogate all control and responsibility – new and deep level learning still need to be promoted. Neary (1998) suggests that what students want to learn can only be developed if the mentor, through facilitation, directs and gives clear guidelines on expected outcomes of learning. Stenhouse (1975 in Mazhindu 1990) made the contentious point that the quality of the facilitator is either the main weakness or the greatest strength of the learning contract. There is no doubt that the success of contract learning depends not only on the student's own enthusiasm and commitment to the agreement but also on the enthusiasm, commitment and ability of the mentor as facilitator. The mentor needs to assist the student with making a successful transition to this form of learning, if required, and also to help the student sustain the interest and commitment to the contract. One key strategy in maintaining student motivation in contract learning is to provide opportunities for success and to give continuous immediate formative and summative feedback (Neary 1998).

Students must also make a shift in their perceptions of their roles as learners. A traditional learner role is that of dependency. Students are perceived, and perceive themselves to be, dependent on the teacher for planning and evaluating their learning, and are more or less dependent and passive recipients of transmitted content. In contract learning, the role of the student shifts from that of 'more or less passive receiver of transmitted information and submissive executor of the instructor's directives, to that of initiative-taking planner and executor of strategies and resources for achieving mutually agreed [outcomes]' (Knowles 1986:44). As an adult learner, the student should also make use of learning opportunities and resources identified in support of the learning contract. It must be pointed out here that the mentor is ultimately accountable and responsible for student learning and so must accept the ultimate responsibility for the quality of the learning and for ensuring that the requirements of the contract have been met. Some roles and responsibilities of the mentor could be to:

- act as a resource and share ideas and recommend learning resources
- identify and negotiate learning opportunities for the student
- support and encourage the student
- assess and evaluate the student's work, giving regular constructive feedback
- provide stimulating learning experiences.

Some roles and responsibilities of the student could be to:

- seek out and make use of learning opportunities and resources
- take the initiative to seek guidance and feedback regularly
- participate in assessment and evaluation through self-evaluation.

7.   Agreement on a time frame – set review date(s) and a target date

Setting a target date allows the student and mentor to pace the learning and provides the student with a goalpost. It is important to meet at specified intervals to determine progress, make changes to the contract or provide help if needed.

The student should be left with the responsibility of seeking guidance and feedback outside of these scheduled times if required. The frequency varies with the type of contract, the level of the student and the ability of the student for self-direction and discipline. The highly motivated, self-directing and self-disciplined student may require little help and therefore fewer occasions for formal review and feedback. The student who is less motivated or has difficulty in maintaining self-discipline will require more frequent meetings to verify understanding, check progress and to provide encouragement and motivation.

It is useful to identify some specific outcomes from the learning contract to work towards during a specified period so that these can be evaluated at each review meeting. This will provide the direction and the goals for learning for that period. Learning is then divided into chunks and is likely to be more manageable and achievable. Opportunities for success are provided: these act as extrinsic motivators to encourage the student to set sights that are progressively higher (Neary 1998). At these review meetings, the student should participate actively through self-assessment and by the seeking of feedback about performance and learning. The following points may be useful for the review of progress.

■ Review the learning contract. Discuss how far the activities that the student has participated in have contributed to the achievement of the learning outcomes and the range.
■ Discuss any difficulties that the student may be experiencing.
■ Discuss and plan future learning activities.
■ Amend the learning contract if necessary – few learning contracts ever go to plan.

If the learning outcomes and the range have been achieved before the target date, a new learning contract should be drawn up. If the actual clinical experience cannot be provided towards the end of the contracted period, plans should be made to use simulation in the place of naturalistic observation as the alternative method of assessment.

8.   Signatures

It is suggested that both the student and mentor sign the contract, as this strengthens the commitment of both participants.

PERIOD OF SUPERVISED CLINICAL PRACTICE AND FORMATIVE ASSESSMENT

The learning contract and assessment plan formulated will provide the mentor/assessor and the student with the framework for teaching, learning and assessment. The period of supervised clinical practice and formative assessment can now proceed more meaningfully, and with the intent that is required in order to help the student achieve the learning during the precious time spent on clinical placements. During this period the student is learning under supervision and working towards achieving the competencies that the training requires.

This learning may occur as a result of interacting with patients/clients, giving patient/client care and being taught by yourself and other staff members. With reference to the learning outcomes and range of context identified in the contract above, it is clear what the types and nature of learning experiences are that are required. Arrangements should be made so that the student and the mentor/assessor work together and with other members of the team as necessary to enable the student to engage in the necessary clinical experiences.

Assessment activities are informal: you may observe activities, evaluate care given, give feedback, pose questions or discuss care given in a planned systematic or ad hoc way. The information which you obtain may be partial or fragmentary in the early days and will not allow you to make a firm evaluation of the student's competence. But repeated assessments of this sort, over a period of time and in a range of contexts, will allow you to build up a solid and broadly-based assessment of your student's attainment.

Phillips et al (2000) found that where assessors are only able to work with students for short intermittent and ad hoc stretches they are not able to collect reliable assessment evidence. This in turn reduces the validity of the assessment. They recommend that there should be a minimum time prioritized for assessment-only activities involving working and observing alongside the learner as part of a specified minimum overall learner entitlement. The ENB (1997) recommends that the assessor directly observes and supports the student for a minimum period equivalent to 2 days per working week for full-time students and pro rata for part-time students.

The formative assessments that take place as you work with the learner and give feedback on performance are generally ad hoc and informal. However, there needs to be occasions when formative assessments are more formalized to enable you and the student to review and reflect on experiences, identify learning that has taken place and plan further experiences. Remember that the aim of formative assessments is to motivate your student and maximize learning. These formalized sessions should be planned, and dates specified in the learning contract. Bedford et al (1993) recommend allocating protected time for these discussions. The number of formal meeting/discussion sessions you hold altogether during the student's placement would be dependent on the length of the placement and the progress the student is making. There should be at least one formalized meeting/discussion session. As a guide, try to hold a formal meeting/discussion session at least every 2 weeks so that you can formally review with your student the progress that is made and identify any difficulties at an earlier rather than a later stage of the placement. Work on learning tells us that shorter units of work with linked assessment are more motivating for many students (Gipps 1994).

At the end of each interim meeting/discussion session, you and your student should jointly decide to what extent the competencies and learning outcomes in the learning contract/assessment plan have been achieved. As indicated in Figure 6.1, if all learning outcomes in the learning contract/assessment plan have been achieved, a new learning contract/assessment plan will be drawn up and a further period is arranged for practice and ·assessment. Likewise, if the student requires more clinical experience to enable the outstanding learning outcomes to be achieved in the existing assessment plan and contract, a further period for practice and assessment will also need to be arranged. It is important to record in writing the discussion that has taken place, as this record should be filed in the student's portfolio for future reference. The student's assessment of practice record is completed as required, e.g. signing those competencies which have been achieved. This will serve to motivate the student.

THE FINAL MEETING/DISCUSSION SESSION AND SUMMATIVE ASSESSMENT

The final meeting/discussion session to perform the summative assessment is done at the end of the placement. As a guide, this meeting should be done during the last week of the student's placement, preferably on the last day. During this final meeting/discussion session, additional time should be allocated to review and analyse fully the evidence of competence. It is important to record the discussion and complete the student's assessment of practice record to be filed in the student's portfolio, so that it can be available to the student for future reference and to other mentors/assessors in subsequent placements. Time should also be spent in preparing the student for future placements. As the mentor/assessor, you can see evidences of changes in the student that provide specific information for fostering future development. Through your guidance learning can be influenced. Glaser (1990) makes the case that assessment must be used in support of learning rather than just to indicate current or past achievement. Assessment must be looked at not only in terms of outcomes measurement but also in terms of the learning process.

Suggestions on how you might conduct these meeting/discussion sessions, the summative assessment meeting, analyse assessment evidence and give feedback more effectively are made in Chapter 7.

In summary then, the stages of the continuous assessment process are as follows:

1. Arrange and conduct the first meeting/interview. Be clear about what you want to include in the learning contract and the assessment plan.
2. Arrange clinical experiences to enable your student to practise and achieve the assessment plan and the learning outcomes in the contract. During this period, arrange to work with and assess your student in practice.
3. Arrange and conduct interim meeting/discussion sessions – formalized formative assessments – throughout the placement. Complete assessment documentation.
4. Arrange and conduct the final meeting/discussion session – summative assessment. Complete assessment documentation.

CONCLUSION

It is acknowledged that outcome measurement in the health care professions is important in order to achieve fitness for practice and fitness for purpose. This chapter has considered that assessment should not be looked at just in terms of outcome measurement but also as part of the learning process. Assessment should be, and can be, facilitative and constructive and should never be used as a punitive tool. It should be used to identify what students have learnt, what they have not learnt and where they are having difficulty. In this way, it supports the teaching–learning process: this form of assessment is known as formative assessment. Assessment in the caring professions also needs to be used for accountability purposes to confer competence and certificate students: this form of assessment is known as summative assessment.

The continuous assessment of practice allows the mentor/assessor to work closely with, supervise and assess the student in the everyday working environment. Assessments that take place in these 'natural' surroundings are more likely to reflect the real abilities of the student. There has been much emphasis that assessments should be of this nature so that they are 'authentic' (Govaerts et al 2001, Gipps 1994) – authentic assessments allow us to test those performances we want students to be good at. It is important to plan assessments carefully so that these time-consuming assessment activities result in high-quality assessment.

If we could work with students all the time they are in clinical practice we would be in a very good position to tell whether they are any good. As a general rule, however, we make judgements on rather small amounts of evidence (Wolf 1995), which is why it is important that assessments should be as well designed as possible. Wolf reminds us that the prime responsibility for assessment planning lies with the assessor. This is particularly the case with assessments in professional education which confer professional qualifications: e.g. a nursing or midwifery qualification is taken to guarantee safe and competent practice for the public that these professions serve.

REFERENCES

Bailey J (1998) The supervisor's story: from expert to novice. In Johns C and Freshwater D (eds) *Transforming Nursing through Reflective Practice*, pp 194–205. London: Blackwell Science.

Bedford H, Phillips T, Robinson J and Schostak J (1993) *Assessment of Competencies in Nursing and Midwifery Education and Training*. London: The English National Board for Nursing, Midwifery and Health Visiting.

Benner P, Tanner CA and Chesla CA (1996) *Expertise in Nursing Practice*. New York: Springer.

Bigge ML (1982) *Learning Theories for Teachers*, 4th edn. London: Harper and Row.

Chambers M (1998) Some issues of assessment of clinical practice: a review of the literature. *Journal of Clinical Nursing*, 7(3), 201–208.

Chan SW and Chien W (2000) Implementing contract learning in a clinical context: report on a study. *Journal of Advanced Nursing*, 31(2), 298–305.

Crooks TJ (1988) The impact of classroom evaluation practices on students. *Review of Educational Research*, 58(4), 438–481.

Donaldson I (1992) The use of learning contracts in the clinical area. *Nurse Education Today*, 12, 431–436.

English National Board (1997) *Standards for Approval of Higher Education Institutions and Programmes*. London: The English National Board for Nursing, Midwifery and Health Visiting.

English National Board (1996) *Regulations and Guidelines for the Approval of Institutions and Courses. Section 5 – Regulations and Guidelines Relating to Assessment*. London: The English National Board for Nursing, Midwifery and Health Visiting.

English National Board (1986) *Guidelines to Preparing Continuous Assessment*, Circular 1986 (16) ERBD. London: The English National Board for Nursing, Midwifery and Health Visiting.

Falchikov N and Boud D (1989) Student self-assessment in higher education: a meta-analysis. *Review of Educational Research*, 59(4), 395–430.

Fish D and Twinn S (1997) *Quality Clinical Supervision*. Oxford: Butterworth-Heinemann.

Gerrish K, McManus M and Ashworth P (1997) *Levels of Achievement: A Review of the Assessment of Practice*. London: The English National Board for Nursing, Midwifery and Health Visiting.

Gipps CV (1994) *Beyond Testing: Towards a Theory of Educational Assessment*. London: The Falmer Press.

Glaser R (1990) Toward new models for assessment. *International Journal of Educational Research*, 14(5), 475–483.

Gomez DA, Lobodzinski S and Hartwell West CD (1998) Evaluating clinical performance. In Billinge DM and Halstead JA (eds) *Teaching in Nursing: A Guide for Faculty*, pp 407–422. Philadelphia: WB Saunders.

Gonczi A, Hager P and Athanasou J (1993) *The Development of Competency-Based Assessment Strategies for the Professions*. National Office of Overseas Skills Recognition, Research Paper No. 8. Canberra: Australian Government Publishing Service.

Govaerts MJB, Schuwirth LWT, Pin A et al (2001) Objective assessment is needed to ensure competence. *British Journal of Midwifery*, 9(3), 156–161.

Harlen W, Gipps C, Broadbent P and Nuttall D (1992) Assessment and the improvement of education. *The Curriculum Journal*, 3, 3.

Hinchliff S (1999) *The Practitioner as Teacher*, 2nd edn. London: Baillière Tindall.

Jarvis P and Gibson S (1997) *The Teacher Practitioner and Mentor in Nursing, Midwifery, Health Visiting and the Social Services*, 2nd edn. Cheltenham: Stanley Thornes (Publishers).

Jessup G (1991) *Outcomes: NVQs and the Emerging Model of Education and Training*. London: The Falmer Press.

Jones PR (1995) Hindsight bias in reflective practice: an empirical investigation. *Journal of Advanced Nursing*, 21, 783–788.

Knowles M (1990) *The Adult Learner: A Neglected Species*, 4th edn. Houston: Gulf.

Knowles M S (1986) *Using Learning Contracts*. San Francisco: Jossey-Bass.

Koretz D, Linn R, Dunbar S and Shepard L (1991) The effects of high stakes testing on achievement: preliminary findings about generalization across tests. Paper presented to the AERA/NCME, April, Chicago.

Linn RL (1993) Educational assessment: expanded expectations and challenges. *Educational Evaluation and Policy Analysis*, 15(1), 1–16.

McAllister M (1996) Learning contracts: an Australian experience. *Nurse Education Today*, 16, 199–205.

Mazhindu GN (1990) Contract learning reconsidered: a critical examination of implications for application in nurse education. *Journal of Advanced Nursing*, 15, 101–109.

Neary M (2001) Responsive assessment: assessing student nurses' clinical competence. *Nurse Education Today*, 21, 3–17.

Neary M (1998) Contract assignments and change in teaching, learning and assessment strategies. *Educational Practice and Theory*, 20(1), 43–58.

Nicklin PJ and Kenworthy N (1995) *Teaching and Assessing in Clinical Practice*, 2nd edn. London: Baillière Tindall.

Paul N (1988) *Constructive Criticism*. Ely, Cambridgeshire: Wyvern Business Training.

Phillips T, Schostak J and Tyler J (2000) *Practice and Assessment in Nursing and Midwifery: Doing it for Real*. London: The English National Board for Nursing, Midwifery and Health Visiting.

Refshauge K and Higgs J (2000) Teaching clinical reasoning. In Higgs J and Jones M (eds) *Clinical Reasoning in the Health Care Professions*, 2nd edn, pp 141–147. Oxford: Butterworth-Heinemann.

Reilly DE and Oermann MH (1990) *Behavioural Objectives: Evaluation in Nursing*. New York: National League for Nursing.

Rogers C (1983) *Freedom to Learn for the 80's*. Columbus, Ohio: Charles E. Merrill.

Rowntree D (1987) *Assessing Students: How Shall We Know Them*, 2nd edn. London: Kogan Page.

Sadler R (1989) Specifying and promulgating achievement standards. *Instructional Science*, 18, 119–144.

Stenhouse L (1975) *An Introduction to Curriculum Research and Development*. London: Heinemann.

Stoker D (1994) Assessment in learning: (i) Understanding assessment issues. *Nursing Times*, 90(11), Section 7 (i), i–viii.

Sutton FA and Arbon PA (1994) Australian nursing – moving forward? Competencies and the nursing profession. *Nurse Education Today*, 14, 388–393.

Tompkins C and McGraw M-J (1988) The negotiated learning contract. In Boud D (ed) *Developing Student Autonomy in Learning*, 2nd edn, pp 172–191. London: Kogan Page.

Torrance H and Pryor J (1998) *Investigating Formative Assessment*. Buckingham: Open University Press.

UKCC (2000a) *Requirements for Pre-registration Midwifery Programmes*. London: United Kingdom Central Council for Nursing, Midwifery and Health Visiting.

UKCC (2000b) *Requirements for Pre-registration Nursing Programmes*. London: United Kingdom Central Council for Nursing, Midwifery and Health Visiting.

UKCC (1999) *Fitness for Practice*. London: United Kingdom Central Council for Nursing, Midwifery and Health Visiting.

White E, Riley E, Davies S and Twinn S (1994) *A Detailed Study of the Relationship between Teaching, Support, Supervision and Role Modelling in Clinical Areas within the Context of P2000 Courses*. London: The English National Board for Nursing, Midwifery and Health Visiting.

Wolf A (1995) *Competence-Based Assessment*. Buckingham: Open University Press.

Wolf A, Kelson M, Silver R (1990) *Learning in Context: Patterns of Skills Transfer and Training Implications*. Sheffield: The Training Agency.

7 Monitoring progress, managing feedback and making assessment decisions

INTRODUCTION

Monitoring progress, managing feedback and making assessment decisions are interrelated activities that are integral to the continuous assessment of practice. These activities are central to and essential in helping students learn through their practice to develop clinical competence. Using the continuous assessment process enables us to monitor progress continually and give feedback informally and constantly as we work with the learner – even over one working shift, feedback is an activity that occurs many times. There are, however, specific times when formal feedback should be given based on a more detailed examination of progress. As discussed in Chapter 6, when we conduct pre-scheduled and preplanned 'formal' formative and summative assessments, we have time and opportunities to discuss progress with the student, formally give feedback and make assessment decisions based on the analysis of assessment evidence. The mentor/assessor is in a 'unique position in being able to provide precise feedback to individual students on all aspects of practical professional development' (Stengelhofen 1993:153). However, if assessment is to be a true learning process, the student should be an equal partner in these activities – progress is monitored jointly through the formative assessment process set up, and the student participates actively during feedback and assessment decision-making sessions. It is important that these activities occur, not only to maintain the integrity of the assessment process itself but also to meet the rights of the student as a learner and the standards laid down by the English National Board (1997). Torrance and Pryor (1998) believe that assessment is only truly formative if it involves the student directly in self-assessment.

MANAGING FEEDBACK

'Managing feedback' is used in this chapter to signify the activity of holding constructive discussions with the student about clinical experiences that the student and the mentor/assessor have been involved in. Feedback can take place informally as the mentor/assessor works alongside the student, or more formally during pre-arranged feedback sessions. Rowntree (1987:24) considers that this essential learning activity is the 'life-blood of learning'. There is research evidence which suggests that this 'life-blood' is not well sustained – feedback is either not done well or as frequently as needed, or worse still, not at all (Neary 2000, Fish and Twinn 1997, Bedford et al 1993). Bedford et al (1993:107) quoted one assessor on assessment feedback:

> . . . I shy away from having to give criticism anyway. I'll always go to great lengths not to give criticism, so I'm not a good assessor from that point of view as I'll always highlight the positive aspects and I'll tend . . . not to go into too many details if a student isn't doing terribly well in certain areas.

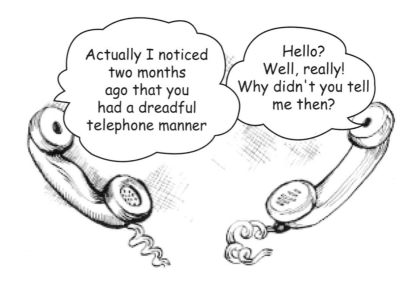

Often, feedback is not done well or as frequently as needed, or not at all

As noted in Chapter 6, it is knowledge of the results of performance provided by detailed factual constructive feedback that enables students 'to monitor strengths and weaknesses of their performances, so that aspects associated with success or high quality can be recognized and reinforced, and unsatisfactory aspects can be modified or improved' (Sadler 1989:120). Feedback therefore contributes directly to learning through the process of formative assessment.

Constructive feedback has an impact not only on the teaching/learning process but also gives messages to students about their effectiveness and worth – their self-esteem (Gipps 1994). Feedback, therefore, has an indirect effect on learning by how the academic self-esteem of the student is affected. Coopersmith (1967 in Gipps 1994:132) defined self-esteem as:

> the evaluation which the individual makes and customarily maintains with regard to himself – it expresses an attitude of approval or disapproval and indicates the extent to which an individual believes himself to be capable, significant, successful and worthy.

A major determinant of self-esteem is feedback from significant others. Consequently, students look to and, indeed, expect and welcome constructive feedback from significant others such as their teachers and assessors (Neary 2000, Phillips et al 2000, Gipps 1994, Bedford et al 1993). Other authors found that students view good clinical experiences to include receiving constructive feedback (Kotzabassaki et al 1997, Bedford et al 1993, Neville and French 1991). What we know about the effects of assessment on motivation tells us that students give up trying if they do not see themselves as capable of success. If they feel relatively worthless and ineffectual they will reduce their effort or give up altogether when work is difficult (Child 1997). On the other hand, people who hold positive self-perceptions usually try harder and persist longer when faced with difficult or challenging tasks.

There are therefore many challenges for the assessor on how to manage feedback so that it has a positive impact on learning, and more importantly, on the self-esteem of the student. Some detailed suggestions of how this may be done are made in Chapter 6.

MONITORING PROGRESS

Monitoring the progress of students is an essential part of the continuous assessment process. Progress can be monitored most accurately if the mentorship is stable. The same mentor/assessor is in a better position in keeping abreast of the clinical activities the student has had and will therefore know the amount of learning the student has achieved and how the competence of the student is developing. Monitoring progress is an ongoing assessment activity and takes place throughout the duration of the student's placement. Monitoring in this context, and not 'policing', is viewed as a process to help student learning, development and progression. We need to keep track of whether the student is developing competence and achieving the statutory competencies for professional practice. We therefore need to consider carefully what the student is learning, the clinical activities the student has been participating in and how further learning can be facilitated. When monitoring the progress of the student it is important to consider the prior clinical experiences of the student, the competencies and learning outcomes that the student needs to achieve during the placement and the stage of training the student is at. Curriculum documents will frequently state the expected level of performance at a specified stage of training.

When monitoring progress, the role and responsibilities of the assessor centre around answering these key questions:

- What has the student done and learnt so far? How will I know?
- Is the student having any difficulties? How will I know?
- What can be done to facilitate further learning and development?

To obtain answers to these questions, the assessment activities shown in Figure 7.1 are suggested.

Observation of practice for developing levels of competence

In Chapter 4 there is a detailed discussion of how observation may be used as a method of assessment to obtain direct evidence of the ability to perform care activities. When monitoring the progress of students during observation of their practice, the assessor needs to gather evidence of:

- continuing safe and accurate performance of care activities with increasing speed and dexterity as the student has more clinical experiences and gains confidence
- the development in the level of a student's competence between the outset of a placement and its conclusion (Bedford et al 1993).

What we know about the nature of expertise tells us that there are well-defined characteristics, across domains, that differentiate the performances of experts from novices (Benner et al 1996, Glaser 1990, Benner 1984). Glaser (1990: 477) sums up the situation thus:

> As proficiency develops, knowledge becomes increasingly integrated, new forms of cognitive skills emerge, access to knowledge is swift, and the efficiency of performance is heightened.

FIGURE 7.1   *Assessment activities to monitor progress.*

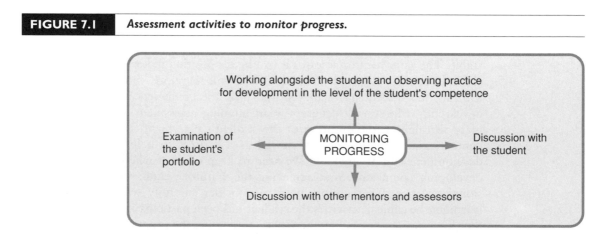

Glaser puts forward the case that, with growing proficiency, the changes in a person's cognitive ability and psychomotor performance can define criteria by which competence can be assessed. The Dreyfus model (in Benner 1984) considers that, in the acquisition and development of a skill, a learner passes through five levels of proficiency: novice, advanced beginner, competent, proficient and expert. As a learner passes through these levels, there are corresponding changes in three general aspects of performance. First, there is a move away from reliance on rules and principles to the use of past experience to guide practice. Secondly, the learner begins to see a situation less and less as a combination of equally relevant bits but more and more as a complete whole in which only certain parts are relevant. Thirdly, the learner becomes an involved performer and engages in the situation.

Benner (1984) and Benner et al (1996) applied the Dreyfus model to the study of *skills* acquisition in the practice of qualified nurses. They are careful in stating that skills in the nursing context refer exclusively to skilled nursing interventions and clinical judgement skills in actual clinical situations and not to psychomotor skills or to other skills learnt in the laboratory setting. For the purposes of this discussion, a summary of the performance characteristics from the work of Benner (1984) and Benner et al (1996) at the levels of development of the novice, advanced beginner and competent will be made here. Although these characteristics are derived from the performance of qualified nurses, it is my view that they can be extrapolated to the developing performance of pre-registration students. Following this exposition, the characteristics of the knowledge base with increasing proficiency described by Glaser (1990) are summarized.

The novice

- Nursing students enter a new clinical area as novices with no experience of the situations in which they are expected to perform
- They must be given rules and explicit detailed instructions to guide their performance; procedural lists are important for successful performance
- They focus on getting individual tasks done; novices generally do not see beyond the task at hand and may not recognize underlying problems of the patient
- They have little understanding of how to use classroom-acquired theory to guide practice.

The advanced beginner

- The advanced beginner can demonstrate marginally acceptable performance
- As a result of prior experiences, they are able to identify the recurring components of situations but are unable yet to sort out what is most important
- They cannot order information into a meaningful whole
- Their concern for good care is almost exclusively related to physical and technological support and to completing all the ordered treatment and procedures.

Competent

Competent nurses have:

- increased clinical understanding and are able to focus on clinical condition and management and less on getting tasks done
- increased technical skill – performance is more fluid and coordinated and they can predict the outcomes of their performance
- increased ability to handle busy complex situations and they can make decisions and solve problems
- improved time management skills
- improved organizational ability – they can prioritize care and manage care for several patients
- increased awareness of the appropriateness of their actions and are able to ask questions about what they have to do.

Knowledge base

Glaser (1990) notes that as competence in a domain grows, the person displays a knowledge base that is increasingly *coherent* and *useful*. The characteristics underpinning these descriptors are described briefly here.

The coherence of knowledge

The beginner's knowledge is spotty with superficial understanding: only fragments of information can be accessed for use. As competence develops, elements of knowledge are integrated with past organizations of knowledge so that information becomes increasingly interconnected and structured. Proficient individuals are able to access 'chunks' rather than fragments of information from memory.

Usable knowledge

Novices generally possess theoretical knowledge without knowing the conditions where that knowledge applies and how it can be used most effectively. More proficient individuals are able to access relevant knowledge to inform practice.

Criteria for assessing development in the novice, advanced beginner and competent levels of performance

The following criteria for assessing the development in the level of a student's competencies are based upon, and extended from the work of Benner et al (1996), Glaser (1990) and Benner (1984). When using these criteria to assess the level of performance and monitor progress, it is important to remember that the change from the novice level to competent level is incremental (Benner et al 1996) and on a continuum. The criteria below have been developed to reflect this.

Novice level

These conditions of practice of the novice along the following continuum can be used as the criteria to monitor the progress of novice level practice.

Conditions of practice

- Requires very detailed and explicit instructions
- Requires less detailed and explicit instructions
- Requires some detailed and explicit instructions
- Performs activities with few prompts
- Performs activities (x, y, z) in a fully integrated way
- Leads activities (a, b, c) with few prompts
- Beginning to assess, plan and implement care
- Within level of practice, responds appropriately in situations requiring urgency.

It is important for each clinical area to identify which activities the student is expected to be able to achieve competence in. The reader is directed to the discussion of 'competence' in Chapter 3.

Knowledge

- Has a grasp of theory underpinning most practices
- Can explain rationale underpinning some practices
- Can discuss pertinent research underpinning some practices.

Advanced beginner level

These conditions of practice of the advanced beginner along the following continuum can be used as the criteria to monitor the progress of advanced beginner level practice.

Conditions of practice
- Performs activities with few prompts
- Performs activities (x, y, z) in a fully integrated way
- Leads activities (a, b, c) with few prompts
- Able to assess, plan and implement care
- Beginning to evaluate effectiveness of care
- Beginning to involve clients in their care
- Within level of practice, responds appropriately in situations requiring urgency.

It is important for each clinical area to identify in which activities the student is expected to be able to achieve competence.

Knowledge

- Can explain rationale underpinning practice
- Can discuss pertinent research underpinning practice
- Beginning to implement evidence-based practice.

Competent level

These conditions of practice of the competent practitioner along the following continuum can be used as the criteria to monitor the progress of competent level practice.

Conditions of practice

- Performs activities (x, y, z) in a fully integrated way, without prompting
- Able to assess, plan and implement care
- Able to evaluate effectiveness of care and make changes in care plans
- Able to plan, prioritize and manage care for a group of clients within a time span
- Actively involves clients in their care
- Is organized and efficient
- Within level of practice, responds appropriately in situations requiring urgency.

Knowledge

- Critiques evidence-based research and its implementation.

During the early stages of a pre-registration programme, a student who is new to a clinical area is likely to start practice at the novice level but may achieve competent practice in some aspects of care by the end of the placement. The rate of progression is dependent on many factors, such as opportunities for practice and debriefing and reflection with the mentor/assessor, the prior experience of the student, the student as a learner and so on. In each new clinical area the 'junior' student may perform at novice level for a longer period before advancing. The 'senior' student who may have been to similar clinical areas, however, would be able to, and indeed would be expected to move more rapidly to advanced beginner and competent level practice. The assessor is reminded that it is a requirement of pre-registration education to prepare students to be able to apply knowledge, understanding and skills to perform to the standards required in employment when registered (UKCC 1998, 1999). It is suggested here that the ability to perform at the competent level is the required level to enable the student to achieve the requirements of statutory training, and to enable them to make the transition to registered practitioner. The criteria for assessing competent level practice should thus be used when monitoring the progress and assessing the practice of students who are at the stage of being prepared for professional practice, e.g. in the last 6 months of training. In its report *Fitness for Practice*, the UKCC (1999) recommends that all students should undertake a period of supervised clinical practice of at least 3 months towards the end of the pre-registration programme. This period of consolidation is intended to assist the student to make the transition to registered practitioner.

When monitoring the progress and assessing the practice of students, it is also important to consider the amount and level of supervision/support required by the student as well as the amount and level of participation in care you expect of the student. When students are at the novice level, they should initially observe care followed by participating and assisting in giving care. When giving care, they should be supervised closely and be supported. Students at the novice level, as discussed above, will require detailed and explicit instructions initially and may not be able to explain the rationale underpinning practice. As they learn and progress in their practice, less prompting is required for practised activities and they should be able to explain the rationale underpinning these practices.

As students progress, they should be encouraged to participate more actively. This should include the joint planning of activities. They should also be allowed to lead those activities they are confident in performing. The transition from novice level practice to advanced beginner level is on a continuum. The amount of supervision required starts to decrease and mentors may be able to 'let go' as they learn to trust the performance of the students. From performance that requires to be prompted because it lacks completeness, performance starts to become smooth and complete as students start to internalize activities. Prompting is generally not required. The rationale underpinning practice is understood.

As students move from advanced beginner level practice to competent level practice, the amount of supervision required becomes minimal, with indirect supervision only required towards the end of the training programme. Students should be taking an active role in giving care. They should be able to plan all practised activities and be leading most of them. They become organized and efficient and can carry out their own workload without having to be reminded of what to do.

Discussion with other mentors and assessors

If it is not possible for the named mentor/assessor to work with the student on enough occasions to monitor the progress of students with validity and reliability, it is important and only fair to the student that the mentor/assessor seeks the views of other practitioners who have worked with the student. In the real world of the busyness of clinical practice, Phillips et al (2000) and Bedford et al (1993) found that assessors are unable to be with assessees for any length of time. These research teams recommend that assessment should be a team effort to obtain a stronger and wider evidence base on which formative and summative assessments may be made. Phillips et al (2000) further recommend the following actions as part of good assessment practice:

- assessment should include discussion that occurs as part of the working day
- evidence and issues should be contributed, where possible, by all members of the team, including the assessee
- this occasion may be during a handover, a 'case' conference or some other event.

When discussing the performance of students as part of the process of monitoring progress, it is important to consider whether the quality and quantity of clinical experiences the student has had are sufficient to help development and therefore progress. Knowledge of the length of the placement, and the stage of training the student is at, will assist mentors and assessors in deciding how much progression, within and across each of the levels (novice, advanced beginner, competent), can be expected.

Discussion with the student

Talking, questioning and listening are crucial to assessment (Phillips et al 2000) and they can be used as instruments for ongoing review of the student's progress. There is a discussion of how questioning can be used to facilitate and assess student learning during clinical practice in Chapter 4. As the assessor and student work together, inviting the student to suggest how best to carry out care in clinical situations in which the student has been involved previously will give the assessor opportunities to consider what the student has learnt from similar past caregiving experiences. Whenever you spend time with your student in care activities, use every opportunity for discussions, using what is going on in front of you as the focus. What the student is able to articulate will indicate the amount of progress made. Subsequent discussion and questioning to explore further the quantity and quality of learning, and any difficulties the student may be having with performing particular care activities, will add to this source of evidence of student progression. In putting forward the case for using 'dialogue in assessment', Bedford et al (1993:136) note that through 'discussion about a particular event, students can demonstrate the knowledge, understanding and values that have informed their actions in the clinical area on a given occasion'. This enables the assessor to ascertain the understanding and the values held by the student about care given. There is further discussion of using dialogue as a vehicle for pre-activity discussion and post-event reflection in Chapter 9.

Progress reviews should also include student self-assessment and constructive feedback from the mentor/assessor. When engaging in self-assessment, students may need help in looking at themselves as they are, to judge realistically what they could become, while at the same time helping them to hold in mind the vision of how they would like to be, perhaps modelled on observations of more experienced practitioners. Assessors should not assume that students are able to self-assess independently (Maloney et al 1997). Boud (1992) contends that self-assessment skills need to be facilitated. On the other hand, students are aware of the standards against which to measure themselves. Woolliscroft et al (1993) suggest that accurate professional self-assessment requires individuals to be realistic about how their performance would be judged by others using valid performance-monitoring tools. Self-assessment schedules like the one devised by Woolliscroft et al (1993) can be of great value as they appear to prompt students to apply ideas to their own practice and reflect on their learning. Such schedules can be given to students prior to clinical activities and meeting sessions to discuss progress. Students can then use them to assess their own performance immediately after the clinical activity. The schedule used by Woolliscroft et al (1993) is modified and adapted for nursing and midwifery and reproduced here in Box 7.1.

Such self-assessment schedules, if used throughout the students' placement, will help them make specific judgements about their own performance and monitor their own progress in a range of clinical activities. Those clinical activities, specified in the learning contract and assessment plan (see Chapter 6), could be the topics for self-assessment schedules.

The crucial role of constructive feedback for learning is discussed at some length in Chapter 6. Feedback sessions should be designed to help

| BOX 7.1 | *Self-assessment by students for patient admission and care planning (modified and adapted from the questionnaire by Woolliscroft et al 1993)* |

Admission history/interview
1. I elicit an appropriate admission history
2. I am able to elicit the main nursing/midwifery problems
3. I accurately interpret the significance of these problems

Initial patient write-ups
4. I accurately document appropriate data in my initial patient/client write-ups, including all major and minor problems

Plan of care
5. I develop an appropriate plan of care

Implementation of care
6. I implement the plan of care I developed in the most appropriate ways

Daily patient/client progress
7. I am aware of my patients'/clients' daily developments
8. I accurately document all patient developments in my daily progress notes

Evaluation of care
9. I am able to evaluate the effectiveness of care given
10. I am able to modify the care plan after such evaluations

Application of knowledge
11. I apply my knowledge base in a well-integrated manner to patient/client problems

Supervision required
12. I require little direction to perform my patient care responsibilities

Interpersonal interactions
13. I interact with patients/clients and their families in a professional manner
14. I interact with other members of the health care team in a professional manner

students grow in their clinical skills and professional competence. Beginning level students have been found to be anxious about their ability to perform basic clinical skills (Robertson et al 1997). They often fail to focus on the patient/client as they have to concentrate their attention on developing clinical skills. Robertson et al (1997) suggest that feedback for these students should be designed to prompt them to think of the client holistically and to build self-confidence to enable the shift of focus to the patient/client. Advanced level students, on the other hand, may feel confident about their clinical skills but anxious about becoming a fully fledged professional in the near future (Robertson et al 1997). These students would benefit from feedback designed to promote the growth of professionalism and confidence in their professional personae to enable them to make the transition to registered practitioner.

Examination of the student's portfolio

In the case of nursing and midwifery students, the ENB (1997) stated that the student's portfolio should contain the following:

1. cumulative information about the student's achievement of outcomes and learning through reflection, demonstrating the interrelationship of theory and practice
2. the outcomes of assessment of both theory and practice
3. issues raised in discussion, including causes for concern between the assessor, the student and the personal/named lecturer as part of the formative process of development
4. the action plan or learning contract agreed between the assessor, the student and the personal/named lecturer
5. key issues from the student's experience which will inform the preparation for subsequent experience.

Additionally, the UKCC (1999) now requires pre-registration students to maintain an evidence-based portfolio during clinical practice. In *Fitness for Practice* (UKCC 1999) recommendation 14 states:

> The use of a portfolio of practice experience should be extended to demonstrate a student's fitness for practice and provide evidence of rational decision making and clinical judgement

In 1993, Bedford et al found that there was much diversity about the contents of portfolios of pre-registration students and how portfolios were used for the assessment of practice. It would appear that the same degree and amount of ambiguity still exists (Phillips et al 2000, Gerrish et al 1997). Appendix 15 gives an example of the contents of the student portfolio of a pre-registration midwifery programme devised by one higher education institution. Pre-registration midwifery students have to maintain a range of practice evidence in their portfolios to demonstrate that they are making progress in meeting both course and professional requirements to fulfil the above UKCC recommendation.

Recording evidence

The use of different methods of assessment in order to gain a comprehensive picture of the skills, knowledge, attributes and attitudes (see Chapter 4) will clearly produce a fairly big range and different kinds of evidence. If several methods are used on a day-to-day basis, how can we possibly keep track of all the evidence that is produced? Even over 1 week there will be more evidence than either the learner or assessor can remember. Memory is also dangerously selective (Jones 1995). So, unless we can record this evidence on a fairly frequent basis, we can lose track of the quantity and quality of learning achieved. The ENB (1997) *Standards for Approval of Higher Education Institutions and Programmes* state that assessment evidence should be documented. Now, try Activity 7.1.

Those of you who have worked alongside NVQ (national vocational qualification) candidates will have seen these learners recording details of achievement in what is known as an *evidence log*. Box 7.2 (p. 172) is an example of

ACTIVITY 7.1

Consider the types of learners in your area. How do they make ongoing records of evidence of what they achieve?

the evidence log of a learner performing blood sugar monitoring on the ward. This example of an evidence log compiled by a learner indicates the occasions when blood sugar was monitored and the aspects learnt. It also shows the progress the learner made. These evidence logs are usually filed with other documented evidence of learning in a portfolio.

The assessor or co-assessor may also provide written evidence logs of learning. Figure 7.2 is an example of the evidence log for a learner in the operating theatre. This evidence log shows the areas of difficulties experienced by the learner and the facilitation of further learning which led to progress and subsequent achievement of learning outcomes. It is of course not possible or feasible to compile evidence logs of every learning task, but crucial aspects of learning can be identified in each clinical area so that such logs of learning can be compiled.

Using the documented evidence to monitor progress

Phillips et al (2000) found that portfolios are most often constructed as collections of evidence of practice – they provide evidence of the student's repertoire of clinical activities. The portfolio can then be used by a range of people to consider the achievement of the student. This summative function of portfolios that has come to assume greater importance than its formative function of facilitat-

| FIGURE 7.2 | *Evidence log compiled by the assessor.* |

Date	Clinical Activities and Teaching/Learning Support
27.10.98	Difficulty with scrub technique. Trolley setting met performance criteria. Asepsis and uses of equipment discussed using question and answer with prompting from observer Discussed time for private study to review asepsis policy. Scrub poster and policy manual used to discuss equipment
2.11.98	Difficulty with scrub technique Trolley setting satisfactorily met performance criteria Highlighted scrub technique as major problem. Further session to be instigated
2.11.98	Practised scrub technique – applying gloves and gown
4.11.98	Practised scrub technique and applying gloves and gown. Improvement made
9.11.98	Improvement in scrub technique. Trolley setting satisfactory. Standard achieved. Further practice required. Asepsis and equipment usage discussed
13.11.98	Demonstrating competent performance. All learning outcomes achieved

| BOX 7.2 | *Evidence log compiled by a learner* |

16.12.98 – 11.30 hours

Today I was asked to perform a BM Stix recording, on a pleasant 72-year-old gentleman; we chatted away, while I explained the procedure to him. He was quite *au fait* with what was happening, having been diabetic for some years. Between us we chose the finger which I would be pricking. I gathered the equipment I needed, washed my hands and put on some gloves. I carried out the procedure as I have been taught. I chatted to this gentleman throughout the procedure giving reassurance. I discarded all the used equipment in the appropriate places. After washing my hands and recording the measurement, I checked that the gentleman was alright and the site was not bleeding.

21.12.98 – 13.50 hours

This afternoon I was asked by staff to perform a BM Stix measurement on a pleasant young lady; having explained to her what I was going to do, she appeared quite relaxed about it. After gathering the equipment that I needed, I washed my hands and put on gloves. After I pricked her finger, she bled a little more than usual, I asked her to press on with the cotton wool I had given her and assured her it would stop shortly, as it did, by the time I had timed the reading, which was within normal range, recorded the measurement and informed the staff nurse.

I discarded all the used equipment in the sharps bin, washed my hands, and checked once more that the lady was feeling alright, she said her finger was a little sore.

21.1.99

I gathered together the equipment that I needed to perform a BM test on a 75-year-old client. I washed my hands and put on some gloves. I then explained to him what I was going to do. I pricked his finger with a multistix, drew enough blood to cover the teststix and gave him some cotton wool to hold on the bleeding point.

After 1 min I wiped the end of the stick with cotton wool and waited a further minute, then recorded the result on the chart and told staff nurse what it was. I cleared away all the equipment and disposed of it in the appropriate places, and washed my hands.

I asked the gentleman if he was alright and checked that the bleeding had stopped.

Reflection

Today I performed a BM test on a 75-year-old gentleman. Having known this gentleman for quite sometime, as he has been staying with us for a while, I felt comfortable in performing this task. He, too, I think had confidence in me. I felt bad about having to stab his finger and maybe cause him pain, but this didn't seem to bother him too much. Having completed the test, recorded the outcome and passed on the information to staff nurse, I made sure that the gentleman was alright with the procedure and the bleeding had stopped and he was comfortable.

ing learning and development. Phillips et al (2000) warn that if the emphasis is on the portfolio's summative function there is frequently no engagement in any discussion and critique of the written evidence – this limits and narrows the usefulness of portfolios as a source of learning. In any case, most portfolios do not tell us how well prepared the student is for practice. An examination of the evidence in the portfolio is therefore only one way of assessing and monitoring progress. The portfolio needs to be complemented by other ways of assessing practice.

Potentially, portfolios are most useful for assessing theoretical understanding and intellectual capacities, such as the capacity to critically analyse the values and issues inherent in the context of the practice situations, leading to the construction of alternative ways to practise. Phillips et al (2000: 110) suggest that good portfolio assessment must capture the following aspects of learning and development:

- critical analysis of the way things are currently done
- identification of the values inherent in current practice
- critical appraisal of the context of current practice
- imagination of alternative ways of practice
- imagination of alternative ways of promoting better care and core values
- envisioning strategies to make changes.

In my view, portfolios should be used as a *process* tool as well as a tool to measure achievements. When reviewing the progress of the student using the portfolio, the documentation within it needs to be considered in terms of:

1. what the student has learnt so far
2. what can be done to facilitate a greater depth and breadth of learning based on what is documented in the portfolio.

The following steps may help you review progress using the portfolio evidence.

- Review the previous action plan or learning contract. Decide how far the activities planned have helped the student in participating in care delivery which have contributed to the achievement of the plan or contract.

- If an evidence log is kept, discuss the nature and amount of clinical experiences the student has participated in which have contributed to the achievement of statutory competencies. (The statutory competencies are usually contained in the student's assessment forms obtainable from the higher education institution of the student.)

- If a learning journal is kept, help the student to analyse critically specific care experiences you have both shared so that the most important issues emerge in order to increase the depth and breath of learning. (See Chapters 4, 6 and 9 for guidelines on the facilitation and assessment of learning through reflection.)

- Ask questions to help the student explain the rationale behind care, thereby enabling the student to apply theory to practice.

- Help the student to consider how practice could change as a result of learning through the specific clinical experiences. Explore alternative practices and strategies with the student.

MAKING ASSESSMENT DECISIONS

Formative assessment – Is the student progressing?

As discussed above, the assessment activities of working alongside the student and observing practice, discussion with other mentors and assessors, discussion with the student and examination of the student's portfolio are done both informally and formally to monitor progress. During the formal sessions, which should be planned and timetabled (Phillips et al 2000), the assessor should formally review with the student the progress that is made and identify any difficulties at an earlier, rather than a later, stage of the placement. The number of formal progress review meetings you hold altogether during the student's placement would be dependent on the length of the placement and the progress the student is making. There should be at least one formalized session (Bedford et al 1993). As a guide, try to hold a formal progress review session at least every 2 weeks. To decide whether the student is progressing, ask the following questions:

- Is the student achieving statutory competencies?
- Is there a demonstration of a growing level of skill?
- Is performance consistent (Maloney et al 1997)?
- Is there a demonstration of a growing understanding of the rationale underpinning practice?
- Is there a demonstration of development of the attitudes and values appropriate to professional practice?
- Is there a demonstration of a developing ability to engage in evidence-based and reflective practice?

It is important for assessors to remember that many factors can affect a student's progress and to explore reasons for the student's difficulties. Phillips et al (2000) made the point that any judgement of a student's capabilities must take into account the circumstances in which that student is performing.

Summative assessment – Should the student be passed?

The summative assessment is done at the end of the placement. A final meeting/discussion session should be arranged to take place during the last week of the student's placement, preferably on the last day. Additional time should be allocated to review and analyse fully the evidence of competence. The following questions may assist in helping you judge and analyse evidence to establish whether there is sufficient assessment evidence to confer competence.

1. Has the student achieved the statutory competencies?

Examine the student's assessment forms, which contain the statutory competencies. Statutory competencies have been set at the point of registration such that the student is able to fulfil the requirements of the practitioner as laid down by the UKCC. In order to prepare the student to practise safely and effectively so that, on registration, the student can assume the responsibilities and accountability for practice as a nurse or a midwife, all competencies for that placement must be achieved in order to pass.

In recommending the use of the competence-based approach for pre-registration nursing and midwifery education, the UKCC (1999) requires students, on qualification, to be able to practise safely and effectively without the need for direct supervision. If these training requirements are to be realized, only *competent* or *not competent* judgements can be made. Wolf (1995:22) states that in competence-based assessment 'either the person has consistently demonstrated workplace performance which meets the specified standards [in the competencies] or they are not yet able to do so'. Using the pre-specified levels of supervision and practice (see Chapter 6), and conditions of practice discussed earlier in this chapter, criteria are put forward to make 'competent' or 'not competent' decisions in Figure 7.3. Levels 1, 2 and 3 correspond to students during years one, two and three of the pre-registration programme, respectively.

Is there sufficient performance evidence to confer competent practice? Performance evidence would have been gathered by the assessor throughout the period of supervised practice or generated from the testimonies provided by other members of the team.

Has the student reached the required level? You may wish to review the section on 'Criteria for assessing development in the novice, advanced beginner and competent levels of performance'. Related to this is discriminating power. When making the final decision either to pass or fail the student, consider carefully whether your assessment has identified the correct standard to be achieved and the correct level of ability of the student for the stage of the training.

2.   Does the assessment evidence achieve validity of assessment?

Examine the student's portfolio. Has the learner engaged in a sufficient number and range of care situations for you to be confident that validity has been achieved? Does the student have 'the ability to actually care for patients?' (Gerrish et al 1997:70). Remember that the narrower the base of evidence for the inference of competence, the less generalizable it will be to the performance of other tasks. The reader is referred to Chapter 5 for a discussion of validity.

3.   Does the assessment evidence achieve reliability of assessment?

Examine the student's portfolio. Has the learner engaged in a sufficient number and range of care situations for you to be confident that reliability has been achieved? The amount of evidence must be sufficient to ensure consistent performance to the standard required across a range of situations. To ensure reliability, evidence is needed of repeated performances or we may be able to draw upon a number of different sources of evidence. It is dubious that a single correct performance is sufficient to confer competence for assessment purposes (Gonczi et al 1993). Maatsch et al (1987 in Gonczi et al 1993) considered that assessments on five to seven cases were required for the casualty physician to achieve general competence.

FIGURE 7.3	*Criteria for assessing the achievement of clinical competencies.*

LEVEL 1

Competence Achieved	Close to minimal supervision required Participates and assists in care Performs with few prompts in practised activities Can explain the rationale underpinning practice
Competence NOT Achieved	Close and direct supervision required Has difficulty participating and assisting in care Requires detailed and explicit instructions Cannot explain the rationale underpinning practice

LEVEL 2

Competence Achieved	Minimal supervision required Active participation in care Planning most activities and leading some Performance is smooth and complete Does not require prompting in practised activities Can explain rationale underpinning practice and discuss pertinent research
Competence NOT Achieved	Close supervision required Participates and assists in care Performance lacks completeness Requires to be prompted Cannot explain rationale underpinning practice

LEVEL 3

Competence Achieved	Indirect supervision required Active participation in care Planning all activities and leading most Does not require prompting Is organized and efficient Critiques evidence-based practice and its implementation
Competence NOT Achieved	Close supervision required Participates and assists in care only Requires prompting Unable to organize care Does not consider evidence-based practice

4. Is there a demonstration of a sound understanding of the rationale underpinning each competency?

Knowledge and understanding underpin competent practice. Students must be able to demonstrate that they understand the rationale for care activities. It is likely that the assessor will have assessed the student's understanding through the use of questioning throughout the period of formative assessment. This may require to be supplemented through further questioning when assessment evidence is being reviewed and analysed. Additionally, at Level 2, can the student discuss pertinent research underpinning evidence-based practice? and at Level 3, can the student discuss and critique pertinent research underpinning evidence-based practice?

5.   Is the student developing the attitudes and values appropriate to professional practice?

The assessment of attitudes and values is not easy. Although several methods of assessment can be used to 'assess' the attitudes and values of another (see Chapter 4), it nonetheless leaves this crucial aspect of competent professional practice open to personal biases and subjectiveness. It also stands in danger of not being assessed at all (Fraser 2000, Bedford et al 1993). A tool termed the 'professional behaviours inventory' to assess pre-specified behaviours expected of a professional exhibiting the accepted conduct of practitioner is proposed in Chapter 4. These behaviours are assumed to be underpinned by the attitudes, values and beliefs of the person.

MANAGING SOME ASSESSMENT PROBLEMS

Students experiencing problems learning during clinical practice

Although 'poor' students were found to be typically in the minority, the issue is nonetheless an important one as these students are a 'cause for concern' (Bedford et al 1993). Any student who is either not progressing or failing to meet the required standard needs identification by assessment systems so that opportunities can be provided for the student to improve. It is suggested here that the use of the assessment activities to monitor progress as discussed above will help the assessor identity those students who require extra help and support. Maloney et al (1997) provide some criteria for recognizing these students early. They remind us that although some of these behaviours are exhibited by many students at some time during clinical practice, the student who is either not progressing or failing exhibits these behaviours to such a degree and extent that learning is interrupted. These behaviours are listed here:

- is inconsistent in meeting the required level of competence for expected stage of training
- is inconsistent in clinical performance
- does not respond appropriately to constructive feedback
- appears unable to make changes in response to constructive feedback – therefore clinical skills do not improve
- exhibits poor preparation and organizational skills
- has limited interactional and poor communication skills
- may experience continual poor health, feel depressed, angry, uncommitted, withdrawn, sad, emotionally labile, tired or listless.

How can the assessor manage the situation when a student is either not progressing or failing? In Chapter 2 there is a discussion of the professional responsibility and accountability of the assessor in these situations. It is acknowledged here that people are generally reluctant to pass negative judgements on fellow workers. Assessors also experience the handling of the assessment of weak students as great challenges, both professionally and personally (Bedford et al 1993). But the implications of poor students 'slipping through the net' to become registered practitioners are grave if the situation is not managed appropriately. Appropriate management, I believe, includes using 'intelligence, sensitivity, understanding and insight' when dealing with these students, as suggested by Maloney et al (1997). It is reiterated here that the use of the strategy of triangulation to collect assessment evidence (see Chapter 4) will increase the confidence of the assessor when dealing with these students. Although the following plan of action is offered, the assessor should be clear of the policy laid down by the higher education institution of the student for dealing with these situations so that the correct procedure is followed:

- Concern is documented in the assessment forms at an early stage, and certainly no later than the point at which formative mid-placement assessment takes place (Bedford et al 1993). The nature of the problem should be carefully, clearly and explicitly documented.

- Discuss the situation with the senior practitioner with overall responsibility for student learning. Following this, inform the student's personal teacher and/or the clinical link lecturer (ENB 1997). Support from the higher education institution is essential in these situations.

- It is important to establish clear and open communication between the student, assessor and the higher education institution.

- Arrange to have a meeting with the student as soon as possible. Explain the reason for the meeting to the student.

- Consider and discuss the evidence which has led to concern. Maloney et al (1997:204) found that some students reacted positively and were relieved when their shortcomings were openly discussed with them, saying: 'It's so good not to pretend, now I feel I can say I don't know and extend my learning and increase my clinical skills'.

- Make sure the student understands the nature of the problems – has the student heard accurately what you are saying? The most difficult cases are those students who are clearly not succeeding but do not recognize this. Students should be provided with the opportunity to give their own perception of their performance. Help students identify what they already know and what they need to focus on in order to learn and overcome their weaknesses. Help students identify resources they can utilize to improve knowledge and skills. Jointly, draw up a targeted detailed action plan:

    1. Provide a clear and unambiguous assessment plan (see Chapter 6) to retrieve the situation
    2. Set deadlines and make sure the student understands these
    3. Make arrangements to work closely with the student

4. Arrangements should also be made for the student to work with other assessors so that testimonies can be provided: this will increase the validity and reliability of the assessment. Furthermore, students have the right to be protected from unfair or biased assessment and should not be failed until they are judged by another assessor (Gomez et al 1998).

- Make arrangements to conduct a progress review in 1 week. If, despite remedial action, there is little or no improvement, make arrangements for the clinical link lecturer to be present at a tripartite meeting to discuss the situation and develop another action plan.

- A weekly progress review is advisable for as long as the student's difficulties persist.

- It is also important to keep careful notes of all discussions: there may come a time when you have to use these as evidence that you may have pointed out the same things again and again and that the student has repeatedly failed to meet the goals you have set.

If, despite the actions and opportunities provided for the student to improve, development does not occur and standards are not achieved, failure decisions can be made fairly and on the basis of a fully documented evidence base.

Managing the situation when a student has to be failed

There comes a time when you may have to fail a student. Before making this critical decision, you must have followed the plan of action outlined above for helping the student who is not progressing. These situations are demanding and sensitive to handle. Notwithstanding that, assessors have professional responsibilities and accountability to make sound and accurate assessment decisions which include failing students who have not met the standards of training. The legal and ethical issues surrounding *not* failing a student who has not met the training standards and is unsafe to practise are discussed in Chapter 2. Suffice here to remind ourselves by asking the following question: *Would I want such a nurse or midwife to look after me or a relative or a friend of mine?* Bedford et al (1993) say that considerable skill and confidence are required to manage these situations effectively. I would also suggest that the assessor requires the courage and strength to fail a student – a conviction that the right assessment decision has been made will vest the assessor with this courage. This conviction will ensue if assessment processes to ensure fair assessments are followed. The assessor, then, will have no fear that there will be reprisals for failing a student.

Having to fail a student causes many of us considerable anguish. This may be a particularly difficult task for the assessor who has a self-image of that of a caring and nurturing person (Stengelhofen 1993). There is also the dichotomy for the assessor who is also the student's teacher – the assessor may feel that when the student fails it is a reflection of standards of supervision and teaching provided. Bedford et al (1993) and Lankshear (1990) outline some personal and professional dilemmas faced by assessors who had to fail students, which contributed to the 'failure to fail' scenario. At the other end of the continuum is to abuse the power to fail and use it as a tool to exert control and punish 'difficult' or unpopular students (Wolf 1995).

ACTIVITY 7.2

Staff Nurse Jack Jones is the named assessor to a student called Mary who has struggled considerably to achieve the required standard in three of the competency statements. He has been reviewing progress with her weekly. She is now approaching the end of the placement and has not achieved the required standard and, in Jack's opinion, should be failed. A fellow registered nurse who has also worked with Mary argues strongly that Mary's practice is up to standard and she should be passed. What should Jack do?

Consider the scenario shown in Activity 7.2. How would you deal with it?

The decision to fail a student is never an easy one to make (Stuart 2002, Lankshear 1990). When another assessor disagrees with your decision, it becomes even more tricky. The starting point is perhaps to consider both sets of assessment evidence objectively – Are both of you using the same criteria for assessment, so that assessment evidence is *reliable*? Therefore, evidence of achievement or non-achievement is based on the same criteria. The next question you may wish to consider is the *validity* of the assessment – e.g. Have both of you been assessing what you should be assessing? Has too much or too little been expected of the student? Other aspects of validity will also need to be considered (see Chapter 5).

Assuming that individual personal biases are not implicated and feasibility (see Chapter 5) within the assessment process has received due attention, and you still cannot agree with each other, as the named assessor you may wish to take the following action(s):

- arrange a meeting with your senior nurse/midwife with overall responsibility for student learning to discuss the situation
- arrange a meeting with your clinical link teacher or the student's personal teacher to discuss the situation
- arrange a joint meeting with your senior nurse/midwife and clinical link teacher to discuss the situation.

The final point to remember is that, as the named assessor, you are responsible for making the final assessment decision and are accountable for passing or failing the student at the end of the period of practice placement. The grade you award should reflect the student's standard of practice in the latter part of the placement.

Student reactions to being failed and how to manage them

Failing students may react in a number of ways (Gomez et al 1998). These behaviours need to be recognized for what they are, i.e. the student's reactions to the news of failure and not a personal vendetta against the assessor. Gomez et al (1998:420) recommend giving extra time to these situations, as the student needs time to 'grieve the loss of what was, perhaps, a dream'. Students need time to process the information and should not feel rushed. Assessors should listen attentively, show concern and provide the appropriate support.

- Students may respond with *denial* – their own perception of their competence contradicts that of the assessor. They may also deny situations where their performance was observed to have been unsafe or the attitude they exhibited was inappropriate. They may make excuses for their behaviours. The conversation needs to be steered to learning outcomes not being met.

- Students may respond with *anger* – they may become abusive and accusing, e.g. making accusations of biases against their personal characteristics. If the assessor suspects that this situation could arise, it may be wise to have the presence of a third person, such as the personal teacher of the student. The anger should not be taken personally. Provide guidance about feelings and focus on anger as part of the loss.

- Some students may attempt to bargain for a passing grade. The assessor needs to stand firm and remain focused on the results.

- As the reality of the loss is recognized, students may respond with *sadness* – they may cry over the loss of the right to carry on with the training. Allow them to cry before going on to discuss the reasons for the failure.

- Some students may be quite relieved. A career as a nurse or midwife may not be what they want but they may not have the courage to make that decision.

Failure may be a positive experience for some students. Some learn from the experience and go on to achieve success. Maloney et al (1997) give an example of a student who learned from failure – failure for her was positive (Case study 7.1).

Failure, however, is not a positive experience for many students. For some, it is a devastating experience and can appear to be a scar carried for life. Being able to determine early which students are not progressing, and making use of this information to give the appropriate support and help, may avert this painful situation for these students. The reader is directed to the work of Maloney et al (1997) for a more comprehensive discussion of students who are either not progressing or failing.

CASE STUDY 7.1 When failure is positive (Reproduced from Maloney et al with the permission of Nelson Thornes Ltd from *Facilitating Learning in Clinical Settings*, ISBN 07487 33167, first published in 1997.)

A university medical lecturer was surprised when approached at a social function by a confident young woman, who had recently been making her name in art design. She thanked him for helping her to make 'the most important decision of her life!' To his baffled enquiries, she told him that his 'help' had been failing her in a first-year medical subject, and taking the time to discuss her failure with her. She realized that she had in fact only done medicine because of her high university academic entrance mark and not through deep commitment. The result made her rethink her future, and decide to follow her real area of interest and skill.

CONCLUSION

When working with learners it is important to be able to indicate to them the progress they are making. Progress during clinical practice needs to be carefully tracked and feedback given so that learners may be able to learn and develop further. A discussion of the four assessment activities – working alongside the student and observing practice for development in the level of the student's competence, discussion with other mentors and assessors, discussion with the student and examination of the student's portfolio – shows how they can be used to monitor the progress of learners. Based upon what we know about the nature of expertise (Benner et al 1996, Glaser 1990, Benner 1984), a model that outlines the performance characteristics of novice, advanced beginner and competent practice is proposed here to monitor and assist with progression during clinical practice.

Monitoring progress is not about policing the learner. It is very much about finding out the quality and quantity of learning which has taken place and any difficulties the learner may be experiencing so that further assessment activities can be discussed and planned to further learning and development. It is inevitable that there will be instances when learners do not succeed: for these learners, early identification of difficulties and taking the appropriate action may reduce the trauma of failure for them.

If progress is carefully tracked through the four assessment activities discussed here, and done throughout the student's placement, it becomes much easier to make assessment decisions that are also more likely to be based on a valid and reliable evidence base, which means that students have a fairer deal. It also makes the task of making assessment decisions easier for the assessor – easier, as it is never easy to make fail decisions.

REFERENCES

Bedford H, Phillips T, Robinson J and Schostak J (1993) *Assessment of Competencies in Nursing and Midwifery Education and Training*. London: The English National Board for Nursing, Midwifery and Health Visiting.

Benner P (1984) *From Novice to Expert: Excellence and Power in Clinical Nursing Practice*. Menlo Park, California: Addison-Wesley.

Benner P, Tanner CA and Chesla CA (1996) *Expertise in Nursing Practice*. New York: Springer.

Boud D (1992) The use of self-assessment schedules in negotiated learning. *Studies in Higher Education*, 17, 185–200.

Child D (1997) *Psychology and the Teacher*, 6th edn. London: Cassell.

Coopersmith S (1967) *The Antecedents of Self-Esteem*. San Francisco: Freeman.

English National Board (1997) *Standards for Approval of Higher Education Institutions and Programmes*. London: The English National Board for Nursing, Midwifery and Health Visiting.

Fish D and Twinn S (1997) *Quality Clinical Supervision in the Health Care Professions: Principled Approaches to Practice*. Oxford: Butterworth Heinemann.

Fraser D (2000) Action research to improve the pre-registration midwifery curriculum. Part 3: Can fitness for practice be guaranteed? The challenges of designing and implementing an effective assessment in practice scheme. *Midwifery*, 16, 287–294.

Gerrish K, McManus M and Ashworth P (1997) *Levels of Achievement: A Review of the Assessment of Practice*. London: The English National Board for Nursing, Midwifery and Health Visiting.

Gipps CV (1994) *Beyond Testing: Towards a Theory of Educational Assessment*. London: The Falmer Press.

Glaser R (1990) Toward new models for assessment. *International Journal of Educational Research*, **14**(5), 475–483.

Gomez DA, Lobodzinski S and Hartwell West CD (1998) Evaluating clinical performance. In Billings DM and Halstead JA (eds) *Teaching in Nursing: A Guide for Faculty*, pp 407–422. Philadelphia: WB Saunders.

Gonczi A, Hager P and Athanasou J (1993) *The Development of Competency-Based Assessment Strategies for the Professions*. National Office of Overseas Skills Recognition, Research Paper No. 8. Canberra: Australian Government Publishing Service.

Jones PR (1995) Hindsight bias in reflective practice: an empirical investigation. *Journal of Advanced Nursing*, **21**, 783–788.

Kotzabassaki S, Panou M and Dimou F et al (1997) Nursing students' and faculty perceptions of the characteristics of 'best' and 'worst' clinical teachers: a replication study. *Journal of Advanced Nursing*, **26**, 817–824.

Lankshear A (1990) Failure to fail: the teacher's dilemma. *Nursing Standard*, **4**(20), 35–37.

Maatsch J, Juang RR, Downing SM and Munger BS (1987) Examiner assessments of clinical performance: what do they tell us about clinical competence? *Evaluation in Programme Planning*, **10**, 13–17.

Maloney D, Carmody D and Nemeth E (1997) Students experiencing problems learning in the clinical setting. In McAllister L, Lincoln M, McLeod S and Maloney D (eds) *Facilitating Learning in Clinical Settings*, pp 185–213. Cheltenham: Stanley Thornes (Publishers).

Neary M (2000) *Teaching, Assessing and Evaluation for Clinical Competence*. Cheltenham: Stanley Thornes (Publishers).

Neville S and French S (1991) Clinical education: student's and clinical teacher's views. *Physiotherapy*, **17**(5), 351–354.

Phillips T, Schostak J and Tyler J (2000) *Practice and Assessment in Nursing and Midwifery: Doing it for Real*. London: The English National Board for Nursing, Midwifery and Health Visiting.

Robertson S, Rosenthal J and Dawson V (1997) Using assessment to promote student learning. In McAllister L, Lincoln M, McLeod S and Maloney D (eds) *Facilitating Learning in Clinical Settings*, pp 154–184. Cheltenham: Stanley Thornes (Publishers).

Rowntree D (1987) *Assessing Students: How Shall We Know Them?* 2nd edn. London: Kogan Page.

Sadler R (1989) Specifying and promulgating achievement standards. *Instructional Science*, **18**, 119–144.

Stengelhofen J (1993) *Teaching Students in Clinical Settings*. London: Chapman and Hall.

Stuart CC (2002) An innovation in midwifery education. Proceedings from the 26th Triennial International Congress of Midwives, International Confederation of Midwives (ICM), Vienna.

Torrance H and Pryor J (1998) *Investigating Formative Assessment*. Buckingham: Open University Press.

UKCC (1999) *Fitness for Practice*. London: United Kingdom Central Council for Nursing, Midwifery and Health Visiting.

UKCC (1998) *Guidelines for Higher Education Institutions on Registration for Newly-Qualified Nurses and Midwives*. London: United Kingdom Central Council for Nursing, Midwifery and Health Visiting.

Wolf A (1995) *Competence-Based Assessment*. Buckingham: Open University Press.

Woolliscroft JO, Tentlaken J, Smith J and Calhonn JG (1993) Medical students' clinical self-assessments: comparisons with external measures of performance and the students' self-assessment of overall performance and effort. *Academic Medicine*, **68**, 285–294.

8 The clinical environment as a setting for learning and professional development

INTRODUCTION

Stated simplistically, the clinical environment is where patient/client care and clinical activities take place – it is where the action is. It is the real world of nursing and midwifery. A range of health professionals interact and work together to deliver care using their 'special brand' of professional expertise, making use of available material resources where needed. The clinical environment is unpredictable, volatile and dynamic; it is frequently noisy and teems with human interactions and activities. The clinical environment is the arena where students from the health care professions learn about care and what clinical practice is all about. The clinical experience of students of health care is widely acknowledged as being one of the most important aspects of their educational preparation (ENB and Department of Health 2001a). It is during practice placements that students learn to care for patients and clients, colleagues and others they work and interact with. Qualified professionals further their learning and 'hone up' on skills and competence.

The clinical environment must therefore also be an environment where learning can take place, thus becoming an educational environment. This type of setting is one which is conducive to learning and professional development. Marton et al (1984) make the important observation that learning is a function of the relationship between the learner and the environment and is never something determined by one of these elements alone. Learners do not respond merely to tasks assigned – rather, they adapt to and work within the environment taken as an interrelated whole. They pay close attention to the 'hidden' as well as the 'visible' curricula (Parlett and Hamilton 1977). It is the learner's engagement with the environment which makes the particular learning experience (Boud and Walker 1990).

This chapter examines those factors contributing to a positive clinical learning environment. Strategies for creating this environment are suggested. Chapter 9 examines how the learner can interact meaningfully with this environment in order to learn through clinical experiences.

THE CLINICAL LEARNING ENVIRONMENT

The learning environment of any formal educational setting is complex. It is suggested here that the clinical environment is a formal educational setting. The mentors/assessors are the teachers and the students are required to learn. There are norms and rules of behaviours and the mentors/assessors and students have expectations of each other and others (Boud and Walker 1990). This complexity is captured by Parlett and Hamilton (1977:14–15), who noted that a learning environment in the formal educational setting is:

> the social-psychological and material environment in which students and teachers work together . . . [it] represents a network or nexus of cultural, social, institutional, and psychological variables. These interact in complicated ways to produce, in each [clinical area], a unique pattern of circumstances, pressures, customs, opinions and work styles which suffuse the teaching and learning that occur there. The configuration of the learning milieu in any particular [clinical area] depends on the interplay of numerous different factors . . . there are numerous constraints . . . there are [also] the individual [mentor's] characteristics . . . and there are student perspectives and preoccupations.

In the nursing literature, Dunn and Burnett (1995:1166) say that the clinical learning environment is the 'interactive network of forces within the clinical setting that influence the students' clinical learning outcomes'. Orton (1981) described the clinical learning environment as a group of stable characteristics unique to that setting. These characteristics will impact on and influence the behaviour of individuals within it. The clinical environment as a formal educational setting is thus much more than the physical environment where patient/client care and other clinical activities take place: it is inclusive of the material resources within it, the formal requirements, the culture, procedures, practices and standards of particular clinical areas, the expectations and interactions of all the people who are in it, as well as the personal characteristics of individuals who are part of this environment. The richness of the clinical environment provides a rich texture for learning during clinical practice. This setting provides the context and events within which the student operates and learns (Boud and Walker 1990). However, it also acts as a distraction and competes for the student's attention.

The environment for teaching and learning in the community opens another world for students. Although they do not have to work within the constraints

ACTIVITY 8.1

Think about the clinical area where you work. This can be a ward, your community 'beat', an outpatients clinic, day care, casualty and so on.

1. Make a list of all the people who you think influence the learning ethos of the environment. How do they exert this influence?
2. What other factors influence your clinical environment as a learning environment?

of a hospital environment, students have to learn a different set of factors which influence practice. Professional carers are visitors in the client's own home – caring and teaching/learning activities are carried out in the client's domain. The client's lifestyle, values and health priorities could challenge the student's value systems. Students need to learn to respond sensitively in these situations as they learn about the complex forces that influence health care (White and Ewan 1991).

You may wish to try Activity 8.1.

We need to take into account several groups of factors and the interaction between these factors when considering the clinical environment as an educational environment. These factors can be grouped into the following categories:

1. The people:
   - the leader of the team
   - the members of the team
   - the students
   - the mentors.

2. Learning opportunities and experiences 'provided by':
   - patient/client care
   - other clinical activities.

3. Staff commitment to teaching and learning:
   - support and supervision of learners
   - continuing professional development.

4. Material resources

The people

The leader of the team

Much of the work which explored the direct influences of the leader of the team on the learning environment was done in the 1980s in the UK. Until the mid-1980s in the UK, one of the key roles of the ward sister was to teach, supervise and assess student nurses. The ward sister was the only person who was directly responsible for student learning during clinical practice. Student nurses then trained under the 'apprenticeship system' and were part of the workforce. With the introduction of schemes of continuous assessment of practice (ENB 1986), this role gradually devolved to staff nurses, and students became increasingly reliant on them for support (Ogier 1989). In the 1980s in the UK, the ward sister as the leader of the ward team was seen to be the single most important person in creating a learning climate (Jacka and Lewin 1987, Fretwell 1982, Ogier 1982, Orton 1981, Pembrey 1980). The conclusion which can be drawn from the work of these researchers is that for learning to occur, the clinical area has to be managed by a leader who is in touch with the needs and abilities of her subordinates. The leader should also have the ability to create an atmosphere which is conducive to learning, a point which is developed below. Ogier (1989: 37) has perhaps captured these messages in the following succinct statement: 'facilitating learning cannot be divorced from competent management and humane leadership'.

The reality today is that the team leader as ward manager (Jowett et al 1994) has a wider diversity of roles to fulfil. This has resulted in removing the ward manager from much, if any, direct patient and student contact. The direct influences of the ward manager on the learning climate of the clinical area remain to be evaluated today. Nonetheless, the importance of the ward manager's indirect influences on the learning climate should not be underestimated. With the support of a ward manager, who is committed to the training and development of students and staff, team members are more likely to be motivated in their role of mentor to students, and to the development of the clinical environment into an educational environment.

The members of the team

Each member of the team can contribute to an environment that fosters learning. Orton (1981) found that in wards that were highly rated by students there was a combination of teamwork, consultation and an awareness of the needs of others. In these wards, students' and patients' physical and emotional needs were amply met. A ward team that is committed not only to delivering a high standard of patient/client care but also to learning and assessing activities will contribute much to the creation of an educational climate. In a later study, Fraser (1994 in Gilmour 1999) also found that, where the ward culture was positive, there was good teamwork. Students and staff used terms such as 'friendly', 'happy', 'involving', 'teaching' and 'explaining to students'. Such a ward culture was perceived to be as important or more important than individual mentors in helping students learn.

Remember also that members of the multi-professional team make up the team even though they are not as visible as nurses and midwives in the clinical area. The multi-professional team's philosophy of patient/client care and their attitudes towards learning and students will also greatly influence the learning environment. It is important that they contribute to the educational environment so that not only do all members of the team learn with, and from each other, but also a spirit of teamwork may be created for the benefit of the patient/client. Following the publication of its report Fitness for Practice (UKCC 1999), the UKCC established the Post-Commission Development Group (UKCC 2001). In its report, this group noted that 'inter-professional education is informal and formal opportunities for members of two or more professions to learn from each other . . . with the aims of improving the effectiveness of care delivery and increasing collaborative practice'. This collaborative learning is strongly endorsed by the Department of Health (2001). Students should gain,

ACTIVITY 8.2

How do you help your students fit into the team?
What opportunities are available in your setting to help students fit into the team?

where possible, experience as part of a multi-professional team (ENB and DH 2001a). Now, you may wish to try Activity 8.2.

The health care team is a complex one. Students need to learn to relate and work with the team members: this is demanding, as it is not easy for students to feel valued as good team members (Stengelhofen 1993). In particular, new students may feel anxious even with the simple act of speaking with a professional, especially when that person is viewed as a senior member of the team. Mentors should ensure that students have opportunities to experience team-work through observing different members of the team at work and working as part of a team. The following ideas, based upon and extended from the work of Stengelhofen (1993), are offered to help students fit into the team and to learn about multi-professional team working:

1. *Ensure that the student has opportunities to fit into the nursing/midwifery team – the 'home team'*: Initially, this can be done informally by introducing the student to these team members. Students should be invited to attend staff meetings, journal clubs, training days, seminars, social events and so on. Arrangements can also be made to enable students to observe the nursing/midwifery team members – this need not involve any teaching. It is important that students demonstrate the ability to fit into the 'home team' before they are expected to become a member of the multi-professional team.

2. *Meeting members of the multi-professional team*: Introducing students to members of the multi-professional team informally – in the corridor, during coffee and meal breaks and in the staff room – can help others recognize new students. Later on, students can be gradually introduced to the work of these team members by making arrangements for students to observe them providing care for patients and being involved in situations which do not make any professional demands on the student. These activities will increase the student's understanding of the roles of the multi-professional team and also give students opportunities to interact with these professionals.

3. *Meeting and working with students from other professions*: If your setting has students from the other professions, explore opportunities for these students to meet and perhaps work together, e.g. discussing a patient/client they have looked after. Each student will be able to contribute to the discussion of care given, viewed from the perspectives of that particular professional group. Students will be able to learn about the roles of some of the other members of the team in this way. This strategy sows the seed for good team working, as students who have such positive experiences of the multi-professional team are likely to carry this into their professional practice.

4. *Working with members of the multi-professional team*: Plan graded steps to team involvement. As students' confidence increases they can be placed in situations where they are required to work alongside a member of the multi-professional team. In the first instance, be careful to involve the student with professionals who are patient and cooperative. The student should gradually

become independent in interacting with all team members and participating in the instances when care requires to be given jointly.

5. *Learning actively from members of the multi-professional team*: Encourage students to see these team members to gather information or discuss management of specific patients/clients. The mentor can assist the student to draw up the aims for the meeting and, subsequently, hold a debriefing session on the conduct and outcome of the meeting.

6. *Explore ways information is communicated within the multi-professional team*: As well as the use of formal letters, written reports and documentation in the patient/client's case notes, discuss other ways that communication takes place within the team, such as chats over coffee, telephone calls, during ward rounds and verbal reports.

The students

Students bring their own personalities, dispositions, hopes and aspirations, past experiences and backgrounds, and also worries and anxieties to the clinical setting. For many beginning students, the impact of the clinical environment can be strong (White and Ewan 1991). They have to deal with the unpleasant experiences such as sights, smells and cries of pain and difficult problems such as the abusive or disturbed patient/client. Students who come from an affluent and comfortable home background may have to learn to cope with the realities of social and economic differences, particularly when in the community setting.

Unlike permanent members of the team, students are more likely to feel like a visitor or short-stay resident (Parlett and Dearden 1977). And if they are not made to feel welcomed, or worse, if they are made to feel a burden (Phillips et al 2000), their plans, hopes and aspirations can be thwarted, and any worries and anxieties compounded by an uncongenial environment. Learning is likely to be affected in this type of environment. Learning plans may be abandoned (Boud and Walker 1990).

White and Ewan (1991) think that the differences between learning in the classroom and the clinical setting are profound – in the classroom setting, students can 'hide' behind the mantle of the group, which shields them from the close attention of the teacher. In the clinical setting, students are visible as they work closely with their mentors and members of the team. Patients and clients may be observing their performance. They can feel threatened and vulnerable, as their performance and behaviours are visible and open to the scrutiny of a range of people. It is important to recognize the differing needs of recent school leavers and mature students with, and without, nursing experience. Learners also have different learning styles – these need to be utilized to maximize student learning (McAllister 1997). Each student forms part of the educational environment, enriching it with his or her personal contribution (Boud and Walker 1990). On entry into the environment, students create interactions which become learning experiences for themselves and others. Lincoln et al (1997) believe that students who have chosen to become health care professionals tend to be committed to the ethos of caring and curing. Clinical practice provides the opportunity for students to experience their desires to care and help and to put into practice the theory they have learnt – they will be learning how to care and to develop the competencies required of a professional.

Stengelhofen (1993:48) points out that it is unfortunate if a student is not seen as a student member of the department or team. They should be viewed as valuable student members of the team with specific clinical learning needs, rather than as valuable members of the team with the emphasis on 'getting the work done' and in providing a service contribution (Melia 1987). A clinical environment that is an educational environment will be able to support students so that they achieve their personal and professional goals in the best possible ways. This seems to be in the hands of mentors and assessors – Eraut et al (1995) report that qualified clinical staff exercise a major influence on the quality of pre-registration programmes.

Students become professionals through the process of 'professional socialization', which takes place predominantly in the clinical setting (Lincoln et al 1997, McAllister 1997). They need to acquire that 'set of values, attitudes, knowledge and skills which are displayed within the culture of a profession by practising professionals' (Lincoln et al 1997:75). From their review of the literature on the components of professionalism, Lincoln et al identified the following four components:

■ technical competence
■ professional interpersonal skills, encompassing communication skills, values and attitudes of the professional
■ knowledge of professional standards of conduct
■ Ethical competence, which is essentially about moral obligation to those for whom professionals care.

It is suggested here that the patient/client care practices of a clinical environment will significantly influence the professional socialization of a student. A clinical environment that is also an educational environment needs to espouse a philosophy of care, reflected in practice, which will enable students to develop into professionals who can truly meet the needs of society for care and caring. The ENB and Department of Health (2001a) recommend that the philosophy of care should be in the form of a written statement. High standards of care need to be modelled. As discussed earlier, Orton (1981) found that wards that were highly rated by students amply met the physical and emotional needs of patients. There are other studies which have also found that students value high standards of care being modelled (Kotzabassaki et al 1997, White et al 1994). White and Ewan (1991) make the point that simply setting a good example for students to follow is not enough. Students must be encouraged to be active in experiencing, discussing and evaluating professional behaviours and care in order to extract personal meaning.

The mentors

It has long been accepted that using the 'apprenticeship' system in nursing and midwifery training is educationally unsound (Fretwell 1982, Ogier 1982, Pembrey 1980). What we know about learning in the workplace tells us that learning is ineffective if students are placed in practice environments as part of the workforce where supervision is inadequate and active facilitation of learning does not take place (Jacka and Lewin 1987, Melia 1987). Within the apprenticeship system, the clinical environment for students was in effect a working environment and not an educational environment. Project 2000 challenged the ways that students were expected to learn during clinical practice. As a consequence, students currently undertaking pre-registration programmes enjoy supernumerary status, and are supported and supervised by practitioners acting as mentors.

Much has been written about mentors and mentorship in the nursing literature (Andrews 1999). The ENB and Department of Health (2001b:9) suggest that mentors have the responsibility to:

- facilitate student learning across pre- and post-registration programmes to ensure quality learning
- supervise, support and guide students in practice
- implement approved assessment procedures
- assess competencies to demonstrate the extent to which learning outcomes have been met.

The fulfilment of these responsibilities is not so easy and straightforward and frequently causes dilemmas for the practitioner who is both mentor and assessor to the student (Neary 1997b, Holloway 1985). The ethical and legal implications of mentoring, supervising and assessing students are discussed in Chapter 2. It is well documented that effective supervision, support and facilitation of learning require the mentor to possess certain qualities and skills. Andrews (1999:204) reports that the literature contains a 'comprehensive catalogue of personal and attributes and skills required for effective mentoring'. Students have certain expectations of their mentors and find certain characteristics and behaviours in mentors helpful (Neary 1997a, 1999b, Spouse 1996, Darling 1984). A common theme is the significance of the personal and professional attributes of the mentor such as approachability, good interpersonal skills, self-confidence, respects and shows interest in students and a competent and enthusiastic practitioner. According to Neary (2000:21), the mentor who can contribute to the clinical environment so that it is an educational environment is the person who is:

- prepared to allocate both time and energy to the role
- up-to-date with professional practice and is innovative
- competent in the core skills of coaching, counselling, facilitating, giving feedback and networking
- interested and willing to help others
- willing and able to learn
- able to demonstrate the many characteristics advocated by Darling (1984).

These characteristics are described in full below to enable you to assess yourself.

Characteristics of a mentor. In her research into the characteristics that students perceive as valuable and helpful in a mentor, Lu Ann Darling (1984) has identified the following:

- a *model* the student can look up to, respect and admire
- an *envisioner* who gives a picture of what could be done, is enthusiastic about opportunities and possibilities and interest is sparked
- an *energiser* who is enthusiastic and dynamic and kindles the student's interest
- an *investor* who makes time for the student; spots potential and capabilities; trusts, 'lets go' and delegates responsibility

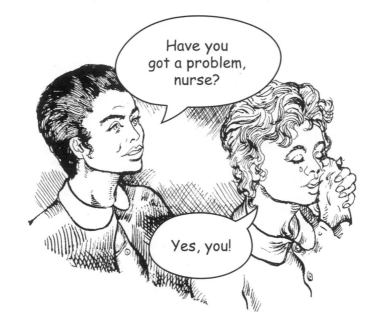

Mentors need good interpersonal skills

- a *supporter* who listens; is warm, caring and encouraging and is available in times of need
- a *standard-prodder* who is very clear about what level of achievement is required and pushes and prods the student to achieve higher standards
- a *teacher-coach* who guides on problem solving and setting priorities, helps in the development of new skills and inspires personal and professional development
- a *feedback giver* who can offer both positive and constructive feedback and helps the student explore things that go wrong
- an *eye opener* who motivates interest in new developments and research, facilitates reasoning and understanding and directs the student into seeing the bigger picture
- a *door opener* who provides opportunities for trying out new ideas and suggests and identifies resources for learning
- an *idea bouncer* who not only discusses and debates issues and ideas but clarifies and stimulates new thoughts
- a *problem solver* who is tolerant of shortcomings and skilfully uses both the strengths and weaknesses of the student to enable further development to take place
- an *educational counsellor* who is trusted; understands the student's needs to achieve and supports and guides towards success
- a *challenger* who questions opinions and beliefs; forces the student to examine choices critically whilst empowering the student towards fulfilment of her/his potential.

Mentors have their own educational experiences, knowledge base, level of competence and history of experiences of caring and practice. These variations will influence the ways individuals practise, their roles and how they view the work environment. Phillips et al (2000) found that many practitioners were enthusiastic about having students in the clinical areas and look forward to sharing knowledge and experiences. Such attitudes will clearly influence the learning climate of the area positively. There were practitioners who were so caught up with the 'busyness' of the workplace that students were viewed as an additional burden. The reality about clinical areas is that pressures, busyness and workloads are continually increasing: there is simply no time to 'teach'. And this is where the individual's beliefs about how learning takes place can influence the learning climate.

Jarvis (1983) and Rogers (1983) believe that teaching is not essential to learning. Many learners acquire knowledge, skills and attitudes independent of any formal teaching. This is not to say that teaching is unimportant but, given certain conditions, most adults engage in much more learning than is often realized and acknowledged. One way that students learn in the clinical setting is by observing their mentors as they work alongside each other. No formal teaching is done here. McLeod et al (1997:54) state that 'students learn most from observing the actions and understanding the reasoning processes of their role models'. The adage 'actions speak louder than words' aptly describes the power of role modelling, as the actions of the practitioner are probably more powerful in influencing the student than what is said, and what is said by the mentor is probably more powerful than what is said by the teacher in the classroom (Stengelhofen 1993). Charters (2000) thinks that this form of facilitating learning has been overlooked or devalued by the very practitioners who employ it. Being a role model is widely recognized as critical in teaching, coaching and shaping as it is the most powerful teaching strategy available to mentors (McLeod et al 1997). 'Attitudes take time to describe or explain, but are quickly demonstrated by every action and word' (Ogier 1989:36) – attitudes are modelled and learnt by the way the patient/client is spoken to; skills and techniques are demonstrated when care is carried out – all are ways of working and learning at the same time.

By working and talking with the student, the practitioner is teaching as well as getting the work done. Read the following extract (Examples 1 and 2) from Ogier (1989:25–26) and then tackle Activity 8.3.

1. Sister: 'Mary (student nurse), can you come here and check this controlled drug with me? Mrs Gavey last had pethidine at 6.00 am, it is now 10.00 am so she can have more.' Sister and nurse can be heard preparing syringes, counting the stock and administering the drug to Mrs Gavey. Following documentation, they clear up and go their separate ways.

2. Sister: 'Mary (student nurse), can you check this controlled drug with me? As you heard at the report, Mrs Gavey had a cholecystectomy yesterday afternoon. She last had pethidine 75 mg at 6.00 am, it is now 10.00 am and the physiotherapist is due to see her at about 10.30 am. If we give her more pethidine now, it will be working by the time the physiotherapist comes to help Mrs Gavey with her deep-breathing exercises.' While sister is talking, the injection is being prepared and the sound of syringes being unwrapped and drug cupboards being unlocked can be heard. They administer the drug and sign the documentation, and, while clearing up, sister asks Mary, 'Are you getting on all right?'

ACTIVITY 8.3

Imagine you are Mary. List what information was imparted in the interaction described in Example 1, and then do the same for Example 2. What types of interaction took place?

Giving the drug took the same length of time in each example, but in Example 2, sister was sharing her decision-making process – Why the pethidine was being given. Mary also gained an insight into the planning of more effective pain relief. She has learnt through experience, which was triggered by sister's full explanation while they worked together. Ask yourself the following questions:

- How can work be planned so that having students is a help rather than a hindrance?
- How can students be involved in care so that they are learning while contributing to the work of the team?

Learning opportunities and experiences

Patients and clients

In practice-based health care professions such as nursing and midwifery, learning must take place in the context of patient/client care. Burnard and Chapman (1990:48) made this important statement:

> The basis of clinical learning should be the process of carrying out nursing with patients. The one thing that is always missing in the School of Nursing and always present in the clinical setting is the presence of patients. Encounters with patients, whatever the clinical setting, should always form the basis of learning.

We have the difficulty of not being able to control these learning opportunities as we cannot prescribe which patients or clients will be in the clinical area. However, we know the nature of the conditions, illnesses or problems of our patients and clients who require our care in any given clinical setting. On this basis, the learning opportunities and clinical experiences which can be provided for students in each setting can be determined. Using these learning opportunities, learning contracts and assessment plans (see Chapter 6) can be developed to meet the needs of the student. Although these plans provide the structure to assist the student achieve learning outcomes, the control and predictability of experiences is unlikely to be possible. Each patient or client is different and each has varied needs that require different care and management. The condition of the patient/client could alter, sometimes dramatically. These differences and the unplanned and unpredictable events are learning opportunities which can be capitalized upon. The way that the mentor responds to an unprecedented clinical event is a learning opportunity in itself. White and Ewan (1991:138) remind us that 'opportunistic teaching is not dependent on the ease of availability of interesting or unusual events but on making opportunities for students to learn'. Opportunistic experiences emerge as the realities of clinical practice unfold. These authors go on to say that the 'ability to see opportunities and use them distinguishes [mentors] as persons with ingenuity and flair' (White and Ewan 1991:138). For example, during the course of performing 'routine' pressure area care with the student, there are opportunities for: involving the student actively in the care of the patient/client by, for example, inviting the student's opinions on the condition of the skin and how the student would manage the situation; pointing out the warning signs of impending practice sore development which the student may not have seen; discussing evidence-based management of pressure areas to prevent pressure sores; the policy of the clinical setting or hospital for the management of patients/clients at risk of developing pressure sores; and so on. If a relative is present who wishes to be involved in the care of the patient/client, involving the relative with caregiving will show the student how this is done and the role of family members when a relative requires care. Subsequently, discussions with the student on this aspect of care will reinforce learning.

You may wish to try Activity 8.4 to help you consider the vast range of activities related to direct patient/client care which are some of the learning opportunities present in your clinical setting.

Remember that it is not only the direct 'encounters' with patients and clients which are the learning opportunities for students. Other examples of learning opportunities provided by patient/client encounters could be the way you plan and manage your workload; the way you plan care; how you make decisions; and how you handle different situations, particularly difficult ones. Chamberlain (1997) found that one strategy student midwives used to obtain information was to listen to their midwives' interactions with each other, clients and doctors.

Total patient/client care gives students the opportunity to observe and participate in the provision and delivery of holistic care. Patient/client and staff satisfaction is generally higher with this method of care delivery, which can only contribute to a positive learning climate. Students can learn, for example, the importance of good team working within a multi-professional team, the range of caregiving activities a patient/client requires and how to coordinate these and how to meet the total needs of a patient/client. These are also opportunities for students to realize that an acquisition of technical competence is not enough for professional practice as a nurse or midwife. It was Virginia Henderson (1966) who very profoundly said that 'nursing is of the head and of the hands and of the heart'.

Other clinical activities

Other than the learning opportunities provided by direct patient/client contact, there is generally a huge range of activities in any clinical setting which are learning opportunities for students to participate in. More often than not, engagement in these activities can generate evidence of competence. Students need to be directed to these activities and assisted to draw up the aims and learning out-

ACTIVITY 8.4

Make a list of the patients/clients you have looked after during your last three spans of duty. Make a list of their conditions, illnesses, and problems that they had presented you with. How did you deal with their range of needs?

The clinical environment 197

ACTIVITY 8.5

Make a list of those activities and events which have taken place during the last 3 days you were on duty. Go on to make another list of those activities and events which you consider to be learning opportunities for students.

comes in order to derive meaningful learning from participating in these activities. You may wish to try Activity 8.5 to help you consider the vast range of other activities which can be learning opportunities for students working in your clinical setting.

White and Ewan (1991) made the observation that students make the surprising but not infrequent comment that they have 'nothing to do' during clinical placements. We need to pause to consider the undertones of this comment. Students frequently equate real learning with actively 'doing'. When the pace is slower and events less dramatic, students may wonder how such experiences contribute to their preparation for competence. Activities which are not directly related to patient/client care may not be viewed as learning opportunities. This is where a list of activities and events with their potential for learning can be useful in directing and guiding students to other sources of learning that contribute to their overall professional development. Some suggestions of activities and events which students can be directed to in most clinical settings and which should be considered to be part of the educational environment – there will be others that will be specific to your own clinical environment – are given below:

1. *Learning and gaining insight about the work of the multi-professional team*: The activities for the student could be to:
   - observe several different professionals working
   - liaise and communicate with a number of different professionals
   - going on ward rounds
   - attending case conferences and seminars
   - attending staff meetings.

2. *Learning communication skills within the nursing/midwifery team, the multi-professional team and with other carers*: The activities for the student could be to:
   - Liaise and communicate with a number of different nurses/midwives, other professionals, including those who provide support services such as pharmacists, and technicians and other carers such as relatives and friends of the patient/client and members of voluntary organizations.
   - Use the telephone to communicate with a range of people. This activity may appear simple but can be anxiety provoking for the student who has to speak in public, to someone unknown to the student, and the student may fear not having the answers and thus feel foolish.
   - Participate in ward handovers, ward rounds, case conferences, seminars, staff meetings. The requirement to speak during these events can be anxiety provoking – students need to be encouraged and supported to develop the courage and skills of speaking and voicing their opinions during these events.
   - Report back to staff on the outcomes of treatment and care given, both verbally and through written reports.

3. *Acquiring administrative and management experience*:   The activities for the student could be to:
   - organize the transfer of patients/clients to other units and agencies
   - organize the discharge of patients/clients, including hospital transport if required
   - order equipment
   - manage own workload. Workload should be incremental and commensurate with the student's experience and stage of training. The aim is to prepare the student so that transition to the role of nurse or midwife is accomplished at the point of registration
   - coordinate the work of the team where appropriate.

4. *Learning about records and record keeping*:   The activities for the student could be to:
   - find out about the handling and storage of case notes
   - retrieve case notes
   - file patient/client reports
   - write in the nursing/midwifery records and other sections of case notes as required
   - extract from and input into computerized record systems.

5. *Learning to use equipment*:   The use of equipment should be demonstrated and followed by immediate supervised practice. Opportunities to handle and use the equipment during patient/client care should be provided as soon as possible. Repeated practice will help the student acquire dexterity, confidence and consistent performance.

6. *Accessing teaching/learning sessions*:   Many clinical areas have these sessions, such as scheduled lectures, seminars, case conferences, demonstration of new equipment by company representatives and teaching ward rounds. Students should be directed to these sessions, as appropriate, and time made available for them to attend these sessions.

When considering the learning opportunities in your clinical setting, it may be useful to remember that 'while students have control over what they want to learn, they have limited control over access to opportunities for learning' (Chamberlain 1997:85). This means that opportunities for learning should be planned so that students can be directed to them and supported while they are learning. This strategy can only contribute to the educational environment in creating an ambience for learning.

Staff commitment to teaching and learning

Support and supervision of learners

Phillips et al (2000) commented that the role of students can be an uncomfortable one – their behaviour and performance are under constant surveillance for what they show about their character and competence. It is widely acknowledged that during clinical placements students experience anxiety and stress for a wide range of reasons. Beginning students are particularly vulnerable. In a Canadian study, Beck and Srivastava (1991) found that when compared with the general population, nursing students were at greater risk of having a physical or psychological illness. Sources of anxiety and stress include:

- Working with dying patients (Parkes 1985)
- Interpersonal conflict with mentors and other practitioners (Jackson and Mannix 2001, Chamberlain 1997, Parkes 1985)
- Insecurity about personal clinical competence (Chamberlain 1997, Parkes 1985)
- Performing intimate care and caring for someone of the opposite sex (Seed 1995)
- Fear of failure (Jones and Johnston 1997, Williams 1993, Parkes 1985).
- Fear of making mistakes (Williams 1993, Kleehammer et al 1990).
- Changes in ward allocation (Phillips et al 2000, Jack 1992). Terms such as 'scary', 'frightening', 'terrified', and 'anxious' were used to describe their early days in practice placements (Phillips et al 2000:71).

Many of the above studies also found that stress and anxiety were heightened when staff were unfriendly, unsupportive and did not make the students feel welcomed. It is important to remember that during clinical placements students are usually removed from their peer support group. Phillips et al's (2000) study showed that the students' chief concern was being made to feel welcome and having time set aside to discuss their learning needs. Students in Jackson and Mannix's (2001) study found the single most helpful behaviour was being recognized as newcomers and shown understanding for their tentativeness and feelings of insecurity. Jackson and Mannix (2001:274) also found students greatly appreciated any interest shown in them and their learning and liked to be given some degree of responsibility. They quoted one student:

> I felt useful, because she loaded me with work that I was capable of doing, such as making beds, observations, assisting with hygiene and communicating with the patients. At the end of the day she would ask me questions about the things she had taught me. I found it very rewarding and helpful to my learning.

It is generally accepted that a degree of anxiety is a healthy basis for growth and development (Lincoln et al 1997). Indeed, we should be perturbed if students had no concerns at all before beginning a placement or throughout a placement. However, there is a curvilinear relationship between anxiety and learning. Decreased learning occurs in the presence of high anxiety (Eysenck 1970 and Spielberger 1966 in Kleehammer et al 1990). In the context of clinical learning, Nolan (1998:626) found that 'until students feel accepted learning cannot proceed, as fitting-in takes up most of their time and energy'. Work on humanistic approaches to facilitating learning tells us that adults learn best in an environment that is psychologically comfortable where there is mutual trust and respect for their own worth and that of others (Knowles 1990, Brookfield 1986, Rogers 1983).

The following are some typical questions that students will ask prior to a clinical placement. These questions are based upon and extended from the work of Stengelhofen (1993) and Boud et al (1985).

ACTIVITY 8.6

Ponder for a few minutes upon the questions below. How do you think a student new to your clinical area might feel?

- What will my role be?
- What will be expected of me?
- How much am I expected to know?
- How will I know how I am doing?
- What are the demands of that setting?
- What will I learn?
- What will the people be like?
- Will they like me? Will I like them? Will I get on with my mentor?

The answers that students seek to these questions could form the basis for the support and supervision that will contribute to the clinical placement being an educational experience for students. You may wish to try Activity 8.6.

Information pack.   Work which has been done into what helps students learn during clinical placements tells us that making students feel welcome is a prerequisite to creating an atmosphere conducive to learning. Ideally, this 'welcome' should start prior to the commencement of the placement in the form of an information pack sent to the student. Stengelhofen (1993:73) makes an important point:

> Providing students with a clear picture of the clinical setting and the cases within that setting, as well as identifying the learning outcomes for them, appropriate to the stage of the course, will be a way of reassuring them that they will not be required to do anything or take responsibility beyond what can legitimately be expected.

An information pack could include, for example:

- A welcome letter. This letter can also contain information to encourage the student to visit the placement prior to starting to meet the mentor and see what learning opportunities are available
- Maps of the locality and/or the hospital
- Facilities such as catering, parking, social and sporting
- Staff profile, including members of the multi-professional team
- The allocated mentor with contact details
- Clinical area profile, such as the philosophy, any nursing/midwifery model in use, the types of patients/clients seen and treatments offered
- A list of learning opportunities
- A list of learning outcomes
- The roles and responsibilities of students in that clinical setting (this may need to be tailored for individual students depending on their prior experiences and stage of training)
- Guidelines on dress.

When pre-placement information packs are provided, important points can be assimilated by the student prior to commencement of the placement. This helps to reduce information overload during the early stages of the placement.

BOX 8.1	*Example of welcome letter (from Stengelhofen 1993)*

Dear

We hope that you will enjoy your placement with us.

The attached information pack is designed to help you understand how our service works, what we have to offer you while you are with us and what we expect from your college. Please read it before your first day. We will go over any queries you may have when we see you, but if you have any urgent questions you can telephone me on _____.

Please confirm that you are starting your placement with us on _____. We suggest that you arrive at _____. Before your arrival it would help us in planning your time if you could send us some information about yourself. We would like to know a little about your background, your academic interests, previous clinical experience and your objectives for this placement.

We look forward to meeting you. Involvement in student training is an enjoyable and stimulating, as well as a time-consuming experience for us. We expect to learn from you as well as with you and we hope that you will be happy with us.

Subsequently, the information is on record for reference. Box 8.1 is an example of a welcome letter extracted from Stengelhofen (1993:68). There are other examples in her text. It is suggested that you draft one to suit your own clinical setting.

Receiving the student.   Some hospitals have student support officers who make arrangements to meet all students on the first day of their placement. A programme of orientation for the day introduces the student to the hospital and its various departments, their key functions and personnel. Arrangements are made for the students to be 'collected' by their mentors or a member of the ward team later in the day, and the students are subsequently orientated to their allocated placement (Hopkins 2000). Hopkins briefs the allocated mentor who has a particular role in receiving the student and orientating the student to the work setting. When the placement is the first one for a student, mentors are reminded to take particular care as the student may be highly anxious. There is no doubt that first impressions will influence the student's enjoyment of the placement (Stengelhofen 1993) and may even shape the student's views of nursing and midwifery. It is important to have a plan for the first day. This might include:

- Setting some time aside to welcome the student. It is sensible to start the student on a first shift at a later time than is the routine, preferably after the hustle and bustle of the shift has been dealt with
- Orientation to health and safety matters (see Chapter 2)
- Orientation to the work place, such as the general layout of the clinical area, working patterns – shift hours, meal breaks
- Introduction to team members
- Showing where information sources are kept, such as placement philosophy and policy and procedure manuals
- Showing communication systems, such as telephones and answering protocols, patient/client buzzer system and emergency call system

- Spending time to discuss the student's learning needs and previous experiences. Students' self-esteem is increased if they feel they can share any previously acquired learning with practitioners (Stengelhofen 1993). It should be made clear to students what their roles and responsibilities are and when they should or should not help or participate. Most beginning students breathe a big sigh of relief when they are told that they are not expected to start to give care and reassured that they will only be asked to do what they are capable of doing
- Taking prior learning into account, jointly develop an action plan for the duration of the placement.

Providing ongoing support and supervision. The mentor who exhibits the characteristics that students perceive as valuable and helpful (Darling 1984) will most certainly be providing the support and supervision desired by students to help them learn. Ongoing support and supervision should aim to facilitate learning. Stengelhofen (1993) and White and Ewan (1991) suggest the following activities for the facilitation of learning in the clinical setting:

1. Answer questions – make students feel free to ask questions and to seek help without loss of confidence or self-esteem.
2. Offer suggestions – be careful to foster students' self-confidence. Rogers (1983) suggested that when the student is moving from exploration into understanding, the facilitator responds directly to the content the student is struggling with, e.g. by giving direct answers. When the student starts to focus on actions that can be taken, the facilitator moves into guiding further development of the student's skills and knowledge.
3. Allow students to make choices about client care – do not limit and constrain the student to your experience.
4. Facilitating desired behaviours – the mentor is reminded that role modelling is one powerful tool for this purpose.
5. Encourage self-monitoring and evaluation – help students identify where they have reached in their learning and help students develop the ability to assess their performance accurately and subsequently set realistic learning goals.
6. Provide opportunities and guidelines for observation (guidelines for observation are discussed in Chapter 9).
7. Learn from the students – listen to the students and facilitate two-way discussions. Rogers (1983) suggested that facilitators need to be able to respond to the feelings of students as they explore learning experiences together.
8. Give students time to reflect on what is happening and has happened – promote discussion about patient/client care.
9. Give students time to prepare – when assigning work to students, spend time briefing them and allocate time for them to prepare to give care. These points are developed in Chapter 9.
10. Allow students to make mistakes in the confines of patient safety – show confidence in students and give positive reinforcement; reinforce the expectation of success. Allow 'hands on' experience even when you think

the task is complex. Manipulate the session to allow students to experience success.

11. Encourage students to think for themselves – structure and sequence questions so that students are led through their own paths of thinking to show how they came to a certain conclusion. Questions should therefore challenge students to trace their own thinking strategies and to explain how they drew inferences or came to certain conclusions.

The following questions may help you evaluate whether students are receiving adequate support and supervision:

1. How do I help students settle into the workplace?
2. What do I do to make their first days more enjoyable?
3. How do I make their placement an educational experience?
4. How do I help students feel confident about their role?
5. Do students in my area feel valued and respected?
6. When students are unhappy at work, do I know the contributory factors?

Continuing professional development

When the clinical environment provides a culture where learning and professional development take place, it becomes a positive learning environment where the atmosphere becomes one where there is a commitment to lifelong learning. Staff develop a commitment to seek to learn for themselves and to share their learning with one another. There is encouragement to undertake further formal education through accredited courses and informal in-house training. 'Lifelong learning' is the term used to refer to the planned or unplanned learning that occurs throughout the life, usually the working life, of an individual (Hinchliff 1998). The undertaking of further education is indeed necessary as professional nurses and midwives cannot hope to practise safely and effectively in a context of continuous change without undertaking updating activities. The importance of continuing professional development (CPD) was recognized by the UKCC and endorsed by the NMC (2002a) in the *Code of Professional Conduct*. In paragraph 3 of *The Scope of Professional Practice*, the UKCC (1992) stated:

> Pre-registration education prepares nurses, midwives and health visitors for safe practice at the point of registration . . . [It] is therefore a foundation for professional practice . . . This foundation education alone, however, cannot effectively meet the changing and complex demands of the range of modern health care. Post-registration education equips practitioners with additional and more specialist skills necessary to meet the special needs of patients and clients.

In its post-registration education and practice project (PREPP), the UKCC (1990, endorsed by the NMC 2002a) saw CPD as fulfilling three functions:

1. updating and extending the professional's knowledge and skills on new developments and new areas of practice so as to ensure continuing competence in the job
2. training for new responsibilities and for a changing role, such as developing new areas of competence in preparation for a more senior post

3. developing personal and professional effectiveness and increasing job satisfaction.

One of the UKCC's (1997) statutory post-registration education and practice (PREP) requirements is that every practitioner must undertake CPD and maintain a personal professional profile containing details of professional development. An important question about mandatory professional development needs to be asked here: Does mandatory professional development serve to inculcate the sense of what Houle (1980:124) termed a 'zest for learning' possessed by an individual, which ultimately controls the amount and kind of education that is undertaken? Depending on their zest for learning, practitioners can be placed in one of four groups:

- *innovators*: a small but highly active group who constantly seek to improve their job performance; they try out new ideas, regularly take up educational opportunities and enjoy independent learning and full-time study
- *pacesetters*: they are not the first to try out new ideas, but are strongly committed to professional ideals and continuing education
- *middle majority*: the bulk of practitioners, whose attitudes to continuing education vary from enthusiasm to apathy
- *laggards*: those practitioners who do the minimum necessary and resist both learning and new ideas.

Factors which determine an individual's zest for learning are invariably complex. It is suggested here that a clinical environment that provides a positive ambience for learning will contribute greatly to the motivation of staff for life-long learning and CPD. It is important to question how CPD can be encouraged in the clinical setting. Are there activities in your clinical area that you think would contribute to the CPD of staff? It is important to utilize learning opportunities in the workplace – not only is such learning directly relevant to practice but also there can be many constraints on the availability and accessibility of formal courses in a resource-limited system. It is my belief that you and your colleagues, including members of the multi-professional team and unqualified staff members, are the most important teaching and learning resource in your work area. The following questions are intended to help you explore how the 'human resource' for learning can be used to contribute to your clinical setting as one that motivates staff to engage in CPD:

- How can you contribute? How much do you contribute? Remember that your contributions such as developing a teaching/learning pack can be used as evidence of continuing professional development for PREP.
- How can your colleagues and members of the multi-professional team contribute? How much do they contribute? Do not forget unqualified staff members – someone may have a personal health experience which they can talk about.
- Are there planned teaching programmes? When this is an established routine, staff will be encouraged to contribute and attend.
- After staff have been on study days and courses, is there a mechanism for the dissemination of information? This can serve several purposes – it helps the individual learn further through teaching or preparing a paper, and brings what is learnt to the clinical area to improve professional practices.

- Are there staff support groups where staff get together to debrief and reflect? Sharing ideas and experiences in a group is an effective way of developing practice wisdom – wisdom being the distillation of knowledge and experience (Hull 1998).
- Are there activities such as case discussions and conferences and seminars? If you have cared for the patient/client featured in the case you will be able to contribute to the discussion. Subsequently, if what you have learnt is written up, preferably supported by literature, it is again evidence of continuing professional development.

Material resources

Having examined how the human resource can make direct contributions to the learning environment of the clinical setting, we now need to consider those non-human resources which can contribute to the learning environment. You may wish to try Activity 8.7. The following questions may guide you in your 'walk-about':

- Do you have a resource room/area where text material such as books and journals can be housed? If not, is it possible to make space for one? This resource area could also house contributions such as learning packages and posters developed by staff after they have been on study days and courses.
- If you have a resource room/area, is the area conducive to reading, browsing and study? For example, is text material shelved and filed in some kind of order; is it up-to-date; is the area generally tidy; is there some fairly comfortable seating; and so on?
- Is there someone who is designated to 'maintain' this area? Staff could take it in turns and be given time out to perform this function, such as going to the library to seek out relevant journal articles and do the general 'housekeeping'.
- Are there places such as notice boards where information such as flyers about courses, teaching/learning events and so on can be displayed? If not, is it possible to find a suitable wall space for a notice/pin board to be installed? These are generally not too costly.
- Are policy and procedure manuals up-to-date? Are they in an accessible location?
- Is there a collection of material such as health promotion leaflets and so on from both charitable and government organizations relevant to your clinical area? These are frequently free and provide useful information for both patients/clients and staff.

- If there are audiovisual aids such as videos and cassette tapes, are they still up-to-date? Is the equipment for using these aids in good working order?
- Are there other teaching/learning aids such as models and mannequins? Are they in good order?
- Are information technology facilities available to access electronic sources of information from the Internet, databases or CD-rom teaching/learning packages? If these are available, are staff conversant with the usage of information technology?

QUALITY ASSURANCE

As can be seen from the exploration of the clinical setting as an environment for learning, there are many factors which influence and interact with each other to impact on this learning environment. These factors and the concomitant processes arising consequent to the interaction of these factors should not be left to chance – they need to be worked at to ensure that there are positive influences. Higher education institutions, in partnership with their service colleagues, need to work together to ensure that high-quality practice placements, in a supportive environment, help students achieve the learning outcomes of their educational programme and ensure that they are able to provide the care needed by patients and clients (ENB and Department of Health 2001a). The ENB and Department of Health (2001a:8) go on to point out that higher education institutions and service providers are 'responsible for the quality of learning opportunities provided for students'. To this end, the ENB has already made it a requirement that assessment of the quality of practice placement experience is incorporated into every quality assurance process within the quality assurance framework that guides the educational practices of higher education institutions (ENB 1998).

Quality assurance can be viewed simply as comprising all those activities in an organization which help to identify and promote good practice and prevent poor practice (ENB 1993). It is now widely accepted that quality can be achieved and maintained through the use of audit, which has become the most prominent and important mechanism for improving the quality of health and education sector services (Nicklin and Kenworthy 1995). In its publication on educational audit, the ENB (1993:12) went on to say that 'educational audit involves monitoring, measuring and evaluating educational provision'. Thus, the educational audit of clinical placement areas should be in terms of 'the standards of care and service provision and the learning environment, to facilitate their continuing suitability for students' practice experience' (ENB and Department of Health 2001a:11). The ENB and Department of Health go on to say that the outcomes of audit and monitoring should lead to the dissemination of good practice and joint action planning between placement providers and higher education institutions to address any areas of concern or those needing enhancement. When we attempt to judge the quality of the students' experiences, White and Ewan (1991:160) say that 'only the students are capable of judging the value of the experience since they are the ones having the experience'. The ENB and Department of Health (2001a) reinforce the importance of actively solicit-

ACTIVITY 8.8

Obtain a copy of the tool for the educational audit of your clinical area. What are the aspects of the clinical environment that are audited? How well do they reflect the clinical environment that is an educational environment?

ing student feedback, which should contribute to the ongoing evaluation of the learning environment.

Criteria for educational audit

You may wish to try Activity 8.8.

In 1993 the ENB proposed the use of the following eight aspects, with their associated criteria, for auditing practice placements. Although published in 1993, these aspects are still relevant today.

1. *Ethos of the placement*:
   - general climate
   - channels of communication
   - approachability of staff
   - relationships between the higher education institution and the placement
   - commitment to teaching and learning.

2. *Organization of care*:
   - philosophy and approach to care
   - the organization of workload so as to promote continuity, e.g. team nursing
   - involvement of students in multi-professional teamwork.

3. *Supervision and mentorship*:
   - effectiveness of supervision and mentorship by first-level practitioners
   - contribution by academic staff
   - fulfilment of clinical contact hours
   - compliance with regulations in supervision and assessment of students.

4. *Teaching programme and assessment*:
   - planned programmes
   - opportunities for students to achieve competencies through continuous assessment
   - learning outcomes set at appropriate academic and professional levels
   - patient/client groups support achievement of learning outcomes.

5. *Research basis of care planning and delivery*:
   - evidence of the application of research in teaching and implementation of care

6. *Academic and professional qualifications of staff*

7. *Staff development programmes*

8. *Physical environment*

To these should be added the following three aspects.

9. *Teaching/learning resources and strategies*:
- a designated study area
- a range of teaching/learning resources are provided
- there is availability of information technology with access to electronic sources of information
- teaching/learning strategies practised to help students relate theory to practice and reflect on care given.

10. *Management of the learning environment*: There is a designated learning environment manager who:
- has overall responsibility for all teaching/learning activities and the learning environment
- liaises with the clinical link lecturer
- supports mentors and assessors.

11. *The clinical link lecturer*. There is a designated clinical link lecturer from the higher education institution who liaises with placement staff to ensure effective implementation of the curriculum by:
- providing support and guidance for staff and students
- acting as a resource for educational activities such as compiling a profile of learning opportunities.

In a later publication, the ENB and Department of Health (2001a) provide what I see as a useful checklist containing key questions which address the planning, provision and evaluation of practice placement experiences. This checklist is reproduced in Appendix 13.

The process of educational audit

Generally, prior to a clinical area being used as a placement area for pre-registration students, an educational audit of that area is required to ensure that it is able to support student learning. Subsequently, the area is audited formally at least annually. Typically, this is done by the learning environment manager and the clinical link lecturer. However, it should also be conducted whenever the circumstances of the clinical setting changes, such as a reduction of bed numbers and the type of patients/clients cared for. Nicklin and Kenworthy (1995) suggest that when a clinical area is consistently rated negatively by students or if there is a high sickness or absence rate amongst students, an educational audit should be carried out for diagnostic purposes.

You may want to try Activity 8.9.

One higher education institution, in collaboration with its service colleagues, requires students to complete a questionnaire at the end of each placement. Staff

ACTIVITY 8.9

How do you, your colleagues and students contribute to the educational audit of your clinical area? How is your clinical link lecturer involved?

complete a questionnaire once a year. The responses of students are collated half-yearly, and yearly, with the responses from staff. The items on the questionnaire may take the form of that used by Orton et al (1993): she and her colleagues developed an instrument which enables the quality of the learning climate to be assessed quantitatively. In brief, ward learning climate indicators are used to measure six key areas that characterize a good ward learning climate:

- orientation to the placement
- theory and practice
- supernumerary status
- staff attitudes and behaviour
- the mentor
- progressive assessments.

Each key area has several indicators. The indicators are the quality statements which define a good ward learning climate. Each indicator is scored numerically from 0 to 3: 0 represents a low learning climate and 3 represents a high learning climate. The calculation and charting of the scores are done by a software package. The scores of the six indicators and how they are charted for the key area of *orientation to the placement* are shown in Figure 8.1 (the indicators for the other five key areas are shown in Appendix 14).

The sum total of the scores for each key area can also be calculated and charted in a summary chart shown in Figure 8.2.

Responses to Orton's questionnaire will only contribute to the overall educational audit. The overall educational audit requires the clinical environment to be monitored and assessed much more comprehensively. One advantage of being able to see, in chart form, how one's clinical area has scored as a learning environment may serve to motivate staff to carry on the good work or to start to make changes to improve the learning climate.

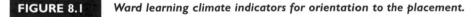

FIGURE 8.1   *Ward learning climate indicators for orientation to the placement.*

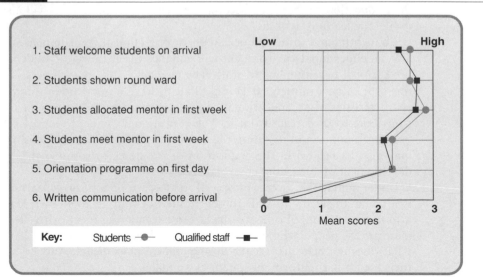

| FIGURE 8.2 | *Ward learning climate indicators for summary.* |

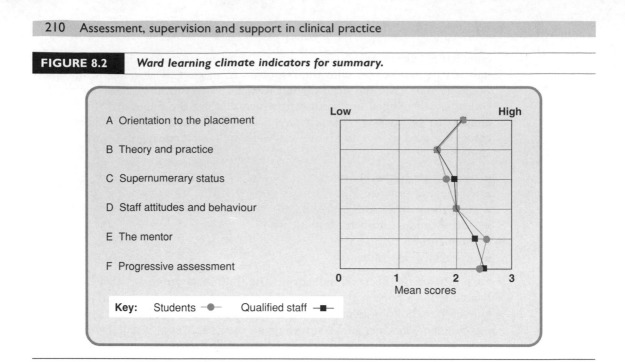

CONCLUSION

What helps students learn and develop into the professional we desire them to be? Clinical settings provide unique learning experiences and opportunities for students – these must be planned, structured, managed and coordinated (ENB and Department of Health 2001a) so that students undergo professional socialization positively and develop the competencies for professional practice which cannot be readily acquired elsewhere. The clinical experience for students should be much more than just learning what to do and how to do it – it should be about the education of students who will one day be our professional peers, colleagues and co-learners. Clinical placements for students should contribute to their education so that they become self-directed learners who will also engage in lifelong learning with us.

Thoughtful and informed development of a clinical environment so that it is also an educational environment will enhance the learning of students and the professional development of staff. The challenge for practitioners is to create this type of environment. It is important to have a good understanding of the characteristics of an educational clinical environment and those factors which contribute to or detract from it. The educational audit of clinical placements helps us monitor and maintain the quality of placement areas. This mechanism may also be helpful in the acquisition of resources to support the continuing development of a learning environment.

Underpinning the success of any efforts to develop a positive learning climate is a commitment by all staff to contribute not only to their own learning but also to the learning of others – the key to engendering this positive learning climate are the people who work in the setting. Students will tell us what does and what does not help them learn during clinical placements. And we should use their feedback to inform any changes we make.

I would like to end this chapter with a short excerpt from Helen Orton's book titled *Ward Learning Climate*. Although her book was published in 1981, I believe that what she wrote in this excerpt is equally true, if not more so, for today's health care climate (Orton 1981:67).

> . . . patient well-being and student well-being have been shown to be inextricably bound together. In terms of potential improvement for either group it is probably not important whether the motive for change stems from a desire to enrich ward experience for patients or for students. What is now certain is that the encouragement and development of 'good' learning climates would bring improvements for all those involved in ward life and that the benefits could be measured not only in economic terms but also by the increase in human happiness and well-being.

REFERENCES

Andrews M (1999) Mentorship in nursing: a review of the literature. *Journal of Advanced Nursing*, **29**(1), 201–207.

Beck DL and Srivastava R (1991) Perceived level and sources of stress in baccalaureate nursing students. *Journal of Nursing Education*, **30**(3), 127–133.

Boud D and Walker D (1990) Making the most of experience. *Studies in Continuing Education*, **12**(2), 61–80.

Boud D, Keogh R and Walker D (1985) Promoting reflection in learning. In Boud D, Keogh R and Walker D (eds) *Reflection: Turning Experience into Learning*, pp 18–40. London: Kogan Page.

Brookfield S (1986) *Understanding and Facilitating Adult Learning: A Comprehensive Analysis of Principles and Effective Practices*. Milton Keynes: Open University Press.

Burnard P and Chapman CM (1990) *Nurse Education: The Way Forward*. London: Scutari Press.

Chamberlain M (1997) Challenges of clinical learning for student midwives. *Midwifery*, **13**, 85–91.

Charters A (2000) Encouraging student centred learning in a clinical environment. *Emergency Nurse*, **7**(10), 25–29.

Darling LA (1984) What do nurses want in a mentor? *Journal of Nursing Administration*, **14**(10), 42–44.

Department of Health (2001) *Working Together – Learning Together*. London: Department of Health

Dunn SV and Burnett P (1995) The development of a clinical learning environment scale. *Journal of Advanced Nursing*, **22**, 1166–1173.

ENB and Department of Health (2001a) *Placements in Focus*. London: The English National Board for Nursing, Midwifery and Health Visiting and The Department of Health.

ENB and Department of Health (2001b) *Preparation of Mentors and Teachers*. London: The English National Board for Nursing, Midwifery and Health Visiting and The Department of Health.

ENB (1998) *Quality Assurance Manual*. London: English National Board for Nursing, Midwifery and Health Visiting.

ENB (1993) *Guidelines for Educational Audit*. London: English National Board for Nursing, Midwifery and Health Visiting.

ENB (1986) *Guidelines to Preparing Continuous Assessment*, Circular 1986 (16) ERBD. London: English National Board for Nursing, Midwifery and Health Visiting.

Eraut M, Alderton J, Boylan A and Wraight A (1995) *An Evaluation of the Contribution of the Biological and Social Sciences to Pre-registration Nursing and Midwifery Programmes*. London: The English National Board for Nursing, Midwifery and Health Visiting and The Department of Health.

Eysenck MW (1970) Anxiety, learning and memory: a reconceptualisation. *Journal of Research in Personality*, **13**, 365–385.

Fraser D (1994) *Evaluation of the non-midwifery placements in a pre-registration midwifery education programme*. M.Phil, Nottingham, University of Nottingham.

Fretwell JE (1982) *Ward Teaching and Learning: Sister and the Learning*

Environment. RCN Research Series. London: Royal College of Nursing.

Gilmour A (1999) *Report of the Analysis of the Literature Evaluating Pre-registration Nursing and Midwifery Educators in the United Kingdom*. London: United Kingdom Central Council for Nursing, Midwifery and Health Visiting.

Henderson V (1966) *The Nature of Nursing*. New York: Macmillan.

Hinchliff S (1998) Lifelong learning in context. In Quinn FM (ed) *Continuing Professional Development in Nursing*, pp 34–58. Cheltenham: Stanley Thornes (Publishers).

Holloway D (1985) Accountability in further education: teachers' perceptions. *Journal of Further and Higher Education*, 9(2), 31–45.

Hopkins S (2000) Support for students. *Nursing Management*, 7(7), 36–37.

Houle C (1980) *Continuing Learning in the Professions*. San Francisco: Jossey-Bass.

Hull C (1998) Open learning and professional development. In Quinn FM (ed) *Continuing Professional Development in Nursing*, pp 182–204. Cheltenham: Stanley Thornes (Publishers).

Jack B (1992) Ward changes and stress in student nurses. *Nursing Times*, 88(10), 51.

Jacka K and Lewin D (1987) *The Clinical Learning of Student Nurses*. NERU Report No. 6. London: Nursing Educational Research Unit, Kings College, University of London.

Jackson D and Mannix J (2001) Clinical nurses as teachers: insights from students of nursing in their first semester of study. *Journal of Clinical Nursing*, 10, 270–277.

Jarvis P (1983) *Adult and Continuing Education: Theory and Practice*. Beckenham: Croom Helm.

Jones MC and Johnston DW (1997) Distress, stress and coping in first-year student nurses. *Journal of Advanced Nursing*, 28, 475–482.

Jowett S, Walton I and Payne S (1994) *Challenge and Change in Nurse Education: A Study of the Implementation of Project 2000*. Slough: National Foundation for Educational Research.

Kleehammer K, Hart AL and Keck JF (1990) Nursing students' perceptions of anxiety producing situations in the clinical setting. *Journal of Nursing Education*, 29(40), 183–187.

Knowles M (1990) *The Adult Learner: A Neglected Species*, 4th edn. Houston: Gulf Publishing.

Kotzabassaki S, Panou M and Dimou F et al. (1997) Nursing students' and faculty perceptions of the characteristics of 'best' and 'worst' clinical teachers: a replication study. *Journal of Advanced Nursing*, 26, 817–824.

Lincoln M, Carmody D and Maloney D (1997) Professional development of students and clinical educators. In McAllister L, Lincoln M, McLeod S and Maloney D (eds) *Facilitating Learning in Clinical Settings*, pp 65–98. Cheltenham: Stanley Thornes (Publishers).

McAllister L (1997) An adult learning framework for clinical education. In McAllister L, Lincoln M, McLeod S and Maloney D (eds) *Facilitating Learning in Clinical Settings*, pp 1–26. Cheltenham: Stanley Thornes (Publishers).

McLeod S, Romanini J and Cohn E et al. (1997) Models and roles in clinical education. In McAllister L, Lincoln M, McLeod S and Maloney D (eds) *Facilitating Learning in Clinical Settings*, pp 27–64. Cheltenham: Stanley Thornes (Publishers).

Marton F, Hounsell D and Entwistle N (1984) *The Experience of Learning*. Edinburgh: Scottish Academic Press.

Melia K (1987) *Working and Learning*. London: Tavistock.

Neary M (2000) *Teaching, Assessing and Evaluation for Clinical Competence*. Cheltenham: Stanley Thornes (Publishers).

Neary M (1997a) Defining the role of assessors, mentors and supervisors: part I. *Nursing Standard*, 11(42), 34–39.

Neary M (1997b) Defining the role of assessors, mentors and supervisors: part II. *Nursing Standard*, 11(43), 34–38.

Nicklin PJ and Kenworthy N (1995) *Teaching and Assessing in Clinical Practice*, 2nd edn. London: Baillière Tindall.

Nolan C (1998) Clinical education: a system under pressure. *Australian Nursing Journal*, 3(9), 20–24.

Nursing and Midwifery Council (2002a) *Code of Professional Conduct*. London: Nursing and Midwifery Council.

Nursing and Midwifery Council (2002b) *The PREP Handbook*. London: Nursing and Midwifery Council.

Ogier M (1989) *Working and Learning*. London: Scutari Press.

Ogier ME (1982) *An Ideal Sister? A Study of the Leadership Style and Verbal Interactions of Ward Sister with Nurse Learners in General Hospitals*. RCN Research Series. London: Royal College of Nursing.

Orton HD (1981) *Ward Learning Climate*. London: Royal College of Nursing.

Orton HD, Prowse J and Millen C (1993) *Charting the Way to Excellence*. Sheffield Hallam University: Pavic Publications.

Parlett MR and Dearden GJ (1977) Experiences of teaching and learning. In Parlett MR and Dearden GJ (eds) *Introduction to Illuminative Evaluation: Studies in Higher Education*, pp 143–146. Cardiff-by-the Sea, California: Pacific Soundings Press.

Parlett MR and Hamilton DF (1977) Evaluation as illumination. In Parlett MR and Dearden GJ (eds) *Introduction to Illuminative Evaluation: Studies in Higher Education*, pp 9–29. Cardiff-by-the Sea, California: Pacific Soundings Press.

Parkes R (1985) Stressful episodes reported by first year student nurses: a descriptive account. *Social Science and Medicine*, **20**(9), 945–953.

Pembrey S (1980) *The Ward Sister – Key to Nursing. A Study of the Organisation of Individualised Nursing*. RCN Research Series. London: Royal College of Nursing.

Phillips T, Schostak J and Tyler J (2000) *Practice and Assessment in Nursing and Midwifery: Doing it for Real*. London: The English National Board for Nursing, Midwifery and Health Visiting.

Rogers C (1983) *Freedom to Learn for the 80's*. Columbus, Ohio: Charles E. Merrill.

Seed A (1995) Crossing the boundary – experiences of neophyte nurses. *Journal of Advanced Nursing*, **21**, 1136–1143.

Spielberger CD (ed) (1966) *Anxiety and Behaviour*. New York: Academic Press.

Spouse J (1996) The effective mentor: a model for student-centred learning in clinical practice. *Nursing Times Research*, **1**(2), 120–133.

Stengelhofen J (1993) *Teaching Students in Clinical Settings*. London: Chapman and Hall.

UKCC (2001) *Fitness for Practice and Purpose*. London: United Kingdom Central Council for Nursing, Midwifery and Health Visiting.

UKCC (1999) *Fitness for Practice*. London: United Kingdom Central Council for Nursing, Midwifery and Health Visiting.

UKCC (1993) *PREP and You*. London: United Kingdom Central Council for Nursing, Midwifery and Health Visiting.

UKCC (1992) *The Scope of Professional Practice*. London: United Kingdom Central Council for Nursing, Midwifery and Health Visiting.

UKCC (1990) *The Report of the Post-registration Education and Practice Project*. London: United Kingdom Central Council for Nursing, Midwifery and Health Visiting.

White R and Ewan C (1991) *Clinical Teaching in Nursing*. London: Chapman and Hall.

White E, Riley E, Davies S and Twinn S (1994) *A Detailed Study of the Relationship between Teaching, Support, Supervision and Role Modelling in Clinical Areas within the Context of P2000 Courses*. London: The English National Board for Nursing, Midwifery and Health Visiting.

Williams RP (1993) The concerns of beginning nursing students. *Nursing and Health Care*, **14**(4), 178–184.

9 Learning through clinical practice: unearthing meaning from experience

INTRODUCTION

There are some who see the initial preparation of health care practitioners as providing would-be professionals with a set of prescribed theory, rules, routines and behaviours in a prepackaged and predetermined curriculum. The argument for preparing practitioners in this manner is that it reduces the risks of professionals failing to provide a reliable service. This so called 'technical-rational' view of professionalism has received much criticism from writers such as Schön (1983, 1987) who stated that such simple offerings do not prepare practitioners to meet the real situations of practice, as this model makes assumptions that practice is a relatively simple interaction in which the practitioner gives and patients and clients receive. Schön emphasized that practice is messy, unpredictable, unexpected and requires the ability to improvise – this ability is often diminished by training and routines.

One important 'hallmark' of the health care professional is generally acknowledged to be the need to be aware of, and to deal with, complex human issues as part of practice (Fish and Twinn 1997). These essential human interactions between professionals and patients/clients make the detailed knowledge and skills needed in each interaction unpredictable. Fish and Twinn (1997:38–39) take this point further:

> Professional practice involves complex decision making and elements of professional judgement and practical wisdom guided by moral principles but that these [cannot] be set down in absolute routines.

> A professional needs to be able to operate professional judgement and select or even create knowledge necessary to the unique situation.

Practitioners need to be prepared so that they are able to engage in these processes not only through their initial pre-registration preparation but also through continuing post-registration education. The technical-rational model of professional preparation, and its consequent influences on how the practitioner practises, does not fully equip the practitioner to deal with what Schön (1983:3) termed the 'swampy lowlands' of practice – those aspects of professional work which cause the greatest human concern and yet defy the use and application of rules and routines. Furthermore, professional knowledge and practices change constantly: this requires the practitioner to be motivated in order to refine and update knowledge and practices so that professional expertise and thus practice wisdom (Hull 1998), is continually developing.

What is also needed is a model of preparation for professional practice that does not rely slavishly on the use and application of rules, schedules and pre-scriptions. A holistic model for the initial preparation, and the continuing professional development of health care practitioners, will have clinical experiences as one of its key foci. This chapter proposes and explores the use of a *model for learning from experience* as the framework to consider experience-based learning and how the student can be assisted to interact with the clinical environment in order to learn through practice and unearth meaning from experiences. This model has four phases. Each phase of the model focuses on several factors and skills/strategies which influence how the learner engages with the experience. The phases, factors and skills/strategies are:

1. *The preparatory phase.* The preparatory phase focuses on:
   - the student as a learner
   - developing noticing skills
   - developing intervening skills.

2. *The experiencing phase.* During this phase the student 'reflects-in-action'. Several teaching/learning strategies influence how the learner engages with, and reflects during, the experience:
   - sharing, explaining and 'pointing out'
   - questioning and challenging
   - allowing to experiment
   - giving feedback on performance.

3. *The processing phase.* The experience is systematically reflected on during this phase. There are three key stages in reflecting on experience:
   - description of the experience
   - processing through critical analysis
   - synthesizing and evaluating.

4. *Outcomes and action*:
   - linking learning to action.

EXPERIENCE-BASED LEARNING

In 1926, Lindeman made the point that experience is the richest resource for adults' learning and put forward the case for the core methodology of adult education to be the analysis of experience. Despite Lindeman's counsel, the dismal picture was that more than half a century later student nurses were still learning clinical practice 'by doing' only (Alexander 1982a, 1982b). A recent study by Phillips et al (2000) suggests that the 'analysis of experience' called for by Lindeman in 1926 is still predominantly absent in the learning of student nurses and student midwives during their clinical placements. Work on experience-based learning (Boud et al 1993, Boud and Walker 1990, Kolb 1984, Dewey 1938) tells us that learning from clinical experience is not the simple 'learning by doing' as has been accepted for too long. What students see, hear and do during clinical placements can often remain at a superficial level unless they are stimulated to analyse critically their observations and to question the meaning of their experiences and their implications for future learning. They also need to be stimulated to apply theory to practice. The implications of all this for nursing and midwifery education are that students need to learn to relate theoretical material to a variety of clinical problems from the earliest days of training. Twenty years ago, Alexander (1982a, 1982b) made it clear that student nurses need help in learning how to learn from their everyday work with patients, to apply theory to practice and to use facts learned in the classroom in a variety of clinical experiences with individual patients.

For students, learning during clinical practice is a complex activity. The student has to contend and learn to deal with the complex, unstable and uncertain worlds of practice (Schön 1987). At the same time, the student needs to be able to synthesize theoretical content from various fields, become familiar with the patients/clients and their needs and problems, learn to analyse those needs and problems, and, during the course of needs analysis and problem solving, attempt to apply theories learnt and experiences gained previously. Subsequently, the student has to learn to evaluate the effectiveness of care given and make the appropriate changes that may be required. Learning through clinical experiences is far more diverse and pervasive than is conceived. Effective facilitation of learning in the clinical setting and the supervision and assessment of clinical practice are challenging roles for the mentor/assessor. If students are to learn to 'think', then we need to determine what thought patterns are required by the practitioner as successful clinical practice requires the highest level of intellectual functioning – namely that of application, synthesis and evaluation (Stengelhofen 1993).

Boud et al (1985:7) ask the following questions about experience-based learning:

- What is it that turns experience into learning?
- What specifically enables learners to gain the maximum benefit from the situations they find themselves in?
- How can they apply their experiences to new contexts?
- Why can some learners appear to benefit more than others?

In practice-based professions like nursing, midwifery and other health care professions, it is particularly pertinent that attempts are made to answer these questions so that students can be best assisted to extract maximum learning and achieve personal and professional development as a result of their experiences during clinical placements.

In order to explore the 'model for learning from experience' in detail, each phase is considered in turn, focusing on those issues which in my view are important in ensuring that the process of learning through experience is an effective one. First, I consider some of the characteristics of the nature of experience for learning.

The nature of experience for learning

It is perhaps appropriate to start by considering what the word 'experience' could mean in the context of learning and the role of experience in learning. In trying to describe the nature of experience for learning, I am mindful of the difficulty of the task. Within the clinical context, is it what a student has observed, encountered or undergone or is it what a student has done? Or is it all of these? Dewey (1925 in Boud et al 1993:6) considered that experience is not simply an event which happens but that the event has meaning, pointing out that 'events are present and operative *anyway*; what concerns us is their meaning'.

Following on from Dewey's ideas of experience, Boud et al (1993:6–7) consider meaning to be an essential part of experience. They suggest that:

> Experience is a meaningful encounter. It is not just an observation, a passive undergoing of something, but an active engagement with the environment . . .

They go on to point out that experience is not singular or limited by time and place, as much experience is 'multifaceted, multi-layered and so inextricably connected with other experiences, that it is impossible to locate temporally or spatially'. Indeed, in 1938, Dewey pointed out that educational experiences have continuity and integrate with one another so that 'every experience should do something to prepare a person for later experiences of a deeper and more expansive quality. That is the very meaning of growth, continuity, reconstruction of experience' (Dewey 1938:47). Work on the cognitive learning theory (see, for example, Ausubel 1968) also tells us that learning always relates in some way to what has gone on before. Boud and Walker (1990) refer to the 'personal foundation of experience' of a learner, which is the accumulation of previous experiences. Contributory sources to this personal foundation of experience may be the social and cultural environment of the learner, prior clinical placements and experiences. The social, cultural and professional norms and mores assimilated contribute to the formation of the perceptual lenses through which the learner views, and acts, in the world of work. The response of the learner to new experiences is determined significantly by these past experiences, as presuppositions and assumptions have been developed – the past creates expectations which influence the present. The present context can serve to reinforce or counterbalance this.

What students bring to the clinical area – their expectations, knowledge, attitudes and emotions – will influence their construction and interpretation of what they experience. The way one learner reacts in a situation will not be the same as another. Boud et al (1993) believe that, in general, if an event is not related in some way to what the student brings to it, whether or not they are conscious of what this is, then it is not likely to be a productive opportunity. Even when starting a first clinical placement in a hospital, students will bring memories, feelings and knowledge of hospitals, whether or not they have been in one. It will be a rarity to have a clean slate on which to begin – unless new experience and ideas link to previous experience to form 'new wholes' (Ausubel

1968), they will exist as abstractions, isolated and without meaning (Boud et al 1993). Planning clinical experiences is therefore important: they should provide continuity rather than being separate and discrete. Furthermore, students should be assisted to make links and connections between experiences to provide new meanings and enable them to 'see' new whole pictures. This encourages a deep approach to learning (Marton and Säljo 1984) in which students seek an understanding of the meaning of what they are learning, relate it to previous material and interact actively with the material at hand.

Most people would agree with Boud et al (1985:7) when they state that 'experience alone is not the key to learning'. Dewey (1938:15) was critical of how experiences were offered to students. He asked this question:

> How many acquired special skills by means of automatic drill so that
> their power of judgment and capacity to act intelligently in new situations
> was limited?

Students were then rendered callous to ideas and lost the impetus to learn. Does this still happen in nursing and midwifery education today? Boud et al (1993) believe that experience cannot be considered in isolation from learning – it is the central consideration of all learning. Although experience is the foundation of, and the stimulus for learning, it does not necessarily lead to learning unless there is active engagement with it. Aitchison and Graham (1989 in Critocos 1993:161) state that:

> Experience has to be arrested, examined, analysed, considered and
> negated in order to shift it to knowledge.

Working with experience in the manner suggested by Aitchison and Graham is the key to learning from experience. For learning to take place, the experience need not be recent. We may return to the same experience again and again and draw different meanings from each 'visit'. Boud et al (1993:9) believe that 'learning occurs over time and meaning may take years to become apparent . . . learning from it can grow, the meaning can be transformed, and the effects of it can be altered'. The meaning of experience is not a given: it is subject to interpretation. Only the person who experiences can ultimately give meaning to the experience. It is the learner's interaction with the learning milieu which creates the particular learning experience (Boud and Walker 1990). No matter what external prompts there might be – mentors, interesting opportunities, resources – learning can only occur if the learner chooses to engage in the experience.

The emphasis in experiential learning is thus on the process of learning. It proceeds from the assumption that ideas are not fixed and immutable elements of thought but are continuously derived from, and tested out, through experience (Kolb 1984). Kolb's well-known model of the learning process is termed an 'experiential learning model' to emphasize the important part that experience plays in the learning process. Learning is conceived of as a four-stage cycle, as shown in Figure 9.1. The here-and-now personal experience is real and concrete, and forms the focal point for learning 'giving life, texture and subjective personal meaning to abstract concepts' (Kolb 1984:21). The core of the model is the translation of experiences into concepts through reflective activities. These concepts are subsequently used to guide and inform new experiences.

FIGURE 9.1 *The Lewinian–Kolb experiential learning model. (Experiential Learning: Experience as the Source of Learning and Development by Kolb, D., reprinted by permission of Pearson Education, Inc., Upper Saddle River, NJ.)*

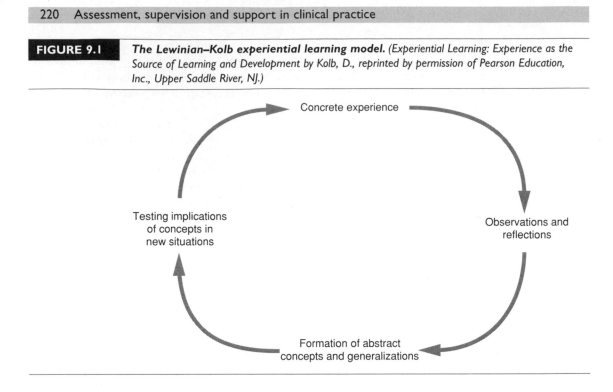

THE 'MODEL FOR LEARNING FROM EXPERIENCE'

Each phase of the 'model for learning from experience' (p. 216) will now be considered in detail.

The preparatory phase

Advanced preparation helps address some of the challenges that students will encounter. The quality of the preparation before the experience also potentially determines the learning extracted during the experience and from later reflection and exploration. The preparatory phase at the start of a clinical placement would normally consist of a number of elements:

- An outline of the aims of the placement and a broad structure of what is to take place. These should be agreed jointly between the mentor/assessor and the student after the first meeting/interview has taken place, as discussed in Chapter 6.
- An introduction to staff, resources and learning opportunities that are available to help the student during the placement. Suggestions on how these may be used to help the student learn are discussed in Chapter 8. Those resources and learning opportunities which are specifically required to enable students to achieve their learning intent should be identified.
- Students should have the opportunity to seek clarification.

Subsequent preparation for experience focuses on *the student as a learner* and on helping the student develop *noticing* and *intervening skills*, as these are two of the prerequisite skills required for learning through clinical experience.

Focusing on the student as a learner

As discussed in an earlier section, what the learner brings to the clinical setting has an important influence on what is experienced and how it is experienced: these factors, including the individuality of the student, should be taken into account during the preparatory phase. The other important element to consider is 'learning intent' (Boud and Walker 1990:64). Intent can be regarded as a personal determination – there is a clear reason for being there, which prompts learners to take steps to achieve their goals. The learning outcomes of a formal educational programme may influence the learning intent. Boud et al (1985) believe that intent to learn for a particular purpose can assist in overcoming many obstacles and inhibitions. Intent can only be determined by direct reference to the learner. For example, during a particular placement the student's intent may be to develop communication skills with very ill patients and their relatives. This intent will influence how the student is likely to experience these types of care situations – it acts to focus and intensify, or play down, perceptions in relationship to these experiences. 'The intent can act as a filter, or magnifier' (Boud and Walker 1990:64): they give the example of the photographer who, when using a zoom lens, will see certain things more clearly but in the process of doing so eliminates other things from the frame.

Students may arrive to a clinical placement with little conscious learning intent or even commitment to being there. Unless the mentor can assist the student form an intent during the preparatory phase, opportunities for learning will not be well utilized due to a lack of focus: this is likely to result in superficial learning. Mentors can play an important role in helping students clarify their intent and guide and direct students to the appropriate learning opportunities in the clinical setting. Mentors should be careful that they do not impose their own intents on the student. A discrepancy in intent between the mentor and student may lead to unproductive experiences and considerable frustration for both parties (Boud and Walker 1990).

Typically, during the preparatory phase there will be a high level of anxiety. Based on the well-documented evidence of student anxiety and stress in clinical settings (see Chapter 8), time should be spent in assisting students to identify and voice their concerns so that you may find ways to reduce their stress and anxiety and increase their confidence. Knowledge that they will not be alone and will not be expected to do more than they are able to will provide reassurance and make students feel less vulnerable. Boud et al (1993) believe that support, trust and confidence in the student can help overcome past negative influences and allow the student to act and think differently from the past. Similarly, conditions of threat or lack of confidence in the student are usually antithetical to any new motivation the student may have and serve to reinforce any negative images the student may already hold.

During the preparatory phase, when students start to focus on their learning intent they start to explore what is required of them, how they can contribute, what their role might be, what the demands of the setting are, what they can learn and how they can use their own resources such as knowledge, skills and what they have learnt from prior clinical experiences.

Focusing on noticing and intervening skills to help students learn through clinical experience

Asking the following questions may prompt both mentor and student to focus on how best to prepare for learning through particular experiences:

- Why has this particular experience – e.g. the care of a certain patient, a visit to another department – been arranged?
- What can be learnt through this experience?
- How can learning from previous experiences be linked to this experience?
- How can students be assisted to plan thoughtfully so that they '[act] deliberately, [observe] the consequences of actions systematically and [reflect] critically on the situational constraints and practical potential of the strategic action being considered' (Carr and Kemmis 1986:40).
- How can students be assisted to engage in the clinical experience so that it means 'living through actual situations in such a way that it informs [them] of the perceptions and understandings of [other similar] subsequent situations' (Benner and Wrubel 1982:28).

Answers to these questions are of course not straightforward, as each clinical situation is different. However, if 'coaching' (Schön 1987:20) of the students starts during the preparatory phase, they can be assisted to extract maximal learning through their experiences. Boud and Walker (1990) believe that there are two aspects of experience-based learning which are necessary to enhance the working of the processes for learning through experience. The first aspect is *noticing*, by which the student becomes aware of the event, or particular things within it. The second aspect is *intervening*, in which the student takes an initiative and is active in the event. I see noticing and intervening as two prerequisite skills for learning through experience.

Developing noticing skills

Boud and Walker (1990:68) define noticing as 'an act of becoming aware of what is happening in and around oneself'. It is active and seeking and involves a continuing effort to be aware of what is taking place in oneself and in the learning experience. As well as paying attention to the happenings around the caregiving situation – the experience – it is equally important that students pay attention to what is happening in themselves. They need to be aware in three areas:

- how they are acting
- what they are thinking
- how they are feeling.

Being aware of *how they are acting* and *what they are thinking* can alert students to what might be influencing them in the event. Being aware of *how they are feeling* will make students more aware of their emotional responses to the event in order for these to be attended to. Attending to feelings involves being sensitive to the situation: seeking to detect the nuances and the affective climate, as well as what is overt. Neglect of emotions can lead to a build up of 'stress and a numbing of awareness which can inhibit the ability to act and distort learning' (Boud and Walker 1990:69). Stuart (2000) gave the example of midwives being in constant contact with women in pain during labour without acknowledging their own feelings and thoughts. This may eventually lead them to become less sensitive to the needs of women during this time.

Noticing provides students with the basis for becoming more fully involved in a caregiving situation and enables them to 'reflect-in-action' (Schön 1983) as they become more aware of the processes of how decisions are made to inform actions taken. It is essential to the initiation of the reflective processes during the third phase of the 'model of experience' so that sufficient information is retained for retrospective analysis and interpretation of practice after the event. Noticing seems to be a skill which has to be present to cause the experience to be the basis for learning (Stuart 2001). Stuart (2001) found that students in her study who did not know 'how' and 'what' to notice were unable to enter into experiences and subsequent reflective interactions with their experiences. As two frustrated student midwives said:

> I think it is very routine . . . what they did, I learnt in the first week . . . It's just like in the morning she [the community midwife] goes round and does the visits, and in the afternoon she does the clinics, and the clinics are all the same, and then going to houses is pretty much the same . . . (p. 178).

> I think on community all your days are very much the same . . . so, no, basically I have nothing to talk about . . . (p. 180).

The starting point for the learning process in order to unearth meaning through experience is *noticing* – paying close systematic attention to detail, noticing exactly what occurred, including any thoughts, feelings, actions and reactions. Developing the skills of noticing will help students utilize their 'observer' status to benefit – how this status can be used for learning is poorly understood and has robbed students of valuable learning opportunities (May et al 1997). This

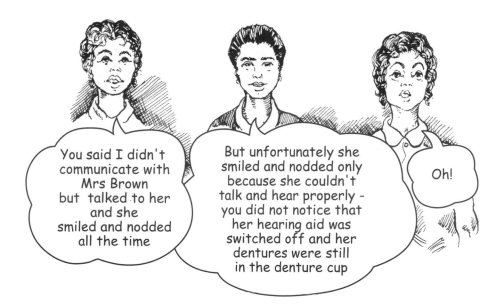

Students have to learn how *and* what *to notice*

| BOX 9.1 | *Aspects to be considered for the development of noticing skills* |

NOTICING while engaging in an experience:

- the context of the episode, such as the history of the patient/client; time of day; location; and team members involved
- other factors in the environment, such as sights, smells and sounds
- what were the patient/client's needs/problems
- what care was given
- how were the patient/client, family and significant others involved
- personal thoughts during, and after, the episode
- personal feelings during, and after, the episode
- personal concerns at the time
- what was noticed about yourself and others, such as the verbal and body language; what you said; what others said; how you behaved; how the patient/client behaved; how the practitioner/s behaved; the approach used by the practitioner(s)
- what was the immediate aftermath of the event

has contributed to the unpopularity of the observer status (Neary 2000). Paying attention to those aspects suggested in Box 9.1 will assist in the development of noticing skills.

Learners can be directed to use these aspects in a general way, which will lead them to notice things that might have gone unnoticed otherwise. Alternatively, the mentor can indicate specific aspects to be noticed to help the learner achieve particular learning intents. For example, if a student wishes to learn how to assess the needs of clients at home following major orthopaedic surgery, the student could be directed to notice specific aspects about individual clients visited. The following example is based upon and extended from the work of Stengelhofen (1993).

The setting. We are visiting Mrs Jones for the first time today since her discharge from the general hospital 3 days ago following internal fixation of her fractured neck of femur, which she sustained after a fall 6 weeks ago. She is 84 and lives on her own in a terraced house.

Aspects for noticing

1. Start observing when we reach the house:
   - How long does she take to answer the door?
   - Note the use of any walking aids – is she using them correctly?

2. During discussion with her:
   - How does she appear to be coping?
   - Is she anxious/confident/confused?

3. What does she feel are her major concerns/difficulties?
4. What do you think are her major concerns/difficulties? What do you think could be causing these concerns/difficulties?

5. Observe her functional activities. Can she manage important manoeuvres such as using the stairs, sit-to-stand and vice versa, independently?

6. How does she get her food supply? Can she manage activities of living such as washing, dressing, preparing a meal, cleaning the house, independently?

7. What are your thoughts and feelings about someone like Mrs Jones living on her own?

Students should be encouraged to keep written records of what they have noticed, as these serve as valuable 'memory joggers' for later critical reflection.

Developing intervening skills

Intervening is when the learner takes an initiative and is active in the event (Boud and Walker 1990). This can be any verbal or physical action taken by the learner within the learning situation. Learning through experience is an active process which involves the learner not only in noticing but also in taking initiatives to extend and test their knowledge. Looking on is no substitute for active involvement, as the learner who intervenes is adopting an active approach to the experience and is therefore more likely to make more of the potential for learning from the event.

The learner's personal foundation of experience will influence interventions taken – it can be either limiting or act as a trigger for further actions. Boud and Walker (1990) believe that the greatest barriers to intervention are past failure and feelings of inadequacy or embarrassment which inhibit clear thinking. These negative self-images can paralyse learners so that they are unable to perform or they act so maladroitly that learning opportunities are lost. On the other hand, past success and feelings of confidence and willingness to 'give it a go' can carry the learner through initial periods of discomfort. During the preparatory phase the best way to help learners to intervene is to attend to those feelings which are blocking their ability to act (see for example, Rogers 1996, for strategies for unblocking blocks to learning).

Learners need to learn the skills to be players. They need to know how and when to intervene and the nature and content of the interventions. Many clinical situations require the exercise of technical skills. Knowing how to perform these, such as doing a bed bath, changing an intravenous infusion, removing of a urinary catheter, can act as great confidence boosters as the learner can intervene directly. Learning how and what and when to intervene is learning how to cope with the experience, as one major concern of students is knowing 'how to cope in clinical' (White and Ewan 1991:108). Typical care events could be analysed and suitable responses rehearsed. The use of role plays, case studies or audio or video recordings of typical events, followed by rehearsal of intervention strategies, will help learners practise appropriate intervention sequences. This will help learners overcome anxieties and uncertainties and develop a degree of confidence before entering unknown situations. Prior to the experience – e.g. before going to the patient/client – it may be possible to predict what common chain of events may arise and a range of strategies are developed and discussed with the learner. The learner could be asked searching questions such as 'knowing what you know about Mr Johns, what problems do you foresee? What care do you think he needs? What actions would you take?' The mentor may suggest particular interventions which the learner could implement or ways in which the learner's own ideas could be put into practice.

Because of the uncontrollable and unpredictable milieu surrounding clinical situations, not all the possibilities available in practice can be anticipated. Boud and Walker (1991) believe that it is neither possible nor desirable to cover every eventuality – part of learning from experience is dealing with the unexpected when it arises. There should, however, be sufficient preparation to ensure that learners can act effectively and that they are able to remain conscious of what they want to learn.

The experiencing phase

During the experiencing phase the key role of the mentor is to facilitate interventions of the learner and reflection within the situation. The learner needs to be assisted to make judgements about when and where to take the initiative and what should be the nature and content of the intervention. Boud and Walker (1990) believe that the most significant influence on the actions of the learner during the situation are the reflective processes that run through it as this active working with the data of the situation by the learner influences actions taken. Reflection within the situation can also lead to a recognition of the feelings and thoughts that accompany intervention, which can significantly influence the quantity and quality of learning extracted from experiences. This, in turn, will influence the learner's ability to transfer learning from this event to other events. As Dewey (1938:51) pointed out:

> We always live at the time we live and not at some other time, and only by extracting at each present time the full meaning of each present experience are we prepared for doing the same thing in the future [a]ll this means that attentive care must be devoted to the conditions which give each present experience a worth-while meaning.

It appears that the 'taking on board of what is going on' while 'performing' needs to be accompanied by the 'thinking' and the 'feeling'. As discussed earlier in this chapter, work on experiential learning theory (Kolb 1984:34) tells us that 'learning involves transactions between the person and the environment'. In their 'model of experience' Boud and Walker (1990) also point out that learners' engagement with, and level of reflection, during an experience are influenced by their personal foundations of experience, learning intent, noticing and intervening skills and the learning milieu. During the preparatory phase, the learner's personal foundation of experience and learning intent would have been explored so that the learner is as 'ready to learn' (Knowles et al 1998) as possible. Although the learner has been prepared to notice and intervene, these learning processes need to be actively facilitated. The mentor also needs to take into account the milieu in which the event is taking place at the time of the experience. The richness of the clinical environment is a facilitating factor for learning, but there are many demands which compete for the learner's attention such as the patient/client condition and even distress, and their need for care and attention, and other disturbing events in the immediate vicinity. At the same time, the mentor may be expecting the learner to listen to an explanation or suggestion for intervention. How can meaningful learning during the 'experiencing phase' be facilitated so that learners' 'power of judgement and capacity to act intelligently in new situations' (Dewey 1938:15) are developed further?

The guiding principles of Schön's three models of coaching for learning during the experiencing phase

Schön's three models of coaching have three distinct yet overlapping styles. The coaching role which mentors might choose to adopt may call on the use of the style of only one or all three models, depending on the level of experience of the student and the complexity of the event. These three models, *joint experimentation*, *follow me* and *hall of mirrors*, are now described.

Joint experimentation. Joint experimentation can succeed only when learners already know what they want to do in order to intervene. The learner must be willing to step into the intervention and 'have a go' with the unfamiliar. The mentor's skill here lies in helping the learner formulate the interventions to be achieved and leading the learner to search for and decide on a suitable way of achieving the intervention. As different interventions are explored together, the mentor works at 'creating and sustaining a process of collaborative inquiry' (Schön 1987:296). The mentor must resist the temptation to tell the learner how to intervene or intervene on behalf of the learner but may generate a variety of interventions and leave the learner free to choose and produce new possibilities for action. Joint experimentation is inappropriate when learners are unable to intervene or when the mentor wants them to grasp a new way of seeing and doing things.

Follow me. When the mentor wants to offer a new way of seeing and doing things, the *follow me* approach is most useful. The mentor provides detailed descriptions of interventions while they are being performed, being careful to give rationales for the interventions. Schön emphatically stated that the 'relations between a whole performance and its parts, between the whole and *aspects* of the whole, are crucial' (Schön 1987:296) and should therefore be emphasized. During this 'analysis-in action' the mentor draws on a repertoire of 'media, languages, and methods of description' (Schön 1987:297), as the ultimate aim is to present images that will 'click' with the learner. During the observation of the mentor, the learner will be attempting to remember the actions and explanations and subsequently trying to derive meaningful learning through personal interventions. As the learner attempts to imitate the mentor, there is great potential for ambiguity and confusion. Guidance and feedback from the mentor is important, as the learner will be 'testing by further words and actions how the meanings she (sic) has constructed are like or unlike his (sic) [mentor] (Schön 1987: 297).

Hall of mirrors. In this model of coaching, there is willing cooperation between the mentor and learner as they try to grasp their own and each other's understandings of the clinical situation. As learners seek to exemplify their proposed interventions in practice, they are assisted to see their interventions from several perspectives. To achieve this, the mentor and learner continually shift perspective – this may be carrying out the intervention proposed by the learner or

FIGURE 9.2   *The coaching strategies during the experiencing phase.*

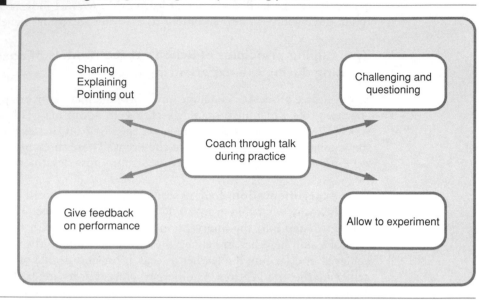

having a dialogue about it or mutually redesigning the intervention. The mentor's skill lies in having the courage to allow the student to experiment and take 'risks'. Schön believed that 'to the extent that he (sic) can do so authentically, he models for his student a new way of seeing error and "failure" as opportunities for learning' (Schön 1987:297).

Using Schön's (1987) three models of coaching to provide the underlying principles for learning during the experiencing phase, several strategies are suggested for use during this phase. These are shown in the framework in Figure 9.2. The strategies in the framework may be seen as 'coaching strategies'. As indicated in Figure 9.2, the central activity which underpins these coaching strategies is 'talk during practice'. This is an essential activity between mentor and learner for meaningful learning to take place during the 'experiencing phase'. Each of the coaching strategies will now be discussed.

Sharing, explaining and pointing out

When mentors work alongside learners, opportunities are provided to engage learners in 'situated negotiation of their practice' (Phillips et al 2000:111). Informal on-the-job conversations take place which allow the sharing of ideas and understanding about care which are then put into practice. These mutual exchanges not only value each other's ideas and understandings but also enable the learner's understandings of practice to be clarified. Phillips et al (2000: 111) give the example of a mentor and her student working together as they make a heavily sedated terminally ill patient as comfortable as possible. As they work, the mentor and student discuss how best to position the patient. The student could see areas of tissue damage which the mentor could not from her position. The position that was planned to be used was modified using the information from the student's evaluation. The mentor in this instance shared how she solved the problem and made the decision by 'thinking aloud' thus:

> Oh well, if you can see that and that's actually happening now, we really can't put her over on her side – well, not completely. If I take her through a bit more this way – I'll not come round to see. It means disturbing her more. So what if we just gently lift her through to me? What if I work your side next time we move her? That way I can get a look at it myself without disturbing her too much.

It can be seen in the above event how the opinion of the student is valued, which can only increase her confidence. As the mentor talked through the rationale for the now better choice of position for the patient, she was also sharing and pointing out other aspects of care that this patient required, such as not being unduly disturbed and the necessity to be gentle. For this student the event would probably have meant much more than merely changing the position of the patient. Through this experience the student may have learnt to 'read' some of the needs that such patients require, thus deriving meaningful learning from what may appear to be the routine task of repositioning a patient.

Most students, even senior ones, need to be alerted to 'signals' from patients and clients. They need to develop skills in interpreting the presenting signs and symptoms of patients and clients so that the physical condition and illness stages can be noted. They also need to become skilled in noting the emotional responses such as fear, distress, withdrawal and other overt indications. White and Ewan (1991) point out that inexperienced practitioners such as students are concerned that their performance should be accurate. They focus on following guidelines and rules. Consequently, they have difficulty in managing the competing demands of the situation. The more subtle cues of response and reactions within a clinical event are often missed. Opportunities for learning through these experiences are thus lost to them. As mentors work alongside students, opportunities are provided for pointing out the messages and signals that patients and clients are overly or covertly giving – teaching them how to handle the 'sensitive moments [which] can be the most difficult aspects of practice to handle' (Open University 2001, Workbook 2:55). Based on such information, explanations can then be given on how care is tailored to meet the needs of the patient/client at the time. Learning through a clinical event is incomplete if a student focuses only on the 'content' of the particular activity – to unearth the real meaning of the experience the student also needs to be aware of its 'extension into the framework of the patient's situation and surroundings' (White and Ewan 1991:132) so that there is awareness of the context of the whole situation for the patient and the carer.

Sharing, explaining and pointing out can be in the form of overt physical guidance of actions such as placing your hand on the student's at times to transfer the amount of pressure to be used in massage, or placing your hand on the student's to transfer the movements and manoeuvres which need to be made to deliver a baby, or 'listening' with the student to body sounds through monitors, or 'seeing' with the student fine discriminations of change in the patient's colour, or 'smelling' with the student to note the odour characteristic of some body fluid or discharges. White and Ewan describe these ways as 'giving away skills – your skills' and guidance is provided by leading 'behind' the student (White and Ewan 1991:135).

Questioning and 'challenging'

The mentor is advised not to give all the answers, which deprives the student of the opportunity of carrying out some of the problem-solving and decision-making activities (Stengelhofen 1993). These cognitive processes foster deep learning, and thus help the student extract more meaningful learning through experiences (McAllister 1997). White and Ewan (1991) state that asking students stimulating and challenging questions helps them to uncover the hidden meaning of their clinical experiences and points them to the 'hidden curriculum' of clinical learning, which may be missed by some students altogether as they are primarily concerned with the task to be completed. Students say they need the mentor to think of things that might never occur to them (Windsor 1987). Skilful questioning and the challenging of thinking help 'awaken' students to the otherwise unrecognized insights and discoveries. Also, we 'need to be challenged so that we do not fool ourselves with our own distorted assumptions or fail to consider new information which is outside our present range of experience' (Boud et al 1993:15).

Some suggestions on how to use questioning and 'challenging' are made below. These are based upon and extended from the work of Stengelhofen (1993) and White and Ewan (1991):

- Ask the student to explain and justify why a certain course of action has been chosen.
- Ask the student why you are proceeding in a certain way.
- Ask the student what actions should be taken in certain situations: e.g. 'What assessment should you be thinking of making? How would you make Mr Johns more comfortable?'
- Place the student in your shoes: e.g. 'I have to make a decision as to whether to treat now or leave. What are some of the considerations which might be going through my head?' (Stengelhofen 1993:97).
- Invite the student to come forward with a diagnosis of what the problem may be and how that problem is best managed: e.g. 'Have a look at Mr Johns then tell me what you think the major problem is and what we can do about it, then you can tell me how we can fix it' (White and Ewan 1991:141).
- Invite the student's opinions about a situation: e.g. 'I would like you to take a look at the patient you looked after yesterday. I think there are some changes . . . see what you think' (White and Ewan 1991:141).

As the student's learning is actively facilitated by questioning and challenging, the mentor needs to be able to facilitate further learning according to the responses of the student as they explore a learning experience (White and Ewan 1991). As the student moves from tentative exploration into understanding, the mentor should respond to the content the student is struggling with. When the student's focus is action, the mentor moves into guiding further development of the student's knowledge and actions.

Questioning and challenging can be threatening for some students – their feelings need to be responded to. Mentors have to be careful not to undermine students' self-confidence. This may be avoided by manipulating situations to allow students to experience success and by giving positive reinforcement.

Allow to experiment

According to Townsend (1990:67) the mentor as facilitator will:

> . . . provide a secure environment in which everyone can experiment, take risks, increase their acceptance for uncertainty and develop mutual trust and commitment. Facilitators are creative, flexible, motivated and involved in mutual goal setting and achievement.

When being allowed to experiment, the student assumes control of clinical care. As in the joint experimentation coaching strategy put forward by Schön (1987), the mentor supports by helping the student formulate the care to be given by prompting the student in searching for, and deciding upon, the most suitable option of care – the final decision rests with the student.

There is prior agreement that the mentor will only intervene if necessary: e.g. when the situation becomes too complex or there could be detrimental consequences for the patient. There is also agreement for the form of support to be given during care delivery: support may be in the form of verbal affirmation of correct performance or nonverbal by the use of body language or just being the 'silent supporting presence' – 'just standing by' – offering neither approval nor disapproval (White and Ewan 1991). Boud et al (1993:15) made the point that as learners we need 'appropriate support, trust and challenge from others. This can enable us to continue our tasks when they seem too much for us or when we get blocked . . . '

If the mentor is present during caregiving, the temptation to take over and assume control must be resisted. Mutual trust must exist, with both the mentor and student accepting any uncertainties. Trust in the student's ability is necessary to enable the student to progress and develop clinical competence. Boud et al (1993:15) found that one of the most powerful factors influencing learning from experience is that of confidence and self-esteem, saying that 'unless learners believe themselves capable, they will be continually handicapped in what they do'. Many students have said that it is a 'nice feeling' to know that they are trusted. The mentor has to 'let go' so that the student can have opportunities to experiment and assume control with confidence. This level of responsibility requires the student to be able to make clinical decisions with the guidance of the mentor. When thus engaged in the thinking and the decision-making processes associated with clinical practice, termed clinical reasoning (Higgs 1997), the student must necessarily use knowledge and higher-order cognitive skills to make clinical decisions. Skilful facilitation of clinical reasoning will help students 'see and read' the depth and breadth of clinical events so that much more meaning can be derived through clinical experiences. The reader is referred to the work of Higgs for a discussion of strategies available to facilitate clinical reasoning.

Give feedback on performance

Giving feedback to students during clinical activities presents invaluable opportunities to enhance learning and meaning derived from care activities. Whereas it is important to time feedback so that errors of care delivery are avoided, it is also important to allow the student enough scope to use individual skill and flair during performance. This requires the mentor to have a degree of trust in the student while being a sensitive observer.

Giving immediate feedback on particularly commendable performances or pointing to where desired improvement could occur will help students extract more learning from clinical events. Remarking on the appropriateness of specific initiatives or praising a demonstration of exceptional caring or indicating to the student that a grasp of principles underlying an action or a behaviour not only reinforces the student's experience of success (White and Ewan 1991) but may also motivate the student to reflect on the actions taken and care given. As the student thinks through these, awareness of the feelings and thoughts associated with a particular action may develop – further learning and meaning may be extracted from the experiences if the student works on these feelings and thoughts to enhance future actions.

If the judgement of the client or patient is also solicited, this source of feedback may act as a direct indicator as to whether care given was appropriate and performed to enhance comfort – this additional information further helps the student to evaluate care skills and rethink clinical decisions and actions if necessary. Some more learning may take place, which can only allow the student to derive more meaning from a particular clinical experience.

The processing phase

Looking back at the preparatory and experiencing phases, we can see that learners have to cope with a considerable amount of new information. Situations force them into active involvement whether they like it or not. They face, and have to deal with, many personal demands. Reflection before and during the experience helps the learner deal with the vast array of inputs and feelings and thoughts generated. Boud et al (1985:26) point out that if 'we are exposed to one new event after another without a break we are unlikely to be able to make the most of any of the events separately'. In the *Four Quartets*, T. S. Eliot spoke of those who 'had the experience but missed the meaning'. Following the experience, it is equally vital, if not more so, to process the experience further through reflection, as reflecting after the event is 'one of the most helpful means of drawing learning from experience' (Boud and Walker 1990:72). What is also significant is that reflection is not an end in itself – the outcome is that knowledge is created through the transformation of experience (Kolb 1984) so that we are 'ready for new experience' (Boud et al 1985:34).

The processing phase is a complex one in which both feelings and cognition are closely interrelated and interactive (Boud et al 1985). Learning is influenced by the socio-emotional context in which it occurs. The role of others in the present, such as support, trust and confidence in the learner, can help overcome negative feelings and allow the learner to act and think differently from the past (Stuart 2001, Boud et al 1993). The climate of the processing phase can act to reinforce or counterbalance both negative and positive experiences – it therefore needs to be planned and managed so that learners may be assisted to extract some more meaning and learning from their experiences. Students are likely to raise many questions and problems which have arisen from their experiences. Generally, it is not possible to 'process' every experience. It may be possible to identify a focus for reflection which addresses several clinical events, e.g. the care of patients who required pressure area care or discussing the cessation of smoking with clients. An alternative is to select discrete experiences identified by the student as significant clinical experiences.

When conducting the session, it is important to remember that this is not another typical group discussion or individual encounter, nor is it a simple reporting back of clinical events, nor an invitation to students to 'rehash' what they did and to receive comment on how well or badly they performed and what to do about it. Particular care has to be taken to prevent a session from turning into a 'moan session' where no learning takes place and feelings of frustration are heightened (Stuart 2001). Students' presentation of their observations, actions and behaviours, feelings and thoughts in their own words need to be acknowledged and actively worked through with the mentor as facilitator. An interactive non-threatening style of questioning and facilitation will assist the student in drawing out the meaning of what has been experienced. As both mentor and student pose questions and attempt to solve problems which have arisen directly from the experience, previously unchallenged assumptions about theory and practice are likely to be explored (Bedford et al 1993, White and Ewan 1991).

Learning through reflection needs to be actively facilitated for many learners (Stuart 2001). The reason may be that certain cognitive skills, which are developed to different stages in different people, are required in order to engage in reflection to learn through this process. Atkins and Murphy (1993) identified these skills as having the abilities to describe, critically analyse, synthesize and evaluate:

- *Description* involves the ability to recollect and replay the experience in its totality. A close attention to detail, noticing exactly what occurred and one's reactions, without making judgements, is required (Boud et al 1985). These authors suggest that this description should be written or verbalized to others.
- *Critical analysis* involves examining the components of a situation, identifying existing knowledge, challenging assumptions and imagining and exploring alternatives (Brookfield 1987, Bloom et al 1956).
- *Synthesis* is the integration of new knowledge with previous knowledge, to form a 'new whole' (Bloom et al 1956). The new knowledge can then be used in a creative way to solve problems and to predict likely consequences of actions.
- *Evaluation*, according to Bloom et al, is the making of judgements about the value of something, for a given purpose. It involves the use of criteria. Mezirow (1981) argues that both synthesis and evaluation are crucial to the development of a new perspective.

These four cognitive skills will now be related to learning through the reflective process during the processing phase. The use of three stages incorporating these cognitive skills are proposed here:

- description of the experience
- processing through critical analysis
- synthesizing and evaluating.

Reflection-on-experience is treated in this format to aid exposition. It is not intended to imply that the stages must take place consecutively. Each stage may be visited and revisited. Reflective exercises within activity boxes are suggested to help the student extract more learning from caregiving experiences – these are offered as a guide and not meant to be a prescription.

Description of the experience

Boud et al (1985) believe that one of the most useful activities for initiating reflection is to recollect what has taken place in as much detail as possible by:

- Replaying and describing the event as it happened chronologically. This replay of the event in the mind's eye may be done verbally or committed to paper.
- Paying close attention to the details of the event.
- Noticing exactly what occurred.
- Noticing one's reactions to it in all its elements. Of particular importance is an observation of the feelings evoked during the experience.

As far as possible, the description should be clear of any judgements, as these tend to cloud our recollections and may blind us to some of the features which may need reassessing. As we 'witness' the event again, it becomes available for us to reconsider and examine afresh; we may begin to realize how we were feeling and how these feelings may have prompted our responses, which in turn influenced our actions.

Those aspects to be considered for the development of noticing skills outlined in Box 9.1 could be used here to assist with the recall of the details of the event. In recalling past events the nature of memory poses problems, as we inevitably forget. To capture the details and nuances of the event, recall should be done as soon as possible.

As students recall and describe their 'lived experiences', it is important for mentors to listen attentively and respond appropriately, without offering any interpretation or analyses of their own. Mentors need to be highly aware of the ways in which language is used by the students to describe or interpret their experience. As the event is replayed and recalled, students will become aware of the feelings that were present during the experience. These feelings need to be acknowledged, as our emotions and feelings can either be a significant source of learning or they can become barriers at times. An examination of our feelings may reveal that our emotional reactions had overridden our rationality to such an extent that we were unaware of our behaviours and our perceptions were blurred. For example, during an emergency situation, feelings of panic may have overtaken rational thoughts and actions so that the chain of events that ensued compromised the well-being of the patient. On occasions, resultant negative feelings become barriers and may inhibit the student from entering into further similar experiences. These negative feelings act as learning blocks, and unless they are recognized and addressed, further learning will not proceed. For example, if a student is overcome with anxiety and fear after encountering an aggressive client or a dying patient, this student is likely to shy away from these situations. There are also occasions when students are hurt and distressed after difficult and painful experiences. Phenix (1964:197) urged educators to take responsibility for 'improving the quality of human meaning at the deepest personal level'. As one student in Stuart's (2001:180) study painfully recounted during the processing phase:

She's got it [terminal cancer] and she's going to die soon. She's only 44. I think because I'd never come into a situation like this before it hit me hard. I don't know . . . I think the imagination goes.

I just feel guilty myself . . . just felt like I should not have been there, just don't know what to do. I don't want to go into a situation like that again.

I went with [the community nurse] for three days and each time she had her on the list, I just dreaded going. It was just so horrible.

It is clear that such feelings must be acknowledged, explored and attended to so that undesirable, and even debilitating, influences are removed or the student may remain disabled. Boud et al (1993:15) emphasize that emotions and feelings strongly influence learning, saying that 'denial of feelings is denial of learning'. An increased awareness of emotions will help students develop the sensitivity required to detect the nuances and the affective tone of the situation so that they can respond sensitively to the needs of the patient/client. In so doing, students will learn to give care as well as *caring* for the patient/client for '. . . care without caring is empty and meaningless . . . ' (Nordman et al 1998:161). And the point when students acquire this form of professional artistry is the point when they have begun to unearth meaning from clinical experiences. Positive feelings should be retained and enhanced so that confidence and self-worth are fostered – these can provide the impetus for students to pursue, or persist with, experiences which they may previously have thought to be too difficult or even insurmountable. Unless we believe in ourselves and our capabilities, we can constrain ourselves to such an extent that we ultimately deny ourselves the learning opportunities for further learning and development.

Processing through critical analysis

During this stage, the experience is thought about and mulled over further to examine and seek relationships among the components of the situation and subsequently to see it as a whole picture within the wider context of the care setting and health care. New knowledge and ideas are identified and related to that which is already known, with the aim of integrating the two sources of knowledge to form a 'new whole'. This 'new whole knowledge' can then be used in creative ways to solve problems and predict likely consequences of future actions. Aspects to be considered to assist processing through critical analysis are suggested in Box 9.2. It is necessary to refer to the information provided from the description of the experience.

As students respond to the issues raised by asking the questions in Box 9.2, their responses and explanations could be prompted at times with further questions to probe more deeply and to expand on 'glib' responses. In addition, they could be asked to reconsider the validity and reliability of their knowledge base and clinical data they have used as the basis for the decisions they have made and the care given. It is important to connect the ideas and feelings which arose during the experience and those which arise during the processing phase with existing knowledge and attitudes. Cognitive theorists such as Ausubel (1968) regard this linking of new information with those relevant elements in our existing cognitive structure as one of the central features of the learning process.

BOX 9.2	*Aspects to be considered for processing through critical analysis*

Consider the following aspects about the experience:

- the rationale for the care given
- the effects on the patient/client/family of the care given
- what aspect(s) of the episode had the most impact on you and why?
- what, if anything, you found demanding
- what you did that was appropriate/inappropriate and the reasons for making that judgement
- what others did that was appropriate/inappropriate and the reasons for making that judgement
- decisions/choices made by yourself and others and whether these were the 'right' ones; what are the reasons for making that judgement?
- in a similar situation, what were your thoughts, feelings and behaviours?
- is there a pattern?

This cognitive process has to be facilitated if we want to encourage learners to develop a deep approach (Marton and Säljo 1984) to learning, an approach characterized by active interaction with the material at hand as the student searches for further meaning from the experience. This results in an integration of formal learning with personal experience and making links between components of knowledge. For example, the student referred to above in Stuart's study (2001) may be assisted to explore her knowledge about the care and support of young clients with terminal cancer and the support services available. The student may then evaluate how such care can influence the quality of life of these clients and start to realize that although it is indeed sad that young people do die of cancer, a quality of life can still be achieved. She has to make connections between the needs of the client, the services available to support the client and her role in meeting the needs of this client and family. This student realized that the client had not had time to come to terms with her illness (Stuart 2001:182):

> These defence mechanisms [referring to the stages of the grieving process] we have – she found out at Christmas that she had cancer and she was given a month to live and it's just come so quickly that I don't think she'd been able to go through these defence mechanisms; she hadn't been able to know that she's got it; she hadn't been able to come to terms that she got it. I think all her feelings are muddled up.

Knowledge and understanding of the stages of the grieving process will assist the student in helping the client work through the grief of having terminal cancer. The student needs to make connections between the formal theory of the grieving process and how this client may be best assisted. The student also needs to make links between what her needs are to enable her to carry out the care required and how she can meet those needs. For example, she may have to learn to come to terms with feelings of guilt and pity for these clients which are present in her existing cognitive and affective structures. The student may realize that she can be a more effective carer if she has an attitude of empathy rather than pity.

The student's feelings of guilt and pity may be a reflection of her assumption that clients with terminal cancer cannot have a quality of life – if this is the case the assumption can be challenged. This challenging may start to take place as the student realizes that, with care and support, these clients can be enabled to experience a quality of life. As the student learns of the strategies she can use to help these clients, and how these strategies may need to be adapted to meet the needs of individual clients, she is beginning to imagine and explore the alternatives for client-centred care.

Synthesizing and evaluating

As students draw conclusions and develop insights into the material they are processing – material from both formal theory and their personal experiences – they develop a set of ideas and perspectives about the management of the clinical situations they were involved with. They have, in effect, developed their own theory of practice through personal experiences. Students can demonstrate the knowledge, understanding and values that have informed their actions. A new set of ideas, concepts and/or 'mindscape' (Bedford et al 1993) may emerge, 'enabling them to appreciate the inherent contradictions within professional caring without incapacitating them to the extent that they are unable to act because of their awareness of those dilemmas' (Bedford et al 1993:141). This will lead to altered ways of giving care. Aspects to be considered to assist further processing through synthesis and evaluation are suggested in Box 9.3.

Boud et al (1985) suggest using the process of validation to test for consistency between the new appreciations and existing knowledge and beliefs and between these and parallel data drawn from others such as those of the mentor and the literature. The literature may be searched for written material which will shed further light on the various facets of the experience, such as data to sup-

---

BOX 9.3	*Aspects to be considered for processing through synthesizing and evaluating*

Students should ask themselves the following questions:

- What made me think, feel and act that way?
- Could I have acted differently?
- Did I have any choice?
- Did I do anything that was different?
- Why was the care given successful/unsuccessful?
- Was the care given an accurate reflection of personal and professional philosophies?
- Were there any conflicts between personal beliefs and values and the care that was given?
- What conclusions can I draw? What ideas, concepts and generalizations can I form?
- How do I know that my conclusions are valid?

port the care given. If there are any contradictions, the situation may need to be reappraised. These authors further suggest that even if our new perception is not consistent with that held by others, it does not imply that we should reject it. Our idea may be breaking new ground or we may wish to hold a certain position regardless of conventional wisdom.

Outcomes and action

The aim of reflecting-on-experience during the processing phase is to make us ready for new experience. However, the benefits gained from reflection could be merely an exercise in abstract thinking if any resultant learning is not linked to action. Students will ask questions such as: 'What do the ideas and concepts mean to me? How can I make use of what I have learnt?' This is an ideal time for assisting students to specify what actions they plan to take so that they can consider the changes in practice and behaviours they want to incorporate into future clinical experiences. The changes may be quite small or they may be large.

In some instances, before changes can be made to practice, students may require to accept the new understanding and approaches into their own value systems. Changing their view of self is involved as well as the values associated with self as practitioner. As students gain a better understanding of self and their professional practices, their confidence is likely to increase. They are then empowered to try out their new ideas in practice. As they do so, their practices are likely to be reshaped and they then enter into new experiences.

Proposed here is a framework (Table 9.1) for assessing learning which has arisen as a result of processing experiences. The treatment of learning in this format is to assist the learner and mentor in deciding the quality of learning achieved and what further learning needs to take place. It is not intended to imply that learning through the processing of experiences can be compartmentalized; nor can such learning be quantified, for example, through the use of grading.

EXPERIENTIAL LEARNING AND CONTINUING PROFESSIONAL DEVELOPMENT

Professional knowledge and practices change constantly and require the practitioner to be motivated in order to refine and update knowledge and practices so that professional expertise and thus practice wisdom (Hull 1998) is continually developing. Furthermore, it is essential to ensure that practitioners can maintain autonomous practice where they are capable of making their own decisions about their actions and the moral bases of those actions (Fish and Twinn 1997). The ability to exercise professional judgement is essential – professional judgement is seen as a complex skill requiring abilities to notice and analyse the patient's/client's problem, deciding what has to be done and evaluating the effectiveness of actions taken. Such ways of managing professional work cannot be laid down as absolute rules of practice and are termed 'professional

TABLE 9.1   A framework to review learning through processing of experience

Stages of processing		Requires further development		Well developed
Identification of learning situations	No appreciation of placement focus	Demonstrates an appreciation of placement focus	Recognizes potential of individual situation for learning	Realizes the potential for exploring individual situation. Situation highly relevant
Description of situation, including personal and others' thoughts and feelings	Relevance of description not demonstrated. Lacks coherence, organization and clarity	Situation described, but lacks focus and omits sufficient detail	Recognizes and recollects key features of situations, including context, feeling and thoughts	High level of perception evident. Subtle nuances in the situation noticed
Critical analysis of situation in relationship to personal and others' involvement	Minimal awareness	Begins to explore thoughts, feelings and behaviour of self and others, triggered by the situation	Constructive exploration of thoughts, feelings and behaviour	Demonstrates insight into situation. Shows an objective appreciation of how and why self and others felt, thought and behaved as they did in situation, and how they affected the situation. Sees the heart of the matter
Synthesizing and evaluating	Relevant underpinning values not identified. No evidence of forming ideas or drawing any conclusions	Identifies some values relevant to the situation. Limited range of ideas formed. Assumptions underlying practice are not explored. Conclusions lack depth	Identifies the values, ideas and concepts relevant to the situation. Explores some assumptions underlying practice and draws some meaningful conclusions	Critically analyses values, ideas and concepts and their relationship to practice. Sees the wider professional implications. Constructively challenges own and others' assumptions
Evidence of learning/outcomes of reflection	No evidence of implications for own practice/learning	Identifies some implications for own practice/learning. Some explicit evidence of learning	Evidence of learning explicit. Identifies implications for practice, and begins to specify how own practice can develop	Integrates 'new' knowledge with previous knowledge to reach new/different perspectives. Specifies where and how own practice will develop. Relates innovative practice development to the wider professional context

artistry' by Schön (1987), which is seen to be well beyond technical efficiency and the use of routine craft skills. The professional artistry view relies on frameworks and rules of thumb rather than rules. The practitioner is not less accountable but is in fact more accountable, as moral accountability for all conduct is exercised (Fish and Twinn 1997). A holistic model for the continuing professional development of health care practitioners, as is the case for pre-registration education, will also have clinical experiences as one of its key points.

Using the 'model for learning from experience' explored so far in this chapter to structure the learning process will help the practitioner use clinical experiences as the key focus for continuing professional development. Although practice is of primary importance, its underlying theory is not set to one side. There is a close interrelationship between theory and practice – no professional action is devoid of theory, for theory involves beliefs, values, ideas and assumptions. Everything we do is thus influenced by theory. What may be absent is awareness of such theories. Many believe that unearthing the meaning of experiences comes after, or at best, during the action. This means that developing expertise (Benner 1984) in professional practice must begin with action. Often, the most useful theorizing for action takes place *during* the activity and the most useful theory develops *after* the activity, if the activity has been carefully reconsidered during the processing phase (Schön 1983, 1987). The experience is the vehicle for enabling practitioners to consider what is involved in learning during and after professional activities, and how this learning can be used to develop professional practice.

The principles of learning from each phase of the model, in particular the experiencing and processing phases, will help the practitioner derive more meaning and learning as professional activities are planned, entered into and reflected upon during and after completion of care. Practitioners enter into a continuum of learning as this model shows; professional activity cannot be separated into the component parts of theory and practice. Using the principles of learning from the model for learning from experience, you may wish to ask yourself the following questions as you go about developing your expertise through continuing professional development activities:

- What is the nature of learning through professional activities? For example, is it a practical problem-solving activity involving people? Is it refining and defining practical wisdom? Is it developing theory? Is it questioning and challenging established practices?

- What sorts of professional/clinical activities should be used for refining and developing professional practice? Should they be every aspect of your working life? Should they be some aspect of practice which catches your attention? Should they be incidents which are outright critical events, such as emergency situations? Should they be aspects of practice which have simply gone unexamined and unchallenged and which are now accepted practices?

- What can you say about yourself as a learner seeking to develop your professional practices? Are you able to get on with it by yourself? Do you find it helpful to bounce ideas off your colleagues? Do your colleagues bounce their ideas off you?

- When was the last time you examined how you practised in a constructive way with others? Bedford et al (1993) believe that as you enter into dialogues with others about your practice, not only do you make your understanding accessible to each other but also you help to develop both the theory and the practice out of each other. If these dialogic debates are of sufficient depth and breadth, you will be able to explore and understand further the moral dimensions and the ambiguity, complexity and uncertainty of the practice settings.

Within its post-registration education and practice (PREP) recommendations, the UKCC requires its practitioners to keep a record of continuing professional development activities by maintaining personal professional profiles (UKCC 1995). The profile is to be created by a 'continuing process which involves *reflecting on* and *recording* what you learn from everyday experiences . . .' (UKCC 1995, Fact Sheet 4, *original emphasis*). It is evident that the UKCC requires written records of these learning episodes to be maintained. It is suggested here that the learning activities in Table 9.1 and those in the section on the processing phase can be utilized to assist you to maintain your portfolio.

CONCLUSION

Dewey (1938) stated that all genuine education comes about through experience. Certainly, in practice-based professions such as the health care professions, clinical experience should be the basis for learning. To extract learning from experience, we need to create meaning from our experiences as we interact with, and react to, them. We cannot allow any experience to be taken for granted: once we do so, actions become routine and habitual, we stop noticing and enter into a rut.

In this chapter, I have attempted to portray some of the complexities of learning through clinical practice which can hinder meaningful learning from experience. Learning from experience is not a simple rational process – not only do we need to know *what* and *how* to do but also we need to know *what* and *how* to think. Impacting on, and influencing these psychomotor and cognitive processes are our feelings, values and beliefs. We therefore also need to exercise our affective self which very frequently dominates our experience and may become either a positive or negative influence for learning. Forces around us also have their influences on how we engage with and extract meaning from an experience, such as the facilitative presence of others and our surroundings. Schön (1987) stated that learning conditions which are not easily met are an awareness of each other's experience, the ability to describe it and a willingness to make it discussable.

Usher (1993) reminds us that experience always says less than it wishes to say: there are many readings of it, it is never exhausted and total clarity may never be reached. Nevertheless, I hope that the discussion in this chapter has provided a range of perspectives to assist the learner and mentor during clinical practice to unearth meaning from clinical experiences.

If professionals are to develop skills in learning through their experience to develop the professional artistry in order to deal with the complex human issues of practice – entering into complex decision making and elements of professional judgement and practical wisdom guided by moral principles – they need to be taught, and encouraged to do so, during their pre-registration training.

REFERENCES

Aitchison J and Graham P (1989) Potato crisp pedagogy. In Criticos C (ed) *Experiential Learning in Formal and Non-Formal Education*, pp 1–13. Durban: Media Resource Centre, University of Natal.

Alexander MF (1982a) Integrating theory and practice in nursing – part I. *Nursing Times*, Occasional Papers, **78**(17), 65–68.

Alexander MF (1982b) Integrating theory and practice in nursing – part II. *Nursing Times*, Occasional Papers, **78**(18), 69–71.

Atkins S and Murphy K (1993) Reflection: a review of the literature. *Journal of Advanced Nursing*, **18**, 1188–1192.

Ausubel DP (1968) *Educational Psychology: A Cognitive View*. New York: Holt, Reinhart and Winston.

Bedford H, Phillips T, Robinson J and Schostak J (1993) *Assessment of Competencies in Nursing and Midwifery Education and Training*. London: The English National Board for Nursing, Midwifery and Health Visiting.

Benner P (1984) *From Novice to Expert: Excellence and Power in Clinical Nursing Practice*. Menlo Park, California: Addison-Wesley.

Benner P and Wrubel J (1982) Skilled clinical knowledge: the value of perceptual awareness, part 2. *Journal of Nursing Administration*, June, 28–33.

Bloom BS, Engelhart MD, Furst EJ, Hill WH and Krathwoll DR (1956) *Taxonomy of Educational Objectives, Handbook 1: Cognitive Domain*. London: Longman.

Boud D and Walker D (1993) Barriers to reflection on experience. In Boud D, Cohen R and Walker D (eds) *Using Experience for Learning*, pp 73–86. Buckingham: The Society for Research into Higher Education and Open University Press.

Boud D and Walker D (1991) *Experience and Learning: Reflection at Work*. Geelong, Australia: Deakin University.

Boud D and Walker D (1990) Making the most of experience. *Studies in Continuing Education*, **12**(2), 61–80.

Boud D, Cohen R and Walker D (1993) Understanding learning from experience. In Boud D, Cohen R and Walker D (eds) *Using Experience for Learning*, pp 3–20. Buckingham: The Society for Research into Higher Education and Open University Press.

Boud D, Keogh R and Walker D (1985) What is reflection in learning? In Boud D, Keogh R and Walker D (eds) *Reflection: Turning Experience into Learning*, pp 7–39. London: Kogan Page.

Brookfield S (1987) *Developing Critical Thinkers*. Milton Keynes: Open University Press.

Carr W and Kemmis S (1986) *Becoming Critical: Education, Knowledge and Action Research*. London: The Falmer Press.

Criticos C (1993) Experiential learning and social transformation for a post-apartheid learning future. In Boud D, Cohen R and Walker D (eds) *Using Experience for Learning*, pp 157–168. Buckingham: The Society for Research into Higher Education and Open University Press.

Dewey J (1925) *The Later Works, 1925–1953, Volume I: 1925*. Carbondale: Southern Illinois University Press.

Dewey J (1938) *Experience and Education*. New York: The Macmillan Company.

Fish D and Twinn S (1997) *Quality Clinical Supervision*. Oxford: Butterworth-Heinemann.

Higgs J (1997) Learning to make clinical decisions. In McAllister L, Lincoln M, McLeod S and Maloney D (eds) *Facilitating Learning in Clinical Settings*, pp 130–153. Cheltenham: Stanley Thornes (Publishers).

Hull C (1998) Open learning and professional development. In Quinn FM (ed) *Continuing Professional Development in Nursing*, pp 182–204. Cheltenham: Stanley Thornes (Publishers).

Knowles MS, Elwood FH III and Swanson RA (1998) *The Adult Learner*, 5th edn. Houston: Gulf Publishing.

Kolb DA (1984) *Experiential Learning: Experience as the Source of Learning and Development*. Englewood Cliffs, New Jersey: Prentice-Hall.

Lindeman EC (1926) *The Meaning of Adult Education*. New York: New Republic.

McAllister L (1997) An adult learning framework for clinical education. In McAllister L, Lincoln M, McLeod S and Maloney D (eds) *Facilitating Learning in Clinical Settings*, pp 1–26. Cheltenham: Stanley Thornes (Publishers).

Marton F and Säljo R (1984) Approaches to learning. In Marton F, Hounsell D and Entwistle N (eds) *The Experience of Learning*, pp 36–55. Edinburgh: Scottish Academic Press.

May N, Veitch L, McIntosh J and Alexander M (1997) *Evaluation of Nurse and Midwife*

Education in Scotland: 1992 Programmes. Edinburgh: The National Board for Nursing, Midwifery and Health Visiting for Scotland.

Mezirow J (1981) A critical theory of adult learning in education. *Adult Education*, 32(1), Fall, 3–24.

Neary M (2000) *Teaching, Assessing and Evaluation for Clinical Competence.* Cheltenham: Stanley Thornes (Publishers).

Nordman T, Kasen A and Eriksson K (1998) Reflective practice – a way to the patient's world and caring. In Johns C and Freshwater D (eds) *Transforming Nursing Through Reflective Practice*, pp 161–176. London: Blackwell Science.

Open University (2001) *Assessing Practice in Nursing and Midwifery (K521 WB2).* Milton Keynes: The Open University for the English National Board for Nursing, Midwifery and Health Visiting.

Phenix PH (1964) *Realms of Meaning.* New York: McGraw-Hill.

Phillips T, Schostak J and Tyler J (2000) *Practice and Assessment in Nursing and Midwifery: Doing it for Real.* London: The English National Board for Nursing, Midwifery and Health Visiting.

Rogers A (1996) *Teaching Adults*, 2nd edn. Buckingham: Open University Press.

Schön DA (1987) *Educating the Reflective Practitioner.* San Francisco: Jossey-Bass.

Schön DA (1983) *The Reflective Practitioner: How Practitioners Think in Action.* New York: Basic Books.

Stengelhofen J (1993) *Teaching Students in Clinical Settings.* London: Chapman and Hall.

Stuart CC (2001) The reflective journeys of a midwifery tutor and her students. *Reflective Practice*, 2(2), 171–184.

Stuart CC (2000) A model for developing skills of reflection. *British Journal of Midwifery*, 8(2), 111–117.

Townsend J (1990) Teaching/learning strategies. *Nursing Times*, 86(23), 66–68.

UKCC (1995) *Post-Registration Education and Practice: PREP and You – Fact Sheets.* London: United Kingdom Central Council for Nursing, Midwifery and Health Visiting.

Usher R (1993) Experiential learning or learning from experience: does it make a difference? In Boud D, Cohen R and Walker D (eds) *Using Experience for Learning*, pp 169–180. Buckingham: The Society for Research into Higher Education and Open University Press.

White R and Ewan C (1991) *Clinical Teaching in Nursing.* London: Chapman and Hall.

Windsor A (1987) Nursing students' perception of clinical experience. *Journal of Nursing Education*, 26(4), 150–154.

Appendix I

UKCC Requirements for Pre-registration Nursing Programmes – Nursing Competencies

36

The UKCC uses the term competence to describe ". . . the skills and ability to practise safely and effectively without the need for direct supervision . . ." (*Fitness for practice, 1999*)

37

The Pre-registration nursing programme should be designed to prepare the student to be able, on registration, to apply knowledge, understanding and skills when performing to the standards required in employment and to provide the nursing care that patients and clients require, safely and competently, and so assume the responsibilities and accountabilities necessary for public protection.

38

The development of nursing programmes arises from the premise that nursing is a practice-based profession, recognising the primacy of patient and client well-being and respect for individuals and is founded on the principles that:

- Evidence should inform practice through the integration of relevant knowledge
- Students are actively involved in nursing care delivery under supervision
- The Code of professional conduct applies to all practice interventions
- Skills and knowledge are transferable
- Research underpins practice
- The importance of lifelong learning and continuing professional development is recognised.

39

The outcomes and competencies expressed will be achieved under the direction of a registered nurse.

TABLE A1.1

DOMAIN	OUTCOMES TO BE ACHIEVED FOR ENTRY TO THE BRANCH PROGRAMME	COMPETENCIES FOR ENTRY TO THE REGISTER
Professional and ethical practice	**Discuss in an informed manner the implications of professional regulation for nursing practice** ■ Demonstrate a basic knowledge of professional regulation and self-regulation ■ Recognise and acknowledge the limitations of one's own abilities ■ Recognise situations which require referral to a registered practitioner. **Demonstrate an awareness of the UKCC's _Code of professional conduct_** ■ Commit to the principle that the primary purpose of the registered nurse is to protect and serve society ■ Accept responsibility for one's own actions and decisions.	**Manage oneself, one's practice, and that of others, in accordance with the UKCC's _Code of Professional Conduct_, recognising one's own abilities and limitations** ■ Practice in accordance with the UKCC's Code of professional conduct ■ Use professional standards of practice to self-assess performance ■ Consult with a registered nurse when nursing care requires expertise beyond one's own current scope of competence ■ Consult other health care professionals when individual or group needs fall outside the scope of nursing practice ■ Identify unsafe practice and respond appropriately to ensure a safe outcome ■ Manage the delivery of care services within the sphere of one's own accountability.
Professional and ethical practice	**Demonstrate an awareness of, and apply ethical principles to, nursing practice** ■ Demonstrate respect for patient and client confidentiality ■ Identify ethical issues in day to day practice. **Demonstrate awareness of legislation relevant to nursing practice** ■ Identify key issues in relevant legislation relating to mental health, children, data protection, manual handling, and health and safety, etc.	**Practise in accordance with an ethical and legal framework which ensures the primacy of patient and client interest and well-being and respects confidentiality** ■ Demonstrate knowledge of legislation and health and social policy relevant to nursing practice ■ Ensure the confidentiality and security of written and verbal information acquired in a professional capacity ■ Demonstrate knowledge of contemporary ethical issues and their impact on nursing and health care ■ Manage the complexities arising from ethical and legal dilemmas ■ Act appropriately when seeking access to caring for patients and clients in their own home.
Professional and ethical practice	**Demonstrate the importance of promoting equity in patient and client care by contributing to nursing care in a fair and anti-discriminatory way** ■ Demonstrate fairness and sensitivity when responding to patients, clients and groups from diverse circumstances ■ Recognise the needs of patients and clients whose lives are affected by disability, however manifest.	**Practise in a fair and anti-discriminatory way, acknowledging the differences in beliefs and cultural practices of individuals or groups** ■ Maintain, support and acknowledge the rights of individuals or groups in the health care setting ■ Act to ensure that the rights of individuals and groups are not compromised ■ Respect the values, customs and beliefs of individuals and groups ■ Provide care which demonstrates sensitivity to the diversity of patients and clients.

TABLE A1.2

DOMAIN	OUTCOMES TO BE ACHIEVED FOR ENTRY TO THE BRANCH PROGRAMME	COMPETENCIES FOR ENTRY TO THE REGISTER
Care delivery	**Discuss methods of, barriers to and the boundaries of effective communication and interpersonal relationships** ■ Recognise the effect of one's own values on interactions with patients and clients and theirs carers, families and friends ■ Utilise appropriate communication skills with patients and clients ■ Acknowledge the boundaries of a professional caring relationship. **Demonstrate sensitivity when interacting with and providing information to patients and clients**	**Engage in, develop and disengage from therapeutic relationships through the use of appropriate communication and interpersonal skills** ■ Utilise a range of effective and appropriate communication and engagements skills ■ Maintain and, where appropriate, disengage from professional caring relationships, which focus on meeting the patient's or client's needs within professional therapeutic boundaries.
Care delivery	**Contribute to enhancing the health and social well-being of patients and clients by understanding how, under the supervision of a registered practitioner, to:** ■ Contribute to the assessment of health needs ■ Identify opportunities for health promotion ■ Identify networks of health and social care services.	**Create and utilise opportunities to promote the health and well-being of patients, clients and groups** ■ Consult with patients, clients and groups to identify their need and desire for health promotion advice ■ Provide relevant and current health information to patients, clients and groups in a form which facilitates their understanding and acknowledges choice/individual preference ■ Provide support and education in the development and/or maintenance of independent living skills ■ Seek specialist/expert advice as appropriate.
Care delivery	**Contribute to the development and documentation of nursing assessment by participating in comprehensive and systematic nursing assessment of the physical, psychological, social and spiritual needs of patients and clients** ■ Be aware of assessment strategies to guide the collection of data for assessing patients and clients and use assessment tools under guidance ■ Discuss the prioritisation of care needs ■ Be aware of the need to reassess patients and clients as to their needs for nursing care.	**Undertake and document a comprehensive, systematic and accurate nursing assessment of the physical, psychological, social and spiritual needs of patients, clients and communities** ■ Select valid and reliable assessment tools for the required purpose ■ Systematically collect data regarding the health and functional status of individuals, clients and communities through appropriate interaction, observation and measurement ■ Analyse and interpret data accurately to inform nursing care and take appropriate action.

TABLE A1.3

DOMAIN	OUTCOMES TO BE ACHIEVED FOR ENTRY TO THE BRANCH PROGRAMME	COMPETENCIES FOR ENTRY TO THE REGISTER
Care delivery	**Contribute to the planning of nursing care, involving patients and clients and, where possible, their carers, demonstrating an understanding of helping patients and clients to make informed decisions** ■ Identify care needs based on the assessment of a patient or client ■ Participate in the negotiation and agreement of the care plan with the patient or client and with their carer, family or friends, as appropriate, under the supervision of a registered nurse ■ Inform patients and clients about intended nursing actions, respecting their right to participate in decisions about their care.	**Formulate and document a plan of nursing care, where possible in partnership with patients, clients, their carers and family and friends, within a framework of informed consent** ■ Establish priorities for care based on individual or group needs ■ Develop and document a care plan to achieve optimal health, habilitation, rehabilitation based on assessment and current nursing knowledge ■ Identify expected outcomes, including a time frame for achievement and/or review in consultation with patients, clients, their carers, family and friends and with members of the health and social care team.
Care delivery	**Contribute to the implementation of a programme of nursing care, designed and supervised by registered practitioners** ■ Undertake activities, which are consistent with the care plan and within the limits of one's own abilities. **Demonstrate evidence of a developing knowledge base which underpins safe nursing practice** ■ Access and discuss research and other evidence in nursing and related disciplines ■ Identify examples of the use of evidence in planned nursing interventions. **Demonstrate a range of essential nursing skills, under the supervision of a registered nurse, to meet individuals' needs which include**: ■ Maintaining dignity, privacy and confidentiality; effective communication and observational skills, including listening and taking physiological measurements; safety and health, including moving and handling and infection control; essential first aid and emergency procedures; administration of medicines; emotional, physical and personal care, including meeting the need for comfort, nutrition and personal hygiene.	**Based on the best available evidence, apply knowledge and an appropriate repertoire of skills indicative of safe nursing practice** ■ Ensure that current research findings and other evidence are incorporated in practice ■ Identify relevant changes in practice or new information and disseminate it to colleagues ■ Contribute to the application of a range of interventions to support patients and clients and which optimise their health and well-being ■ Demonstrate the safe application of the skills required to meet the needs of patients and clients within the current sphere of practice ■ Identify and respond to patients' and clients' continuing learning and care needs ■ Engage with, and evaluate, the evidence base, which underpins safe nursing practice. **Provide a rationale for the nursing care delivered which takes account of social, cultural, spiritual, legal, political and economic influences** ■ Identify, collect and evaluate information to justify the effective utilisation of resources to achieve planned outcomes of nursing care.

TABLE A1.3	(cont'd)

Care delivery	**Contribute to the evaluation of the appropriateness of nursing care delivered** ■ Demonstrate an awareness of the need to assess regularly a patient's or client's response to nursing interventions ■ Provide for a supervising registered practitioner, evaluative commentary and information on nursing care based on personal observations and actions ■ Contribute to the documentation of the outcomes of nursing interventions.	**Evaluate and document the outcomes of nursing and other interventions** ■ Collaborate with patients and clients and, when appropriate, additional carers to review and monitor the progress of individuals or groups towards planned outcomes ■ Analyse and revise expected outcomes, nursing interventions and priorities in accordance with changes in the individual's condition, needs or circumstances.
Care delivery	**Recognise situations in which agreed plans of nursing care no longer appear appropriate and refer these to an appropriate accountable practitioner** ■ Demonstrate the ability to discuss and accept care decisions ■ Accurately record observations made and communicate these to the relevant members of the health and social care team.	**Demonstrate sound clinical judgement across a range of differing professional and care delivery contexts** ■ Use evidence based knowledge from nursing and related disciplines to select and individualise nursing interventions ■ Demonstrate the ability to transfer skills and knowledge to a variety of circumstances and settings ■ Recognise the need for adaptation and adapt nursing practice to meet varying and unpredictable circumstances ■ Ensure that practice does not compromise the nurse's duty of care to individuals or the safety of the public.

TABLE A1.4		
DOMAIN	OUTCOMES TO BE ACHIEVED FOR ENTRY TO THE BRANCH PROGRAMME	COMPETENCIES FOR ENTRY TO THE REGISTER
Care management	**Contribute to the identification of actual and potential risks to patients, clients and their carers, to oneself and to others and participate in measures to promote and ensure health and safety** ■ Understand and implement health and safety principles and policies ■ Recognise and report situations, which are potentially unsafe for patients, clients, oneself and others.	**Contribute to public protection by creating and maintaining a safe environment of care through the use of quality assurance and risk management strategies** ■ Apply relevant principles to ensure the safe administration of therapeutic substances ■ Use appropriate risk assessment tools to identify actual and potential risks ■ Identify environmental hazards and eliminate and/or prevent where possible ■ Communicate safety concerns to a relevant authority ■ Manage risk to provide care which best meets the needs and interests of patients, client and the public.

Appendix 2

UKCC Requirements for Pre-registration Midwifery Programmes – Midwifery Competencies

19 The UKCC uses the term competence to describe " . . . the skills and ability to practise safely and effectively without the need for direct supervision. . . " (*Fitness for practice*, 1999)

20 The pre-registration midwifery programmes shall be designed to enable the student to achieve the competencies under direction of a practising midwife and so to assume on registration the responsibilities and accountability for her practising as a midwife.

21 The outcomes and competencies expressed will be achieved under the direction of a practice midwife.

22 Each competency statement is followed by some specific examples of outcomes, which must go toward the achievement of the competency. The examples are intended to illustrate the intent of the competency and are not an exhaustive list.

TABLE A2.1	DOMAIN	COMPETENCIES TO BE ACHIEVED FOR ENTRY TO PART 10 OF THE REGISTER
	Effective midwifery practice	**Communicate effectively with women and their families* throughout the preconception, antenatal, intrapartum and postnatal stages** Communication will include: ■ listening to women, jointly identifying their feelings and anxieties about their pregnancies, the birth and the related changes to themselves and their lives ■ enabling women to think through their feelings ■ enabling women to make informed choices about their health and health care ■ actively encouraging women to think about their own health and the health of their babies and families, and how this can be improved ■ communicating with women throughout their pregnancy, labour and the period following birth.
	Effective midwifery practice	**Diagnose pregnancy, assess and monitor women holistically throughout the preconception, antenatal, intrapartum and postnatal stages through the use of a range of assessment methods and reach valid, reliable and comprehensive conclusions** The different assessment methods will include: ■ history taking ■ observation ■ physical examination ■ biophysical tests ■ social, cultural and emotional assessments.
	Effective midwifery practice	**Determine and provide programmes of care and support for women which**: 1. are appropriate to the needs, contexts, culture and choices of the women, babies and their families 2. are made in partnership with women 3. are ethical 4. are based on best evidence and clinical judgement 5. involve other practitioners when this will improve health outcomes. This will include consideration of: ■ plans for birth ■ place of birth ■ plans for feeding their babies ■ needs for postnatal support ■ preparation for parenthood needs.
	Effective midwifery practice	**Provide seamless care and interventions in partnership with women and other care providers during the antenatal period which:** 1. are appropriate for women's assessed needs, context and culture 2. promote their continuing health and well-being 3. are evidence-based 4. are consistent with the management of risk 5. draw on the skills of others to optimise health outcomes and resource use.

*The use of the word families in this document may refer to significant others, as identified by the woman

TABLE A2.1	DOMAIN	COMPETENCIES TO BE ACHIEVED FOR ENTRY TO PART10 OF THE REGISTER (CONT'D)

These will include:

- acting as lead carer in normal pregnancies
- contributing to providing support to women when their pregnancies are in difficulty (e.g. those women who will need operative or assisted delivery)
- providing care for women who have suffered pregnancy loss
- discussion/negotiation with other professionals about further interventions which are appropriate for individual women, considering their wishes, context and culture
- ensuring current research findings and other evidence are incorporated into practice
- team working in the best interests of individual women.

Effective midwifery practice

Refer women who would benefit from the skills and knowledge of other individuals:

1. to an individual who is likely to have the requisite skills and experience to assist
2. at the earliest possible time
3. supported by accurate, legible and complete information, which contains the reasoning behind making the referral and describes their needs and preferences.

Referrals might relate to:

- women's choices
- health issues
- social issues
- financial issues
- psychological issues
- child protection matters
- the law.

Effective midwifery practice

Care for, monitor and support women during labour and monitor the condition of fetus and conduct spontaneous deliveries

This will include:

- communicating with women throughout and supporting them through the experience
- ensuring that the care is sensitive to individual women's culture and preferences
- using appropriate clinical and technical means to monitor the condition of mother and fetus, providing appropriate pain relief
- providing appropriate care for women once they have given birth.

Effective midwifery practice

Undertake appropriate emergency procedures to meet the health needs of women and babies

Emergency procedures will include:

- manually removing the placenta
- manually examining the uterus
- managing post-partum haemorrhage
- resuscitation of mother and/or baby.

TABLE A2.1	DOMAIN	COMPETENCIES TO BE ACHIEVED FOR ENTRY TO PART 10 OF THE REGISTER (CONT'D)

Effective midwifery practice

Examine and care for babies immediately following birth
This will include:
- confirming their vital signs and taking the appropriate actions
- full assessment and physical examination.

Effective midwifery practice

Work in partnership with women and other care providers during the postnatal period to provide seamless care and interventions which:
1. are appropriate to the woman's assessed needs, context and culture
2. promote their continuing health and well-being
3. are evidence-based
4. are consistent with the management of risk
5. when undertaken by the midwife, s/he is the person best placed to do them and s/he is competent to act
6. draw on the skills of others to optimise health outcomes and resource use.

These will include:
- providing support and advice to women as they start to feed and care for the babies
- providing any particular support which is needed to women who have disabilities
- post-operative care for women who have had caesarean and operative deliveries
- providing pain relief to women
- team working in the best interests of the women and their babies
- facilitating discussion about future reproductive choices
- providing care for women who have suffered pregnancy loss, stillbirth or neonatal death.

Effective midwifery practice

Examine and care for babies with specific health or social needs and refer to other professionals or agencies as appropriate
This will include those with:
- congenital disorders
- birth defects
- low birth weight
- pathological conditions (such as babies with vertical transmission of HIV, drug affected babies).

Effective midwifery practice

Care for and monitor women during the puerperium offering the necessary evidence-based advice and support on baby and self care
This will include:
- providing advice and support on feeding babies and teaching about the importance of nutrition in child development
- providing advice and support on hygiene, safety, protection, security and child development
- enabling women to address issues about their own, their babies' and their families' health and social well-being
- monitoring and supporting women who have postnatal depression and other major mental illness
- advice on bladder control
- advising women on recuperation
- supporting women to care for ill/pre-term babies or those with disabilities.

TABLE A2.1	DOMAIN	COMPETENCIES TO BE ACHIEVED FOR ENTRY TO PART10 OF THE REGISTER (CONT'D)

Effective midwifery practice

Select, acquire and safely administer a range of permitted drugs consistent with legislation, applying knowledge and skills to the situation that pertains at the time
Methods of administration will include:
- oral
- intravenous
- intramuscular
- topical
- inhalation.

Effective midwifery practice

Complete, store and retain records of practice which:
1. are accurate and legible
2. detail the reasoning behind any actions taken
3. contain the information necessary for the record's purpose.

Records will include:
- biographical details of women and babies
- assessments made, outcomes of assessment and the actions taken as a result
- the outcomes of discussions with women and the advice offered
- any drugs administered
- action plans and commentary on their evaluation.

Effective midwifery practice

Actively monitor and evaluate the effectiveness of programmes of care and modify them to improve the outcomes of women, babies and their families
This will include:
- consideration of the effectiveness of the above and making the necessary modifications to improve outcomes for women and their families.

Effective midwifery practice

Contribute to enhancing the health and social well-being of individuals and their communities
This will include:
- planning and offering midwifery care within the context of public health policies
- contributing midwifery expertise and information to local health policies
- identifying and targeting care for groups with particular health and maternity needs and maintaining communication with appropriate agencies
- involving users and local communities in service development and improvement
- informing practice with the best evidence shown to prevent and reduce maternal and perinatal morbidity and mortality
- utilising a range of effective, appropriate and sensitive programmes to improve sexual and reproductive health.

Professional and ethical practice

Practise in accordance with the UKCC's *Code of Professional Conduct*, within the limitation of one's own competence, knowledge and sphere of professional practice, consistent with the legislation relating to midwifery practice
This will include:
- using professional standards of practice to self-assess performance

TABLE A2.1.	DOMAIN	COMPETENCIES TO BE ACHIEVED FOR ENTRY TO PART10 OF THE REGISTER (CONT'D)
		■ consulting with the most appropriate professional colleagues when care requires expertise beyond one's own current competence ■ consulting other health care professionals when needs fall outside the scope of midwifery practice ■ identifying unsafe practice and responding appropriately.
	Professional and ethical practice	**Practise in a way which respects and promotes individuals' rights, interest, preferences, beliefs and cultures** This will include: ■ offering culturally sensitive family planning advice ■ ensuring that women's labour is consistent with their religious and cultural beliefs and preferences ■ acknowledging the roles and relationships in families dependent on religious and cultural beliefs, preferences and experiences.
	Professional and ethical practice	**Practise in accordance with relevant legislation** This will include: ■ practising within the contemporary legal framework of midwifery ■ demonstrating knowledge of legislation relating to human rights, equal opportunities and access to patient records ■ demonstrating knowledge of legislation relating to health and social policy relevant to midwifery practice ■ demonstrating knowledge of contemporary ethical issues and their impact on midwifery practice ■ managing the complexities arising from ethical and legal dilemmas.
	Professional and ethical practice	**Maintain the confidentiality of information** This will include: ■ ensuring the confidentiality and security of written and verbal information acquired in a professional capacity ■ disclosing information about individuals and organisations only to those who have a right and need to know it once proof of identity and right to disclosure has been obtained.
	Professional and ethical practice	**Interact with other practitioners and agencies in ways which:** **1.** value their contribution to health and care **2.** enable them to participate effectively in the care of women, babies and their families **3.** acknowledge the nature of their work and the context in which it is placed. Practitioners and agencies will include those who work in: ■ health care ■ social care ■ social security, benefits and housing ■ advice, guidance and counselling ■ child protection ■ the law.

TABLE A2.I	DOMAIN	COMPETENCIES TO BE ACHIEVED FOR ENTRY TO PART 10 OF THE REGISTER (CONT'D)
	Professional and ethical practice	**Manage and prioritise competing demands** This will include: ■ working out who is best placed and able to provide particular interventions to women, babies and their families ■ alerting managers to difficulties and issues in service delivery.
	Professional and ethical practice	**Support the creation and maintenance of environments, which promote the health, safety and well-being of women, babies and others** This will include: ■ preventing and controlling infection ■ promoting health, safety and security in the environment in which the practitioner is working, whether it is at women's home, in the community, a clinic, or a hospital.
	Professional and ethical practice	**Contribute to the development and evaluation of guidelines and policies and make recommendations for change in the interest of women, babies and their families** Evaluation policies will include: ■ providing feedback to managers on service policies ■ representing own considered views and experiences into broader health and social care policies in the interest of women, babies and their families.
	Developing the individual midwife and others	**Review, develop and enhance the midwife's own knowledge, skills and fitness to practise** This will include: ■ making effective use of the framework for the statutory supervision of midwives ■ meeting the UKCC's continuing professional development and practice standards ■ reflecting on the midwife's own practice and making the necessary changes as a result ■ attending conferences, presentations, learning events, etc.
	Developing the individual midwife and others	**Demonstrate effective working across professional boundaries and develop professional networks** This will include: ■ effective collaboration and communication ■ sharing skills ■ multiprofessional standard-setting and audit.
	Achieving quality care through evaluation and research	**Apply relevant knowledge to the midwife's own practice in structured ways which are capable of evaluation** This will include: ■ critical appraisal of knowledge and research evidence ■ critical appraisal of the midwife's own practice ■ gaining feedback from women and their families and appropriately applying this to practice ■ disseminating critically appraised good practice.

TABLE A2.1	DOMAIN	COMPETENCIES TO BE ACHIEVED FOR ENTRY TO PART 10 OF THE REGISTER (CONT'D)
	Achieving quality care through evaluation and research	**Inform and develop the midwife's own practice and the practice of others through using the best available evidence and reflecting on practice** This will include: ■ keeping up-to-date with evidence ■ applying evidence to practice ■ alerting others to new evidence for them to apply to their own practice.
	Achieving quality care through evaluation and research	**Manage and develop care utilising the most appropriate information technology (IT) systems** This will include: ■ recording practice in consistent formats on IT systems for wider-scale analysis ■ using analysis of data from IT systems to apply to practice ■ evaluating practice from data analysis.
	Achieving quality care through evaluation and research	**Contribute to the audit of practice to review and optimise the care of women, babies and their families** This will include: ■ auditing the individual's own practice ■ contributing to the audit of team practice.

Appendix 3

The University of Sheffield Academic Diary & Student Handbook (2001–2002) – General Regulations as to Academic Appeals

1. A student may apply under these Regulations for a recommended grade for any unit or Degree classification or examination result to be reconsidered in the light of new evidence.

Grounds for Appeal

2. For these purposes, 'new evidence' is defined as:

   (i) procedural error either by the Examiners or during the recording transcription and reporting of the examination results.

   (ii) extenuating circumstances which the student was unable to place, or for valid reasons did not place, before the Examiners.

   (iii) in the case of higher Degrees by research, evidence of negligence or misconduct on the part of the Examiner.

   (iv) in the case of higher Degrees by coursework and dissertation and by research, evidence of a failure of supervision which significantly affected the candidate's performance and which could not reasonably be expected to have been the subject of complaint by the student to the Head of Department or the Dean of the Faculty before the examination.

   These are the only grounds on which representations can be made. Appeals will not be considered against the academic judgement of the Examiners.

Procedure

3. A student who wishes to place such new evidence before the Board of the Faculty shall apply in writing, setting out clearly the facts which the student wishes the Board to consider and showing how those facts constitute new evidence as here defined in writing. The application must be made to the Dean.

   a. within 28 days of the publication of the examination result in the case of a candidate for a higher Degree by research or

   b. within 10 days of the publication of the examination result in any other case.

   The Dean may extend the time limit imposed by this Regulation.

For the purposes of these Regulations, the date of publication of examination results means the date upon which the examination results are first made available to students in the relevant Department, even though the results are still subject to confirmation by the Board of the Faculty and the Senate.

Academic Appeals Committee

4. There shall be an Academic Appeals Committee of the Board of the Faculty which will be convened if the Dean is satisfied that a prima facie case has been established by the student.

5. The Academic Appeals Committee shall comprise:
   a. in the case of an appeal by a candidate for a higher Degree by research.
      (i) the Dean
      (ii) two other members of the Board
      (iii) one member of the Board of the Faculty of Law
      (iv) one member of the Board of another Faculty; and
   b. in any other case
      (i) the Dean
      (ii) not less than two and not more than four other members of the Board.

6. The student may opt either (a) for the appeal to be dealt with on written submissions or (b) for an oral hearing (at which the student may choose to be accompanied by a friend or adviser).

7. Where the appeal is to be dealt with on written submissions, the Committee shall receive:
   a. the material submitted by the student
   b. any written comments made on that material by or on behalf of the Head of Department and, where appropriate, by the supervisor, and
   c. any written comments made by the student on the material submitted under (b) above.

8. Where there is an oral hearing, the Committee shall hear oral submissions by or on behalf of the student, the Head or other representative of the Department, and where appropriate the supervisor. The student may comment on the submissions made by others. In any case in which factual matters are in dispute, the Committee shall investigate the facts, and may invite appropriate persons to attend to assist; during this process, the student may be present and may ask questions, make comments, and produce other persons who can provide information or testimony.

9. At no other stage during the appeal process does the student have the right to see any examination script bearing marks or comments of an examiner or any report prepared by an Examiner on a thesis or dissertation.

10. The Committee shall reconsider the grade, classification, result or other subject of the appeal in the light of the material available to it. Except as

provided above, no person other than members of the Committee and its Secretary shall be present during its deliberations.

11. The Committee shall report to the Board and may make any recommendation as to the subject matter of the appeal as could, under the relevant Regulations, have been made by the Examiners.

12. The decision of the Board, acting on the recommendation of the Academic Appeals Committee is final.

13. Where the substance of the appeal concerns acts or omissions of the Dean, and in any other case where it is inappropriate for the Dean to act under these Regulations, the Dean shall appoint a Deputy.

Appendix 4

The University of Sheffield Academic Diary & Student Handbook (2001–2002) – General Regulations as to Progress of Students

Conduct of Review

1. A review of the progress of a student registered as a candidate for any Degree or other qualification shall be conducted by the Board under the following Regulations or by the Faculty Student Review Committee to which the Board was delegated this function.

2. A student's progress may be reviewed if the student is reported by a Head of Department to the Dean for review on any one or more of the following grounds:

   a. failure to attend regularly the programme of study for which the student has registered.

   b. failure to perform adequately the work of the programme.

   c. failure to present at the times appointed such written work as may have been required.

   d. failure to pass an examination.

   e. failure to pursue the programme of research or to co-operate appropriately with the appointed supervisor.

   f. failure to demonstrate a satisfactory level of professional competence in dealings with others which form part of the student's programme of study or research.

   Where a student is reported for review on the ground of unsatisfactory attendance, the student's academic progress may be taken into consideration.

3. The Dean or another Officer of the Faculty shall offer any student whose progress is to be reviewed the opportunity to bring before the Board or the Committee considerations affecting the case.

4. The Board or the Committee shall have power:

   a. to exclude or suspend the student from further attendance at lectures, classes and examinations in the Faculty.

   b. to suspend the student from attendance at lectures and classes in the Faculty but with permission to take examinations.

   c. to exclude or suspend the student from candidature for the higher Degree for which the student is registered.

    d. to permit the student to continue the programme of study uncondi-
tionally or subject to such requirements of an academic nature as may
be imposed, provided that, in the absence of special circumstances, an
undergraduate student registered for a full-time programme of study
shall not be permitted to repeat with attendance more than one year of
the programme of study.

5. The despatch of a letter to a student's address last notified to the Registrar
and Secretary shall fulfil any requirements of giving notice or information
to the student under these Regulations.

6. A student who has been excluded from attendance at lectures, classes and
examinations in any Faculty may register in another Faculty only with the
permission of the Board of the latter Faculty.

Right of Appeal

7. The decision of the Board or Committee shall be reported to the Registrar
and Secretary, who shall inform the student of the decision and of the effect
of this Regulation. A student wishing to appeal against the decision to the
Appeals Committee of the Senate shall give notice in writing within 14 days
of the date of the letter of notification and the notice shall contain a brief
statement of the grounds the student has for believing that the decision of
the Board or Committee should be varied or quashed. A Pro Vice-
Chancellor may extend the time-limit imposed by this Regulation.

8. An appeal by the student shall involve a complete re-hearing of the case by the
Appeals Committee of the Senate. The Committee may confirm, vary or quash
the decision of the Board or Committee and may exercise any of the powers
conferred upon the Board or Committee by the foregoing Regulations. The
Committee shall have no power to vary any decision made by Examiners.

Reconsideration

9. The Registrar and Secretary shall notify the student of the decision of the
Appeals Committee and of the student's right to give notice in writing within 14 days of the date of the letter of notification, of a wish to apply for the
decision to be reconsidered by the Appeals Committee of the Council.

10. Such an application for reconsideration shall only be granted if a prima
facie case has been made out to the Vice-Chancellor that some evidence
about the student concerned was not available when the previous decisions
were made, or that there has been a substantial error in the procedure.

Appendix 5

The University of Sheffield Academic Diary & Student Handbook (2001–2002) – Regulations as to the Discipline of Students

Misconduct Defined

1. Misconduct for the purposes of these Regulations is improper interference, in the broadest sense, with the proper functioning or activities of the University, or those who work or study in the University, or action which otherwise damages the University.

2. Subject to the general definition in the preceding Regulation, the following shall constitute misconduct:

   a. disruption of, or improper interference with the academic, administrative, sporting, social or other activities of the University, whether on University premises or elsewhere.

   b. obstruction of, or improper interference with the functions, duties or activities of any student, member of staff or other employee of the University or any authorised visitor to the University.

   c. violent, indecent, disorderly, threatening or offensive behaviour or language whilst on University premises or engaged in any University activity.

   d. fraud, deceit, deception or dishonesty in relation to the University or its staff or in connection with holding any office in the University or in relation to being a student of the University.

   e. behaviour likely to cause injury or impair safety on University premises.

   f. behaviour which puts or is likely to put at risk of harm any person with whom a student has dealings as part of a programme of study or research.

   g. sexual, racial or any other form of personal harassment of any student, member of staff or other employee of the University or any authorised visitor to the University.

   h. breach of the Regulations on the Use of Computing Facilities, of the University's Code of Practice relating to Meetings and Other Activities on University Premises under Section 43 of the Education (No 2) Act 1986 or of any other Regulation which provides for breaches to be dealt with under these Regulations.

   i. the use of any unfair means in examinations of the University.

   j. damage to, or defacement of, University property or the property of other members of the University community caused intentionally or recklessly, or misappropriation of such property.

   k. misuse or unauthorised use of University premises or items of property, including computer misuse.

    l. conduct which constitutes a criminal offence where that conduct:

       (i) took place on University premises or

       (ii) affected or concerned other members of the University community or

       (iii) damages the good name of the University or

       (iv) itself constitutes misconduct within the terms of these Regulations or

       (v) is an offence of dishonesty, where the student holds an office of responsibility in the Union of Students, a Hall of Residence, or a self-catering complex.

    m. behaviour which brings the University into disrepute.

    n. failure to disclose name and other relevant details to an Officer or employee of the University in circumstances when it is reasonable to require that such information be given.

    o. failure to comply with a previously imposed penalty, requirement or undertaking under these Regulations.

Appendix 6

United Kingdom Central Council for Nursing, Midwifery and Health Visiting – Declaration of Good Character to support admission to a part or parts of the Council's professional register

United Kingdom Central Council
for Nursing, Midwifery and Health Visiting

Declaration of Good Character to support admission to a part or parts of the Council's professional register

I...
on the basis of my knowledge of
(full name of applicant) ....
whose UKCC Professional Identification Number is ....
state that she/he is of good character and I support her/his application to be entered in the professional register for nurses, midwives and health visitors.

Signature* ....Date ....

Post Held ....

Stamp of education/
training institution

*The individual signing this form should be the person responsible for directing the educational programme and whose name should appear on the Council's register. In signing the Declaration of Good Character, the individual should take account of the personal responsibilities and accountability that professional registration confers upon those practitioners registered with the Council.

23 Portland Place, London W1N 4JT Telephone 020 7637 7181 Facsimile 020 7436 2924

Appendix 7

General Nursing Council for England and Wales: Record of Practical Instruction and Experience for the Certificate of General Nursing 1969

1969
Reprint 1970

The General Nursing Council for England and Wales
23 Portland Place, London W1A 1BA

PREFACE

The Syllabus sets out in broad terms the subjects to be studied during training for Registration in the general part of the Register maintained by the General Nursing Council for England and Wales.

The concept underlying this syllabus is that of total patient care but for convenience the syllabus is divided into three main sections: nursing, the study of the individual and the nature and cause of disease together with the prevention and treatment. These three aspects of patient care should be learned concurrently throughout training. In this way the various needs of patients will be closely linked together; their needs as individuals and as patients requiring nursing and specialised care and rehabilitation in preparation for return home.

The patient in hospital cannot be considered in isolation from the community and the nurse must be aware of the services provided by local health authorities and voluntary organisations to help and safeguard individuals in their home and work. The nurse also has an important part to play as a health teacher and must have a knowledge of the factors in the environment which give rise to ill health since she will be called upon to advise patients and their relatives on how to care for themselves and their family in a way which will promote a state of physical and mental well-being.

The syllabus includes a section on the elementary principles of management which will form the basis for further post-registration courses.

Learning will take place both in the teaching department and in the wards and departments of the hospital with some experience in the community services. Teaching will be by means of lectures, tutorials, group discussions and project work.

Since nursing is essentially a practical art the majority of the training period will be spent in the wards and departments of the hospital learning and practising nursing skills under the guidance of Registered Nurses. These skills and techniques are to be recorded in Section 1 of the Record and the main types of conditions from which the patients are suffering are to be shown in Section 2. These two sections are to be a guide to the student in planning private study and writing patient care studies. Each student nurse must be responsible for her Record which should be completed regularly in consultation with the Registered Nurses supervising and teaching in the wards and departments and will thus provide a detailed record of training.

The period of training is normally 3 years exclusive of excess sick and special leave and student nurses will be required to pass written and practical examinations prior to Registration.

The General Nursing Council for England and Wales

Record of Practical Instruction and Experience for the Certificate of General Nursing

Section 1 (pages 14 to 28)

Space is provided to record procedures and treatments observed or carried out, columns are provided for each year of training, one for observation, one for practice under supervision. When a procedure is observed the student nurse should place a √ in the appropriate column. When a procedure has been practised satisfactorily under supervision the student nurse should initial and the Registered Nurse who supervised, sign in the appropriate column.

Basic nursing procedures usually undertaken throughout training need not be signed for in each year but if a more specialised procedure is practised in the early part of training and again later, a second entry should be made to indicate a deeper knowledge at this later stage.

Author's note: In the GNC document, these items are shown using the format on page 272. It is reproduced here in list form only.

Section 2 (pages 29 to 66)

This section should provide a record of the types of cases nursed in the various wards and departments. The commoner types of conditions and operations have been listed, others may be added. The initials of the student nurse and signature of the Registered Nurse should be entered against the conditions nursed.

Section 3 (pages 68 to 69)

The clinical experience gained during training is to be verified by the training school authority.

SECTION I

Items	after observation ✔	FIRST YEAR After practise under supervision:- Initials of Student Nurse	FIRST YEAR After practise under supervision:- Signature of Registered Nurse	after observation ✔	SECOND YEAR After practise under supervision:- Initials of Student Nurse	SECOND YEAR After practise under supervision:- Signature of Registered Nurse	after observation ✔	THIRD YEAR After practise under supervision:- Initials of Student Nurse	THIRD YEAR After practise under supervision:- Signature of Registered Nurse
Admission of patients to hospital									
Care of clothing and personal belongings									
Washing and bathing in bed:									
adults									
children									
infants									
Washing and bathing in bathroom:									
adults									
children									
Washing and bathing of infants									
Care of mouth and teeth									
Care of pressure areas									
Use of devices for relieving pressure									
Care of hair									
Treatment of infestation of:									
hair									
skin									
clothing									
Care of:									
ambulant patients									
incontinent patients									
paralysed patients									
unconscious patients:									
post-anaesthetic									
long term									

Section I (*contd*)

Care of the dying

Last offices

Discharge of patients from hospital

Making of:
  beds
  cots

Use of special types of beds and mattresses

Care and use of appliances for providing
  additional warmth

Lifting and moving of patients:
  in bed
  between bed and trolley
  between bed and chair

Feeding:
  serving meals
  feeding helpless patients:
    infants
    physically handicapped
    elderly
  preparation of infants' feeds
  artificial feeding:
    by nasogastric tube
    by gastrostomy

Attending to patient's sanitary needs:
  giving and removing bedpans
  giving and removing urinals
  assisting patients using commode
  assisting patients using W.C.
  changing of napkins

Administration of:
  rectal suppositories
  evacuant enemas
  retention enemas

Rectal washout

Passing a flatus tube

Care of:
  colostomy
  ileostomy

Catheterization:
  female
  male

Care of indwelling catheter

Care of bladder drainage

Irrigation of the bladder

Section I (*contd*)

Vulval toilet

Making observations on and keeping records of:
  temperature
  pulse
  respiration
  apex beat
  blood pressure
  level of consciousness
  weight
  height
  fluid intake and output

Giving and receiving reports of patient's condition:
  oral
  written ·

Interviewing and advising patient's relatives

Preparation of patient and equipment for examination of:
  ear, nose, throat
  eyes
  chest and abdomen
  rectum
  vagina
  nervous system
  locomotor system

Observation and collection of specimens:
  sputum
  vomit
  urine
  faeces
  discharges

Urine testing:
  specific gravity
  reaction
  tests for:
    albumen
    sugar
    acetone
  other tests: [X]

Care and custody of drugs:
  storing
  checking
  recording
  ordering

Administration of drugs by the following routes:
  mouth
  injection:
    subcutaneous (hypodermic)

Section I (*contd*)

    intramuscular
    intravenous (preparation for)
    intrathecal (preparation for)
  skin:
    ointments
    lotions
  vagina

Preparation of patients and equipment for intravenous infusions:
  blood
  other fluids

Care of patients having intravenous infusion of:
  blood
  other fluids

Prevention of cross-infection:
  use of:
    gowns
    gloves
    masks

Disinfection and/or disposal of infected material:
  urine
  faeces
  sputum
  bedding
  clothing
  napkins
  equipment

Isolation nursing technique

Routine preparation of patients for operation

Routine post-operative care

Preparation for sterile procedures

Conduct of dressings

Care associated with methods of drainage:
  underwater seal
  others: [X]

Removal of:
  sutures
  clips

Administration of inhalations:
  steam
  oxygen
  drugs
  others: [X]

Assisting patients with breathing and coughing exercises

Assisting patients having postural drainage

Section I (*contd*)

Assisting patients having leg exercises

Use of suction apparatus:
  pharyngeal tracheal
  others: [X]

Emergency resuscitation:
  assisted respiration
  cardiac massage

Care of tracheostomy

Gastric aspiration

Gastric washout

Ear mopping
  instillation of drops

Nasal drops and sprays

Eye swabbing
  application of heat
  irrigation
  instillation of drops
  application of ointments

Preparation of patient and equipment for application of:
  skin traction
  plaster of Paris

Care of patient after application of:
  skin traction
  skeletal traction
  plaster of Paris

Management of patients and equipment prior to, during and after:
  ear syringing
  antrum puncture
  nasal packing
  lumbar puncture
  abdominal paracentesis
  peritoneal dialysis
  aspiration of pleural cavity
  bone marrow puncture
  renal biopsy
  liver biopsy
  sigmoidoscopy
  other procedures: [X]

Preparation and after-care of patients having special tests and investigations:
  special tests of function of:
    kidney
    liver
    endocrine glands
    others: [X]
  special X-ray procedures:

Section 1 (*contd*)

    barium meal
    barium enema
    cardiac catheterization
    cholecystogram
    intravenous pyelogram
    retrograde pyelogram
    cystogram
    bronchogram
    arteriogram
    ventriculogram
    myelogram
    others: [X]

Any additional procedures: [X]

[X] = list investigations/procedures.

SECTION 2

Items	Signature of Supervisor	Initials of Student Nurse
Surgical Nursing		
Amputation of limbs		
Appendicectomy		
Arterial surgery		
Bowel surgery:		
relief of acute intestinal obstruction		
resection of bowel with:		
internal anastomosis		
colostomy		
ileostomy		
abdomino-perineal excision of rectum		
Gall bladder surgery		
Gastric surgery		
Haemorrhoidectomy		
Herniorrhaphy		
Mastectomy		
Thyroidectomy:		
partial		
total		
Varicose veins (surgery of)		

Section 2 (*contd*)

Genito-urinary Nursing
Circumcision
Cystectomy
Cystodiathermy
Cystoscopy
Hydrocele, excision of
Ileal conduit
Nephrectomy
Nephro-lithotomy
Orchidectomy
Prostatectomy: [X]
Pyelolithotomy
Pyleoplasty
Radon seeds, implantation of
Retention of urine, management of patients with
Undescended testicles, operation for
Urethero-lithotomy
Vasectomy

Orthopaedic Nursing
Amputations
Arthritic conditions: [X]
Congenital abnormalities
Fractures of femur
  other fractures: [X]
Laminectomy
Meniscectomy
Osteomyelitis
Osteotomy
Keller's operation
Patellectomy
Physiotherapy, occupational therapy and rehabilitation, importance of
Spinal disc lesions
Spinal fusion
Tumours

Gynaecological Nursing
Abortion:
  threatened
  inevitable
  incomplete
  therapeutic
Cervix, operations on
Curettage, diagnostic
Colporrhaphy:
  anterior
  posterior
Examination under anaesthetic

Section 2 (*contd*)

Hysterectomy:
  abdominal
  vaginal
Infective conditions: [X]
Myomectomy
Oophorectomy
Ovarian tumours
Radium, insertion of
Salpingectomy
Sterilization
Vulvectomy

Cardio-thoracic Nursing
Cardiac surgery: [X]
Congenital oesophageal atresia
Hiatus hernia
Lobectomy
Oesophageal varices
Oesophagectomy
Pneumonectomy

Ear, Nose and Throat Nursing
Adenoidectomy
Deafness, care, understanding and management of the deaf
Epistaxis
Laryngectomy
Mastoidectomy
Nasal polypi, removal of
Otitis media:
  acute
  chronic
Sinusitis:
  acute
  chronic
Stapedectomy
Submucous resection of nasal septum
Tonsillitis
Tonsillectomy
Tonsillectomy and adenoidectomy
Tracheostomy
Tympanoplasty

Ophthalmic Nursing
Blindness, care, understanding and management of the blind
Enucleation of eyeball
Corneal abrasions and ulcers
Corneal graft
Cataract

Section 2 (*contd*)

Foreign bodies, removal of
Glaucoma
Infective conditions: [X]
Retinal detachment
Strabismus

Burns and/or Plastic Surgery Nursing
Special preparation:
  site for operation
  freedom from infection
  psychological
Post-operative management:
  conduct of dressings
  occupational therapy
  rehabilitation
General care and management of patients with burns and scalds
General care and management of patients having plastic surgery

Medical Nursing *Conditions of*:
Cardio-vascular and reticulo-endothelial system:
  Cardiac failure:
    acute
    chronic
  coronary thrombosis
  endocarditis
  pericarditis
  valvular disease
Cerebro-vascular accident
Hypertension
Anaemia: [X]
Leukaemia: [X]
Haemophilia
Thrombocytopaenia
Hodgkin's disease

Respiratory system:
  asthma
  bronchitis:
    acute
    chronic
  bronchiectasis
  carcinoma
  cor pulmonale
  pneumonia
  pulmonary tuberculosis

Alimentary system:
  carcinoma of:
    bowel

Section 2 (*contd*)

    oesophagus
    stomach
  Crohn's disease
  diverticulitis
  malabsorption
  oesophageal varices
  peptic ulcer
  ulcerative colitis
  liver diseases:
    cirrhosis
    failure
    hepatitis

Urinary system:
  cystitis
  nephritis:
    acute
    chronic
  nephrotic syndrome
  pyelonephritis
  renal colic
  renal failure:
    acute
    chronic

Locomotor system:
  rheumatoid arthritis:
    acute
    chronic
  rheumatic fever

Endocrine system:
  under- or over-activity of endocrine glands
  diabetes mellitus
  obesity

Poisoning by:
  drugs
  other substances: [X]

Neurological and Neuro-surgical Nursing
Cerebral abscess
        tumour
Cerebral embolism
      haemorrhage
       thrombosis
Disseminated sclerosis
Encephalitis
Epilepsy
Head injury: [X]

Section 2 (*contd*)

Hydrocephalus
Meningitis: [X]
Muscular dystrophy
Parkinson's disease
Peripheral polyneuritis
Spina bifida
Trigeminal neuralgia
Laminectomy
Spinal fusion
Spinal injury: [X]

Dermatological Nursing
Dermatitis
Eczema
Herpes zoster
Psoriasis
Varicose ulcer

Geriatric Nursing
General management and care of:
  physically handicapped patients
  mentally confused patients
Habit training
Occupational therapy
Rehabilitation

Conditions nursed:
Arthritis
Carcinoma
Cerebro-vascular accident
Chronic heart disease
Disseminated sclerosis
Fractured femur
Malnutrition
Parkinson's disease
Senility

Radiotherapy Nursing
X-ray therapy; care and management of patients undergoing treatment:
  local care
  general care
Radium, care and management of patients undergoing treatment:
  precautions required
  custody on completion of treatment
  custody on death of patient
Radio-active isotopes, care and management of patients undergoing treatment:
  precautions required
  disposal on completion of treatment
  disposal on death of patient

Section 2 (*contd*)

Psychiatric Nursing Experience
Participation in the management of:
  short stay patients suffering from: [X]
  Long stay patients suffering from: [X]
Nurses' notes on patients
Participation in ward meetings:
  patients and staff
  medical and nursing staff
Nursing care in relation to psychiatric treatment:
  electroconvulsive therapy
  drugs used in psychiatric nursing
Participation in patients':
  occupation
  recreation
  social activities
  educational activities
  resocialisation and rehabilitation

Infectious Diseases Nursing
Diphtheria
Dysentery
Chicken pox
Food poisoning: [X]
Gastro-enteritis
Glandular fever
Infective hepatitis
Influenza
Measles
German measles
Meningitis:
  meningococcal
  tuberculous
  viral
  others
Mumps
Pemphigus
Poliomyelitis
Puerperal sepsis
Scarlet fever
Smallpox
Tuberculosis
Typhoid fever
  paratyphoid fever
Whooping cough
Worm infestation
Wound sepsis

Children's Nursing *Conditions of*:
Cardio-vascular and reticulo-endothelial system:

Section 2 (*contd*)

  cardiac disease: [X]
  cardiac surgery: [X]
  anaemia
  leukaemia: [X]

Respiratory system:
  bronchitis
  pneumonia

Alimentary system:
  appendicectomy
  gastro-intestinal conditions: [X]
  intestinal obstruction: [X]
  pyloric stenosis
  herniorrhaphy

Urinary system:
  conditions nursed: [X]

Nervous system:
  meningitis
  spina bifida

Orthopaedic conditions:
  conditions nursed: [X]

Metabolic disorders:
  diabetes mellitus

Failure to thrive
Repair of hare lip
Repair of cleft palate
Tonsillectomy and adenoidectomy
Other conditions nursed: [X]

Emergency/Accident Department
Reception of patients:
  walking
  stretcher
Management of emergency admissions
Care of relatives
Preparation for minor operations
Minor operations seen: [X]
Reduction of closed fractures
Application of plaster of Paris
Attendance at clinics
Special treatments carried out and prepared for: [X] (other than those in Section 1)
Overnight-stay wards, observations and treatments for: [X]

Intensive Care Nursing
Nursing care of patients with:
  artificial ventilation machine: [X]

Section 2 (*contd*)

endotracheal tubes
tracheostomy
Use of E.C.G. monitoring equipment
  other monitoring equipment: [X]
  defibrillating machine
Venous pressure (measurement of)
Types of conditions nursed: [X]

Operating Theatre

Preparation of theatre
Preparation and sterilization of:
  instruments
  ligatures, sutures, needles
  equipment
Knowledge of rules for safety of patients
Management of theatre table and lighting
Management of diathermy and suction apparatus
Positions used in operations: [X]
General preparation of anaesthetic apparatus
Care of anaesthetised patients
Care of specimens
'Scrubbing' for operations: [X]

Out-patient Department

Reception of out-patients
Attendance at the following clinics:
  Medical
  Surgical
  Cardiac
  Chest
  Dermatological
  Diabetic
  Ear, nose and throat
  Genito-urinary
  Gynaecological
  Neurological
  Ophthalmic
  Orthopaedic
  Paediatric
  Plastic surgery
  Psychiatric

Venereal Diseases Nursing

Special clinic experience
Reception of new cases
Examination, treatment and observation of patients suffering from:
  gonorrhoea
  syphilis

Section 2 (*contd*)

non-specific infections
Special tests: [X]
Social work: [X]

Aspects of Community Nursing
Aspects addressed: [X]

Obstetric Nursing Experience
Case histories: [X]
Ante-natal examinations: [X]
Normal labours: [X]
'Follow-up' nursing care: [X]

Clinical Teaching—Pregnancy
Psychological aspects of pregnancy
History taking
Examination of patient
Changes in pregnancy
Abdominal examination
The foetal heart
Taking of blood pressure
Urine testing
Minor disorders
Minor varicosities
Records in pregnancy
Toxaemia of pregnancy
Bleeding in pregnancy
Breech presentation
External cephalic version
Forms applicable to social services
Mothercraft teaching

Clinical Teaching—Labour
Admission of patient in labour
Records on admission
Administration of inhalational analgesia
Records in labour
Care of patient in labour
Examination of placenta
Trolley setting:
  normal delivery
  repair of perineum-episiotomy
  resuscitation of infant

Clinical Teaching—Lying-in Period
Vulval toilet
Routine care of breasts
Onset of lactation
Breast expression
Cracked and sore nipples

Section 2 (*contd*)

Breast infection
Observation of lochia
Fundal height
Postnatal records
Urinary infections
Pyrexia, notification, etc.

Clinical Teaching—The Baby
Immediate care at birth
Bathing of normal baby
Care of cord
Moulding
Caput succedaneum
Cephalhaematoma
Breast feeding
Management of milk kitchen
Making of artificial feeds
Stools of infant
Test weighing
Vomiting associated with feeding
Special care babies
Incubators, oxygen therapy
Feeding of premature infant

Any Additional Types of Cases: [X]

[X] = list investigations/procedures/type of disorder.

Appendix 8

Central Midwives Board Midwives Rules 1980, First Edition, Part III: Rules Regulating Training, Examinations and Admission to the Roll

Course of Training

The course of training of a student midwife shall consist of:

a. theoretical, clinical and practical instruction in each of the subjects included in Schedule II.
b. practical experience in the nursing and care of the mother and baby.

SCHEDULE II: SUBJECTS TO BE INCLUDED IN THE COURSE OF TRAINING

Physiology and applied anatomy of the body with particular reference to circulatory, respiratory, alimentary, endocrine, central nervous system.

Physiology and anatomy of the female reproductive system; the male reproductive system; the healthy neonate.

Microbiology, its significance in obstetric and neonatal care.

Drugs, modes of administration, indication for use, action, effects and interactions of those in general use in obstetrics and paediatrics; legislation affecting the supply and control of drugs.

Psychology of childbearing; social and environmental influences.

Preparation for parenthood; health education for families.

Nutritional requirements of the baby and of the infant; breast feeding and the preparation of artificial milk feeds.

Human relations and emotional reactions associated with childbirth affecting – the mother and baby; the family.

Pregnancy – physiology, signs, symptoms, diagnosis and management; assessment of maternal and foetal wellbeing; management of minor disorders; preparation for labour and parenthood; family planning counselling.

Labour – physiology, progress and management throughout all stages; assessment of maternal and foetal wellbeing; indications for and methods of induction and acceleration of labour; emotional support of parents; fostering and mother/baby relationships.

Puerperium – physiology, assessment of progress and management in hospital and home; education in infant care, and the initiation and management of breast feeding; family planning counselling; genetic counselling.

Infant – physiology of the newborn; methods of resuscitation; assessment and management of progress in the first month of life; neonatal nutrition and management of infant feeding with special reference to the preparation of artificial feeds and the care of the equipment; disorders, abnormalities and infections which may place an infant at risk, their causation, prevention and treatment.

Applied anatomy – female reproductive system, including the bony pelvis and its contents; the pelvic floor and external genitalia; the male reproductive system; the urinary system; the breasts; development of the fertilised ovum; the foetus, placenta, membranes, liquor amnii and umbilical cord at term.

Drugs – those commonly used in midwifery and neonatal care; obstetric analgesia and anaesthesia; legislation and regulations governing the administration of drugs by midwives.

Health education – principles and methods of teaching health care; maintenance of physical and emotional well-being; psychosexual problems in relation to childbearing; preparation for childbirth and parenthood; family planning; sexually transmitted diseases.

Complications of pregnancy – medical and obstetrical conditions, their aetiology, recognition and treatment and the effect on mother or baby; termination of pregnancy – social and environmental problems.

Complications of labour – the recognition of the potentially abnormal and abnormal conditions which may occur, their management and the midwife's duties.

Complications in the puerperium – the recognition of the potentially abnormal and abnormal conditions which may occur, their management and the midwife's duties.

Social legislation/community health – the development of health and social services; services available to the mother and child provided by legislation and voluntary associations; health care teams – the relationships between the members of the teams and their responsibilities.

Records – statutory requirements; confidentiality.

Central Midwives Board – rules and regulations affecting training and practice.

Statistical indices – with special reference to maternal, foetal and infant mortality and morbidity.

Research – introduction to the methods used, interpretation and application of results in the maternity services.

Appendix 9

Statutory Instrument 1983 No. 873 The Nurses, Midwives and Health Visitors Approval Order 1983, Part III: Nurse Training Rules

Training for admission to Parts 1 to 8 of the register

RULE 18

1. Courses leading to a qualification the completion of which shall enable an application to be made for admission to Part 1, 3, 5 or 8 of the register shall provide opportunities to enable the student to accept responsibility for her professional development and to acquire the competencies required to:

    a) Advise on the promotion of health and the prevention of illness:

    b) Recognise situations that may be detrimental to the health and well-being of the individual:

    c) Carry out those activities involved when conducting the comprehensive assessment of a person's nursing assessment:

    d) Recognise the significance of the observations made and use these to develop an initial nursing assessment:

    e) Devise a plan of nursing care based on the assessment with the co-operation of the patient, to the extent that this is possible, taking into account the medical prescription:

    f) Implement the planned programme of nursing care and where appropriate teach and co-ordinate other members of the caring team who may be responsible for implementing specific aspects of the nursing care:

    g) Review the effectiveness of the nursing care provided and where appropriate, initiate any action that may be required:

    h) Work in a team with other nurses, and with medical and para-medical staff and social workers:

    i) Undertake the management of the care of a group of patients over a period of time and organise the appropriate support services:

related to the care of the particular type of patient with whom she is likely to come in contact when registered in that Part of the register for which the student intends to qualify.

Appendix 10

Nurses Rules: Training Outcomes for Project 2000 (from Statutory Instrument 1989, No. 1456). Preparation for entry to Parts 12, 13, 14 and 15 of the Register

18A. – (1) The content of the Common Foundation Programme and the Branch Programme shall be such as the Council may from time to time require.

(2) The Common Foundation Programme and the Branch Programme, shall be designed to prepare the student to assume the responsibilities and accountability that registration confers, and to prepare the nursing student to apply knowledge and skills to meet the nursing needs of individuals and of groups in health and in sickness in the area of practice of the Branch Programme and shall include enabling the student to achieve the following outcomes:

(a) The identification of the social and health implications of pregnancy and child bearing, physical and mental handicap, disease, disability, or ageing for the individual, her or his friends, family and community

(b) The recognition of common factors which contribute to and those which adversely affect physical, mental and social well-being of patients and clients and take appropriate action

(c) The use of relevant literature and research to inform the practice of nursing

(d) The appreciation of the influence of social, political and cultural factors in relation to health care

(e) An understanding of the requirements of legislation relevant to the practice of nursing

(f) The use of appropriate communication skills to enable the development of helpful caring relationships with patients and clients and their families and friends, and to initiate and conduct therapeutic relationships with patients and clients

(g) The identification of health related learning needs of patients and clients, families and friends and to participate in health promotion

(h) An understanding of the ethics of health care and of the nursing profession and the responsibilities which these impose on the nurse's professional practice

(i) The identification of the needs of patients and clients to enable them to progress from varying degrees of dependence to maximum independence, or to a peaceful death

(j) The identification of physical, psychological, social and spiritual needs of the patient or client; an awareness of values and concepts of individual care;

the ability to devise a plan of care, contribute to its implementation and evaluation; and the demonstration of the application of the principles of a problem-solving approach to the practice of nursing

(k) The ability to function effectively in a team and participate in a multi-professional approach to the care of patients and clients

(l) The use of the appropriate channel of referral for matters not within her sphere of competence

(m) The assignment of appropriate duties to others and the supervision, teaching and monitoring of assigned duties.

Appendix 11

Nurses, Midwives and Health Visitors (Midwives Amendment) Rules 1998 – Midwives Rules and Code of Practice (UKCC 1998)

EDUCATION RULES

33 Outcomes of programmes of education leading to admission to part 10 of the register

1 The content of programmes of education shall be such as the UKCC may from time to time require.

2 Programmes of education shall be designed to prepare the student to assume on registration the responsibilities and accountability for her practice as a midwife.

3 Such a programmes of education shall:

(a) meet the requirements of the midwives directive

(b) be provided at an approved educational institution

(c) enable the student midwife to accept responsibility for her personal professional development and to apply her knowledge and skill in meeting the needs of individuals and of groups throughout the antenatal, intranatal and postnatal periods and shall include enabling the student to achieve the following outcomes:

(i) the appreciation of the influence of social, political and cultural factors in relation to health care and advising on the promotion of health

(ii) the recognition of common factors which contribute to, and those which adversely affect, the physical, emotional and social well-being of the mother and baby and the taking of appropriate action

(iii) the ability to assess, plan, implement and evaluate care within the sphere of practice of a midwife to meet the physical, emotional, social, spiritual and educational needs of the mother and baby and the family

(iv) the ability to take action on her own responsibility, including the initiation of the action of other disciplines, and to seek assistance when required

(v) the ability to interpret and undertake care prescribed by a registered medical practitioner

(vi) the use of appropriate and effective communication skills with mothers and their families, with colleagues and with those in other disciplines

(vii) the use of relevant literature and research to inform the practice of midwifery

(viii) the ability to function effectively in a multi-professional team with an understanding of the role of all members of the team

(ix) an understanding of the requirements of legislation relevant to the practice of midwifery

(x) an understanding of the ethical issues relating to midwifery practice and the responsibilities which these impose on the midwife's professional practice

(xi) the assignment of the midwife of appropriate duties to others and the supervision and the monitoring of such assigned duties.

Appendix 12

An example of a professional behaviour with its descriptors

ATTENDING TO CLIENT NEEDS AND REQUESTS WITHIN EXPECTED CAPABILITY

95, 85, 75	68, 65, 62	58, 55, 52	49, 47, 45	40	30	20
Is attentive, considerate and conscientious when attending to client needs and requests at all times	Is attentive and conscientious when attending to client needs and requests at all times	Is attentive and conscientious when attending to client needs and requests most of the time	Is conscientious in attending to client needs and requests most of the time	Occasionally not conscientious in attending to client needs and requests	Usually not conscientious in attending to client needs and requests most of the time	Not at all conscientious in attending to client needs and requests most of the time

95, 85, 75	68, 65, 62	58, 55, 52	49, 47, 45	40	30	20
Outstandingly prompt in attending to client needs and requests at all times	Very prompt in attending to client needs and requests at all times	Prompt in attending to client needs and requests at all times	Very occasional delay in attending to client needs and requests	Occasional delay in attending to client needs and requests	Frequently delayed in attending to client needs and requests	Always delayed in attending to client needs and requests

Note: 40 is the pass mark.

Appendix 13

Checklists for the clinical learning environment

The checklists below contain key questions, which address the guidance for good practice.

Those responsible for practice placements within HEIs and service environments should ensure that all these questions have been considered in the planning, provision and evaluation of practice placement experiences.

1. Providing practice placements

- Is there a jointly developed strategy agreed by HEI and service for the selection, development and monitoring of practice placements?
- Is the strategy for the selection and monitoring of practice placements shared with other health care education providers?
- Does the strategy for the selection of practice placements enable supply to meet demand?
- Is the identification of practice placements a joint exercise between HEI and service providers?
- Does the strategy require a profile of practice placements?
- Do all placement providers have a profile which determines:
  — maximum number and type of students at any time in a placement?
  — the skills required by the student before beginning the practice experience?
  — the learning opportunities available and the learning outcomes expected from the placement?
- Have practitioners working in practice areas received preparation for their role in teaching, supporting and supervising students?
- Do the arrangements for practice placements enable students to have equity of opportunity for their learning experiences?
- Do programme planners take account of any special needs students may have?
- Does the totality of the practice experience enable the student to meet all statutory/professional requirements of the programme?
- Do students and mentors/assessors know what is expected of them through specified practice outcomes?
- Are placement areas designed to enable students to experience the full 24 hours a day, seven days per week nature of health care where necessary?
- Are practice placements introduced at an early stage in the programme so students can see the relevance of related theory?
- Are placements of sufficient length to enable students to achieve the stated learning outcomes?
- Do all students have a period of practice experience to support and consolidate their transition to registered practitioner?

- Does practice experience outside the United Kingdom meet the requirements of the statutory/professional body?
- Are all placement areas audited in line with the requirements of the statutory/professional body as to their continuing suitability for students' practice experience?
- Is the quality of practice placements monitored jointly by service providers and HEIs and is feedback provided to all participants?
- Is good practice disseminated following audit and monitoring and does joint action planning address areas of concern or needing enhancement?

2. Practice learning environment

- Does the practice area have a stated philosophy of care which is reflected in practice and supports curriculum aims?
- Does the practice provision reflect respect for the rights of health service users and their carers?
- Does the provision of care reflect respect for the privacy, dignity and religious and cultural beliefs and practices of patients and clients?
- Is care provision based on relevant research-based and evidence-based findings where available?
- Does care provision involve different models of care commensurate with current practice and encompassing local and national initiatives?
- Are interpersonal and practice skills fostered through a range of teaching/learning methods?
- Does the practice experience enable students to experience the role of the registered practitioner in a range of contexts?
- Do all placements have an infrastructure to support continuing professional development opportunities for practitioners?
- Do students gain experience as part of a multi-professional team?
- Does the sequencing and balance between university and practice-based study promote the integration of knowledge, attitudes and skills?
- Is a learning resources area available in the practice environment?
- Does student feedback contribute to the ongoing evaluation of the learning environment and the student experience and are all stakeholders aware of the feedback?

3. Student support

- Are students given comprehensive programme information and information about their particular placements?
- Do students receive adequate and appropriate preparation for the practice placements?
- Does this preparation include practice in a skills laboratory?
- Do students receive a comprehensive orientation to each of their placements and is the orientation jointly agreed between mentors/assessors and programme teachers?
- Are students given an initial interview during the first week of the placement, to agree the learning outcomes and ways of achieving them, taking into account their prior knowledge and experience?

- Are students' learning needs, achievements and opportunities reviewed regularly?
- Do students receive agreed written learning outcomes for each placement?
- Do practice placements facilitate progression in terms of the learning experience available?
- Does the experience available among clinical staff support the student's achievement of the learning outcomes of the educational programme at the appropriate level?
- Do students receive consistent supervision and support during all practice placements?
- Is there a named mentor/assessor with qualifications and experience commensurate with the context of care delivery and the requirements of the appropriate professional/statutory bodies, which supervises and guides students in all practice placements?
- Are students supported at the appropriate level in successive practice placements?
- Do practice staff have dedicated time in educational activities to ensure they are competent in teaching and mentoring/assessing roles?
- Do lecturers have dedicated time in practice to ensure they are competent in the practice environment?
- Are lecturers involved in supporting student learning in practice areas?
- Are students assisted in linking theory and practice and using a research base for practice, by lecturers and practitioners?

4. Assessment of practice

- Are the periods of practice experience used for summative assessment of sufficient length to enable the agreed learning outcomes to be achieved?
- Is there a named mentor/assessor with the appropriate qualifications and experience to assess students in practice placements?
- Are the assessment methods used rigorous, valid and reliable?
- Are there enough mentors/assessors to assess the student's developing competence and to observe the student's achievement of the intended learning outcomes over a suitable period of time?
- Does the student's demonstration of competence involve the achievement of learning outcomes in both theory and practice?
- Is a portfolio of practice experience included in the assessment of the student's fitness for practice?
- Is the student's practice assessed in the context of a multi-professional team?
- Does the assessment strategy reflect progression, integration and coherence?

REFERENCE

These checklists were reproduced with permission from the English National Board for Nursing, Midwifery and Health Visiting from:

ENB (2001) *Placements in Focus: Guidance for Education in Practice for Health Care Professions.* London: The English National Board for Nursing, Midwifery and Health Visiting.

Appendix 14
Ward learning climate indicators

A. ORIENTATION TO THE PLACEMENT

1. Staff welcome students on arrival.
2. Students shown round ward.
3. Students allocated mentor in first week
4. Students meet mentor in first week
5. Orientation programme on first day
6. Written communication before arrival

B. THEORY AND PRACTICE

7. Students prepared in College for placement
8. Nursing models incorporated into practice
9. Opportunity to observe nursing
10. College theory relevant to placement
11. Students link theory to practice
12. Adequate contact with Link Teacher
13. Opportunity to participate in nursing
14. Gain confidence in nursing skills
15. Staff follow stated pattern of care
16. Relation between staff and Link Teacher
17. Practice reflects relevant research

C. SUPERNUMERARY STATUS

18. Staff share meaning of supernumerary status
19. Students and staff share meaning of supernumerary status
20. Students not used as 'pairs of hands'
21. Students able to negotiate shifts
22. Students able to negotiate outside visits
23. Students able to negotiate study time
24. Students negotiate work with non-mentor
25. Students have clear understanding of role

D. STAFF ATTITUDES AND BEHAVIOUR

26. Staff friendly and approachable
27. Staff well informed about the course
28. Staff in favour of the course
29. Staff support students
30. Staff distinguish learning needs at different stages
31. Staff willing to spend time teaching students
32. Students encouraged to ask questions
33. Students involved in ward activities
34. Students given adequate feedback
35. Staff work as a team
36. Students included in the team
37. Assess staff morale
38. Ratio of staff to students satisfactory
39. Staffing levels adequate
40. Staff respond to students' individual ways of learning

E. THE MENTOR

41. Students have same mentor throughout placement
42. Students have named second mentor
43. Students have no more than two mentors
44. Mentors know stage students have reached
45. Mentors are supportive
46. Mentors make time for students
47. Mentors respond to students' individual ways of learning
48. Mentors help students achieve learning outcomes
49. Students satisfied with balance of ward/outside learning

F. PROGRESSIVE ASSESSMENT

50. Orientation parts 1 & 2 completed in first week
51. Students have preliminary interview with mentor
52. Students have progress interview with mentor
53. Students have final assessment with mentor
54. Mentors correctly interpret Programme Assessment booklet
55. Students achieve learning outcomes

REFERENCE

Orton HD, Prowse J and Millen C (1993)
Charting the Way to Excellence. Sheffield
Hallam University: Pavic Publications.

Appendix 15

Contents of a portfolio for pre-registration midwifery education

1. Curriculum Vitae and Personal Profile
2. Evidence of Achievement of UKCC Competencies, Requirements of the Midwives Directive and Integration of Theory with Practice
    2.1 'Assessment of Practice Record' booklet (inclusive of learning contracts)
3. Evidence of Developing Professional Behaviours
    3.1 'Professional Behaviours' Inventory
4. Supplementary Evidence
    4.1 Evidence of Integration of Theory with Practice, Reflective Practice, Critical Awareness of Care and Evidence-Based Practice
    4.1.1 Reflective accounts of care
    4.1.2 Research critique to support care delivery
    4.2 Other Evidence
    4.2.1 Learning accounts of time spent with members of the multidisciplinary team – these accounts to reflect on the contributions made by these team members to midwifery care
    4.2.2 Learning accounts of activities in the clinical area other than direct client care such as ward rounds, case discussions/conferences, CTG meetings, mandatory update sessions, etc. These accounts to reflect on how these activities have contributed to personal professional development
    4.2.3 Learning accounts of activities and visits to organisations outside direct midwifery care areas – e.g. 'sure start', 'breastfriends', etc. – these accounts to reflect on the contributions made by these organisations to midwifery care
    4.2.4 Analysis of entries in the 'Record of Experience' booklet
    4.2.5 Others, e.g. simulated practice, case studies
5. Evidence of Ability to Perform Clinical Skills and Carry Out Procedures
    5.1 Clinical Skills Inventory
6. Self Assessment at the End of the Placement

Index